Atlas of
Tropical Medicine and Parasitology

Sixth Edition

Acquisitions Editor: Karen Bowler
Development Editor: Joanne Scott
Editorial Assistant: Sven Pinczewski
Project Manager: Gemma Lawson
Design Manager: Andy Chapman
Illustration Manager: Bruce Hogarth
Illustrator: Oxford Illustrators
Marketing Manager(s) (UK/USA): Clara Toombs/Kathleen Neely

Atlas of Tropical Medicine and Parasitology

Sixth Edition

Wallace Peters
MD (London), DSc (London), Docteur Honoris Causa
(Université René Descartes, Paris), FRCP, DTM&H

Emeritus Professor of Medical Protozoology
London School of Hygiene and Tropical Medicine
London
UK

Geoffrey Pasvol
MA (Oxon), MB ChB, DPhil (Oxon), FRCP, FRCPE

Professor of Infection and Tropical Medicine
Director Wellcome Centre for Clinical Tropical Medicine
Imperial College London
Northwick Park and St Mary's Hospitals
London
UK

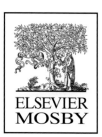

ELSEVIER
MOSBY

ELSEVIER
MOSBY

An imprint of Elsevier Limited

First published 1995 by Mosby-Wolfe, Times Mirror International Publishers Ltd.
Fifth edition 2001
Sixth edition 2007
  Reprinted 2007, 2008, 2009

ISBN-13: 978-0-323-04364-9

British Library Cataloguing in Publication Data
A catalogue record for this book is available from the British Library

Library of Congress Cataloging in Publication Data
A catalog record for this book is available from the Library of Congress

Notice
Medical knowledge is constantly changing. Standard safety precautions must be followed, but as new research and clinical experience broaden our knowledge, changes in treatment and drug therapy may become necessary or appropriate. Readers are advised to check the most current product information provided by the manufacturer of each drug to be administered to verify the recommended dose, the method and duration of administration, and contraindications. It is the responsibility of the practitioner, relying on experience and knowledge of the patient, to determine dosages and the best treatment for each individual patient. Neither the Publisher nor the author assume any liability for any injury and/or damage to persons or property arising from this publication.

The Publisher

Printed in China
Last digit is the print number: 9 8 7 6 5 4

Contents

Preface

The development of a new edition of a book provides the writers with an excellent opportunity to reflect not only on the detailed increase of knowledge of the subject matter, but also on modifications in the manner in which the overall view of the subject has evolved on the larger scale. The specific changes that have emerged over the past five years, which form the detailed content of this new edition, are briefly summarised at the head of each chapter. Here we present a few thoughts on the broader, global factors that are currently in the forefront of the minds not only of those personally concerned in the diagnosis, management and prevention of diseases of primary importance to people living in the warmer and less developed countries of the world, but also of individuals and institutions that devote their efforts to tackling some of our world's most prevalent diseases on a national or international scale. It is especially to the latter audience that some of the following remarks are directed.

Within the past five years an astounding change has occurred in the growing awareness of the importance of the individual countries of the world and their inhabitants of being parts of a 'global village'. The increasing ease of international travel (*see* **Frontispiece**) and the spreading ubiquity of communication through the Internet have facilitated not only the dissemination and knowledge of some old and new and newly emerging pathogens from their traditional homes, especially in the warmer climates, but also an awareness among the more privileged of the world's inhabitants of the relentless burdens of poverty and ill health prevalent among the millions who occupy much of the tropics and subtropics. This awareness is at last generating more

serious national and international measures to redress the balance between the haves and the have-nots than have been forthcoming until recently. Unprecedented funds are promised almost daily for the improvement of the prevention and treatment of the major diseases that afflict mankind through both basic scientific and operational research. The Millennium Development Project (MDP) proposed to the United Nations in 2000 now incorporates major health interventions such as the Global Fund to Fight AIDS, Tuberculosis and Malaria, which is envisaged to require US$7–8 billion by 2010, 60% of which would be directed towards Africa. The provision of expanded water supplies and improved sanitation, as well as mass treatment programmes to reduce the burden of banal intestinal worms, are identified as essential targets of the MDP. Other international interventions aim to reduce or eliminate helminth infections e.g., lymphatic filariasis, schistosomiasis, onchocerciasis and trachoma, as well as the vaccine-preventable diseases e.g., measles, diphtheria, whooping cough, poliomyelitis and tetanus. It is hoped that these ambitions will be realised.

This is not to imply that nothing has been done or achieved in the recent past. Here are some of the pluses and minuses. First there are major universal problems that have to be addressed. Some are of Nature's making, others Man's. Whether the principle is universally accepted or not, the scientific world can no longer deny the existence of the phenomenon of global warming, some of it at least due to our mismanagement of the environment. The implications of global warming are already beginning to be felt and will have increasingly deleterious effects on a large proportion of the poorer peoples of the developing world, as well as those in more privileged circumstances. The spread of canine leishmaniasis to northern Italy from its original distribution along the Mediterranean littoral may well be due to global warming, as may the presence of *Vibrio parahaemolyticus* in oysters in Alaska, a thousand miles north of its normal habitat.

Growing urbanisation in hot countries, with its consequences of overcrowding and inadequate hygiene provisions, poses a special hazard to human health. Natural disasters such as the Asiatic tsunami of 2004 killed 300 000 people and threatened the lives of millions of survivors both with infectious diseases and deteriorating nutrition. Given the will, mankind can take steps to minimise the seemingly inexorable advance of global warming and perhaps even reduce the impact of such unavoidable catastrophes such as major earthquakes and their aftermaths. Uncontrollable aggression in several countries of the developing world has resulted in massive genocide and immeasurable disease and deprivation among surviving communities. Political instability in relatively small areas, which, in some cases, has fed on human fears and inequalities, has given rise to the threat or even conduct, so far fortunately on a limited scale, of biological warfare.

Most of the old and some new infections and parasitic diseases are still with us. The reader will note, for example, an added emphasis in these pages on tuberculosis and on HIV/AIDS. There are some major victories to report, as will be seen in the following pages. However, the gap between control and elimination of a disease is greater than one would imagine. For example, by 2004 the incidence of acute flaccid paralysis caused by the poliomyelitis viruses had come close to zero, down from 350 000 a year in 1988 to 1267 in 2004, thanks to a prestigious international campaign of protection with oral vaccination. As a result of the premature and totally unreasonable interruption of this campaign in one west African country, the wild virus spread again from a residual focus there to contaminate at least 16 African countries previously freed of infection and, beyond Africa, to parts of the Middle East and as far east as Indonesia, thus necessitating a massive renewal of vaccination in those countries.

Two other great success stories are those of the eradication of smallpox (which, however, remains as a potential threat as an agent of biowarfare) and of Guinea worm infection.

On the negative side of the equation are the emergence of pathogens either previously unknown or relatively new in humans. The fact that several of these are essentially zoonoses brings home the importance of disease in animals to the health of humankind, not only in terms of their practical and economic impact on domestic livestock, but also in terms of the possibility of the spread, especially of some viruses, across species barriers. Perhaps for the first time the dichotomy between human and animal medicine is being exposed as a barrier not only to the advance of disease control in humans, but also to its control in their domestic animals and to the traditional subjects of veterinary medicine in the wild. Indeed, the extensive epidemiological veterinary databases now readily available can and should serve as advanced warnings of the threat of epidemics of zoonotic infections in the human population. The rapid global dissemination of the coronavirus that causes severe acute respiratory syndrome (SARS) from its source, among others, in Chinese civet cats, sounded alarm bells. The topical concern with avian influenza lies not only in its threat as a source of a potentially devastating human pandemic, especially if the H5N1 virus should hybridise with an intercurrent human influenza strain – an event that, fortunately, at the time of writing has not yet materialised, but also in the fact that the avian virus is already posing a major economic loss to those concerned with poultry husbandry across the globe. This is especially so in the poorer countries of the tropics where more than 150 million chickens and ducks had died or been culled by the end of 2005. The lethal filovirus infections causing Ebola and Marburg disease in humans have not only arisen as zoonoses from as yet unidentified sources in the African rainforests but have also caused major enzootics among the rare African great apes, such as chimpanzees and gorillas, that threaten the very survival of these species. African trypanosomiasis, traditionally a threat to human welfare when people are infected by the tsetse fly, is even more of a burden on mankind through the devastation it causes among livestock in endemic countries, but we are far from realising a way of eliminating it.

Some of the greatest plagues of mankind remain malnutrition, viral diarrhoea and malaria. To these are added HIV/AIDS and tuberculosis, which is witnessing a massive resurgence, especially in association with AIDS and multiple drug-resistance. Other newly emerging or spreading viral infections include several caused by Hanta viruses, especially in the New World, West Nile encephalitis, Rift Valley fever and zoonotic hepadnaviruses causing encephalitis in domestic animals and humans.

Wallace Peters
Geoffrey Pasvol
2006

Frontispiece
The global pathogen transport network

The expansion of international air travel has enhanced exponentially the hazard of spreading pathogens through human-to-human contact from a limited locality across the continents. The recent experience of the explosive emergence of SARS and its rapid transfer from China to the New World served as a forewarning of the danger that, for example, a localised epidemic of a novel, highly virulent strain of human influenza could very rapidly extend around the world to create a major pandemic. This figure, which represents the intricate network of intra- and international airline routes and the numbers of passengers travelling per day who use those routes, illustrates the ease with which such a potential catastrophe could occur. In this figure each line indicates a direct connection between major airports and the colour coding represents the estimated numbers of passengers transported daily on those lines from 10 (dark red) to 25 000 (light yellow). (Adapted by courtesy of the authors from Hufnagel L, Brockmann D, Geisel T 2004 Forecast and control of epidemics in a globalized world. *Proceedings of the National Academy of Sciences of the USA* 101: 15124–15129 with permission of the National Academy of Sciences of the USA.)

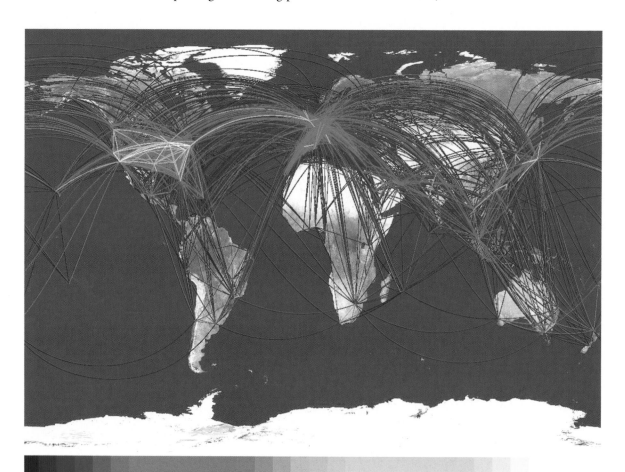

10   25000

1. Arthropod-borne infections

Numerically speaking, mosquitoes are probably responsible for more disease than any other group of arthropods but other insects too are of great importance. While *Anopheles* mosquitoes carry malaria, various viral infections and some types of filariasis, other viruses and filarias are transmitted by culicines. Different types of biting fly transmit African trypanosomiasis, leishmaniasis, bartonellosis and several kinds of filariasis. Fleas carry plague and one species of typhus, lice carry epidemic typhus, and mites and ticks other varieties of typhus. Ticks are also responsible for transmission of some of the haemorrhagic and relapsing fevers as well as Lyme disease and the human anaplasmoses (formerly known as ehrlichioses).

The arthropod vectors of disease are classified in Table 1. It will be noted in the literature that the important vectors in the former subgenus *Aedes* (*Stegomyia*) such as *Aedes* (*Stegomyia*) *aegypti* were to have been reclassified since phylogenetic studies have revealed that *Stegomyia* should be regarded as a genus. Thus *A.* (*Stegomyia*) *aegypti* should strictly become *Stegomyia aegypti* or *S. aegypti*. However, the universal usage of the older name makes it likely that it will be retained for the foreseeable future.

Among the major arthropod-borne (arbo) viruses considered here are yellow fever, dengue, Rift Valley fever, West Nile fever and Japanese encephalitis. These are representative of the arbovirus diseases, which include many other infections of humans in the tropics (Table 2). In spite of the availability of protective vaccination, yellow fever remains a serious public health problem, particularly in sub-Saharan Africa and South America. In those regions some 200 000 cases arise annually in spite of the deployment of mass vaccination in human popula-

tions at risk. As seen in the distribution map (**14**) there was a marked increase in incidence in Africa between the late 1980s and mid-1990s. The incidence and geographical spread of dengue has increased dramatically over the past 30 years. It is estimated that 2.5 billion of the world's population are at risk and that 100 million cases arise annually, including 500 000 cases of dengue haemorrhagic fever. Rift Valley fever made its first appearance beyond the African mainland in an enzootic/epidemic outbreak in the south-west of Saudi Arabia and adjoining territory of Yemen. In spite of an intensive, international programme of insecticiding to destroy potential mosquito vectors, by mid-January 2001 the virus had killed at least 230 people (a mortality rate of 11.5% in about 2000 known to be infected) and more than 3000 sheep, cattle, camels and goats.

In Reunion, an island of the Comoros group in the Indian Ocean, it has been estimated that between March 2005 and February 2006 at least 110 000 people have been infected with Chikungunya fever caused by an *Alphavirus* that is mainly transmitted by *Ae.* (*Stegomyia*) *aegypti*. Of this number about 22 000 were infected during a single week in February 2006 during which over 500 cases occurred in the neighbouring island of Mayotte. Fortunately this infection is relatively mild with a very low mortality rate.

The geographical distribution of West Nile virus is also increasing significantly. Late in 1999 this pathogen was identified as the cause of an extensive epidemic and enzootic in several of the north-eastern states of the USA. A serological survey in the Queens district of New York indicated that as many as 2.6% of the population had been infected. Most cases were mild but seven people died. Local

Table 1 Arthropod vectors of disease

Class	Order	Vectors	Diseases transmitted
Arachnida	Acarina	Hard ticks	Spotted and Q fevers, virus encephalitis, Lyme disease
		Ornithodorus spp. (soft ticks)	Endemic relapsing fever
		Mites	Scrub typhus, Rickettsial pox, scabies
Crustacea	Cyclopoida	*Cyclops* spp. (water fleas)	Guinea worm, fish tapeworm
	Decapoda	Crayfish, freshwater crabs	Paragonimiasis
Insecta	Dictyoptera	Cockroaches	*Hymenolepis diminuta* (rat tapeworm)
	Hemiptera	Reduviidae (assassin bugs)	Chagas' disease
	Phithiraptera	*Pediculus humanus* (body louse)	Epidemic typhus, epidemic relapsing fever
	Anoplura		
	Mallophaga	Chewing lice	*Dipylidium caninum* (dog tapeworm)
	Coleoptera	Beetles	Rat tapeworms
	Lepidoptera	Grain moths	Rat tapeworms
	Diptera	*Anopheles*	Malaria, filariasis (*Wuchereria bancrofti, Brugia malayi*)
		Culicines	Filariasis (*W. bancrofti, B. malayi*), arboviruses (including yellow fever, dengue)
		Culicoides	Filariasis (*Mansonella ozzardi, M. perstans, M. streptocerca*)
		Simulium	Onchocerciasis (*Onchocerca volvulus*)
		Chrysops	Filariasis (*Loa loa*)
		Phlebotomus	Sandfly fever, bartonellosis, leishmaniasis
		Lutzomyia	New World leishmaniases
		Glossina	African trypanosomiases
	Siphonaptera	Fleas	Plague, murine typhus, rat and dog tapeworms

See also Chapter 7 and Table 23.

transmission was by peridomestic *Culex pipiens* mosquitoes. A third of a large sample of birds found dead in the affected areas were positive for the virus. The virus, which spread further during 2000 and was isolated from other species of culicines and birds in a widening geographical area, has become permanently established in North America and had moved as far south as Argentina by April 2006. It has been suggested that one reason for the rapid transcontinental spread of the virus in North America may be that the vector *Culex pipiens* in that region is a genetic hybrid of two populations, one essentially human-biting and the other feeding on birds. A number of vaccines show promise for the protection of humans, that based on the use of DNA from the related Kunjin virus possibly giving crossprotection against West Nile virus.

Usutu virus, a flavivirus closely related to West Nile virus, has been isolated from birds, mammals and culicine mosquitoes. Although it has so far only been reported to cause illness in a few humans, this virus has decimated blackbirds in Austria since its first recognition there in 2001 but does not appear to be highly pathogenic to most avian species in Africa, where it is believed to have its origin.

The worldwide dissemination of a dangerous arbovirus vector, *Aedes* (*Stegomyia*) *albopictus*, poses a possible new threat for the coming years in relation to a number of diseases, including yellow fever and dengue. Fortunately it is not, at least under field conditions, a very efficient vector of yellow fever and has only apparently been responsible to date for some localised epidemics of dengue. Of the rickettsioses, louse-borne typhus due to *Rickettsia prowazekii* is potentially the most important, but tick typhus is fairly common in some areas (e.g. east Africa) and mite-borne scrub typhus (tsutsugamushi disease) in south-east Asia and the south-west Pacific. Several species of rickettsial fever have been identified in South Korea, for example, where scrub typhus and murine typhus also occur. The sandfly-transmitted organisms (*Bartonella bacilliformis*) that cause bartonellosis (Carrión's disease – a disease limited to mountainous areas of western South America) have

Table 2 Arboviruses that infect humans

Family	Genus	Virus or disease	Vectors	Reservoir hosts	Amplifier hosts
Togaviridae	*Alphavirus*	Chikungunya	*Aedes*	Monkeys, ? rodents	
		Eastern equine encephalitis	*Culiseta*	Birds	Horses
		Mayaro	*Aedes, Anopheles*	Wild vertebrates	
		Mucambo	Culicines	?	
		O'Nyong-Nyong	*Anopheles*	Humans	
		Semliki Forest	Mosquitoes	?	
		Ross River	*Aedes*	? Wallabies	
		Sindbis	Culicines	Birds	
		Venezuelan equine encephalitis	*Aedes, Culex* spp.	Rodents	Horses
		Western equine encephalitis	*Culex*	Birds	Horses
Flaviviridae	*Flavivirus* (mainly mosquito-borne)	Banzi	Culicines	?	
		Bussuquara	Culicines	Rodents	
		Dengue 1, 2, 3, 4	*Aedes*	Mosquitoes*	? Monkeys
		Ilheus	Culicines	Birds	
		Japanese encephalitis	*Culex, Anopheles*	Birds	Pigs, equines
		Murray Valley encephalitis	Culicines	Birds	
		Rocio	*Psorophora* spp.	Birds	
		St Louis encephalitis	Culicines	Mosquitoes*, birds	
		Spondweni	Culicines	?	
		Wesselbron	Culicines	Rodents	
		West Nile	Culex, ixodids, argasids	Birds, bats, horses, rodents	Birds
		Kunjin	Culicines	Birds	
		Yellow fever	*Aedes* (*Stegomyia*)	Mosquitoes*	Monkeys
			Haemagogus spp.	Mosquitoes*, rodents	Monkeys
		Zika	Culicines	?	
	Flavivirus (mainly tick-borne)	Absettarov	Ixodids	?	
		Hanzalova	Ixodids	?	
		Hypr	Ixodids	Rodents	
		Kumlinge	Ixodids	Rodents, birds	
		Kyasanur Forest disease	Ixodids, argasids	Forest rodents	Monkeys
		Louping ill	Ixodids	Rodents, birds	
		Negishi	Ixodids	?	
		Omsk haemorrhagic fever	Ixodids	Ticks*,†, rodents	
		Powassan	Ixodids	Rodents	
		Russian spring-summer encephalitis	Ixodids	Rodents, birds	
		Dakar bat virus	?	Bats	
Reoviridae	*Orbivirus*	Colorado tick fever	Ixodids, argasids	Rodents	
Bunyaviridae	*Nairovirus*	Crimea–Congo haemorrhagic fever	Ixodids	Ticks*, birds, leporids, rodents	Sheep
	Hantavirus	Hantaan virus‡	? Ticks	Murine rodents	
	Bunyavirus	California encephalitis group	Mosquitoes	*Aedes*, rabbits	
		Oropuche	Mosquitoes	Monkeys, sloths	
		Brazilian group	Mosquitoes	?	
		Bunyamwere group	Culicines	?	
	Phlebovirus	Rift Valley fever	Mosquitoes	? Rodents	
		Sandfly fever	*Phlebotomus*	Sandflies*	? Sandfly, mites

See also Table 26

* Vertical transmission occurs in vectors. † Infection may occur from handling carcasses or pelts of infected rodents, e.g. muskrats. ‡ One species is the cause of Korean haemorrhagic fever; other viruses in this group, which are spread by murine rodent excreta, cause haemorrhagic fever with renal syndrome (HFRS) and nephropathia epidemica.
?, Not yet known.

recently been shown to have some genetic relationship to the rickettsias.

Plague due to *Yersinia pestis* is still endemic in certain tropical and subtropical areas, and localised outbreaks are not uncommon, especially in the disrupted social and ecological situations brought about by wars. Relapsing fever in Africa is also geographically limited, but may occur in epidemics under wartime conditions, as witnessed in 1991 in Ethiopia.

Among the protozoal infections malaria, African trypanosomiasis and the leishmaniases are widespread and increasing – sometimes in epidemic fashion – in spite of measures to control them. Malaria, to which over half of the world's population is exposed, continues to cause severe morbidity and mortality in many countries. A marked parallel is seen between the burden of poverty in the world and the burden of malaria. The problem is aggravated by factors that include the extension of irrigation for agricultural production (e.g. in Rajasthan, India), the existence, on an increasing scale, of vector resistance to insecticides, and parasite resistance to antimalarial drugs. It was calculated that, in 2002, about 515 million clinical cases of falciparum malaria occurred in the 2.2 billion people exposed to infection throughout the world. Of this number some 70% were in the African region and, among these, it is believed that the infection was involved in the death of 1–2 million, mainly infants and children. The annual incidence of malaria caused by *Plasmodium vivax* was estimated recently to be between 70 and 80 million cases, of whom only 10–20% were in Africa. Fortunately, a new class of drugs based on artemisinin (the active constituent of Chinese wormwood – *Artemisia annua* Linn.) is being developed, and these are proving, for the time being at least, very effective in reducing morbidity and mortality from severe malaria, especially when deployed as part of drug combinations that are designed to impede the selection of further drug-resistant mutant organisms. It is to be hoped that the current, intensive effort to develop vaccines against malaria will, in time, provide new and powerful weapons with which to combat this persistent and deadly disease. This approach, however, carries the risk that the virulence of parasites that

survive in incompletely immunised human populations may actually increase. Novel approaches to immunisation include attempts to modify by genetic manipulation the ability of sporozoites to invade hepatocytes.

In addition to the long-recognised four species of *Plasmodium* that infect humans, new varieties of these, as well as infections by simian species, have been identified by immunological or molecular genetic techniques. Two sympatric variants of *Plasmodium ovale* have been described in Africa and south-east Asia. A malaria parasite resembling a simian species, *Plasmodium simiovale*, which was originally described in a monkey, *Macaca sinica* in Sri Lanka, has been identified by immunological detection of a species-specific peptide sequence in small number of human patients in Papua New Guinea, Indonesia, Madagascar, Brazil and Guyana. It is reported to produce an infection resembling that normally associated with *Plasmodium vivax* but more severe. More recently it has been shown that, in parts of the island of Borneo, *Plasmodium malariae* appears to have been replaced by *Plasmodium knowlesi*, normally a parasite of macaques. This simian parasite has also been identified in humans in Thailand.

African trypanosomiasis is increasing in both west and east Africa but, in numerical terms, was considered to be mainly of importance for its effect on domestic animals. 60 million people in 36 of the 52 countries of Africa are still at risk: up to 0.5 million are believed to be infected by *Trypanosoma brucei* and up to 100 000 new cases may arise each year. In Angola, for example, where control efforts have been disrupted by years of war, cases increased from three recorded in 1975 to 8000 in 1998 and more than 12 000 in 2001. South American trypanosomiasis (Chagas' disease), spread by reduviid bugs, extends through much of the subcontinent and is responsible for considerable ill health in parts of its distribution. Of the 100 million who were estimated to be at risk in 1985, some 18 million were believed to be infected. Two major, multinational vector-control programmes, one in the 'southern cone' countries (Argentina, Brazil, Bolivia, Chile, Paraguay and Uruguay) and the other in the Andean and Central American countries (see **227**), have now made a major impact on transmission. These programmes are based on the use of fumigant canisters and insecticidal paints, together with screening of blood donors, but transfusion infection remains a serious problem. Although the aim was to eliminate Chagas' disease transmission by 2005, about 5 million people even today are assumed to carry clinical changes caused by *Trypanosoma cruzi*.

The leishmaniases, especially the visceral forms (VL), continue to pose a high burden on health. Some 350 million people are exposed to VL in 88 countries, in which 500 000 new cases are estimated to arise yearly. A global estimate of 59 000 deaths from VL in 2002 was probably an underestimate. Associated HIV infection frequently exposes cryptic infections with parasites such as *Leishmania infantum*, for example in southern Europe. Between 1 and 1.5 million new cases of cutaneous infection (CL), both anthroponotic and zoonotic, arise each year. In Afghanistan between 2002 and 2004 67 500–200 000 new infections were caused by *Leishmania tropica* each year. VL in particular has long been infamous for its ability to give rise to massive epidemics, such as one that occurred in southern Sudan as recently as the early 1990s, when it killed roughly 10% of the population of 1 million. The existence of a large range of animal reservoirs, vector species and parasites renders the control of the leishmaniases especially difficult and demands an exceptional level of political and financial commitment, which is rarely forthcoming. Novel vaccines and drugs are urgently needed.

Of the more than 1 billion people in 80 endemic countries of the tropics who are exposed to lymphatic filariasis, more than 120 million are believed to be infected and of these about 40 million are incapacitated or disfigured, especially by *Wuchereria bancrofti* and *Brugia malayi*. A new major international programme, the Global Alliance to Eliminate Lymphatic Filariasis, based mainly on mass chemotherapy, was launched in 2000 with the objective of interrupting transmission of and relieving suffering from infection with *W. bancrofti*, *B. malayia*, *Brugia pahangi* and possibly *Brugia timori* by 2020. Already by 2004 over 400 million of those at risk in 39 countries had been targeted for mass drug administration. Infection with the skin-dwelling parasite *Onchocerca volvulus* remains a problem in parts of tropical Africa and Central America. However, thanks to an extensive control campaign, the Onchocerciasis Control Programme (OCP), which was launched in 1974 to destroy the aquatic stages of the vectors of onchocerciasis (species of *Simulium*), and to the introduction of the macrofilaricide ivermectin, the most serious complication, blindness, is being conquered and should become a thing of the past. By 2002 when this programme ended it was estimated to have prevented more than 200 000 cases of blindness at a cost of about $556 million. From 1995 the OCP, which was based essentially on the elimination of the blackfly vectors, was complemented by a new venture, the African Programme for Onchocerciasis Control (APOC), which aims at mass drug therapy with the microfilaricide ivermectin. However, by 2010 when this programme is due to close, there will remain the danger that transmission may recur, since there will remain a significant residue of people carrying living adult *Onchocerca* as well as foci of potential *Simulium* vectors. The current focus is therefore the search for a macrofilaricide that will eradicate this potential source of resurgence of onchocerciasis in Africa. Meanwhile, in the New World, the Onchocerciasis Elimination Program for the Americas, based essentially on the mass administration of ivermectin two and four times a year, is expected to end by 2007.

While the diagnosis of the viral and bacterial infections must be confirmed by appropriate serological and cultural techniques, most protozoal and helminthic infections are readily recognised, if not on clinical grounds alone then by fairly simple techniques designed to demonstrate the presence of the causative parasites. Powerful new diagnostic agents in the form of highly sensitive and specific, simple monoclonal antigen and antibody detection tests have been developed. In addition, whereas novel molecular procedures using DNA probes and polymerase chain reaction (PCR) primers are increasingly gaining acceptance, especially for epidemiological studies, most of them are likely to be of limited practical application for the foreseeable future in many developing countries, except where sophisticated central laboratory facilities are available.

THE ARBOVIRUSES

The main differential characters of the principal families of mosquito vectors of disease are shown in the next figures (see also **107, 316–325** and **327.**)

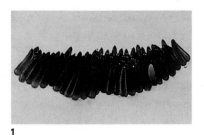
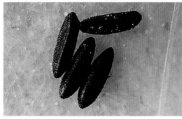
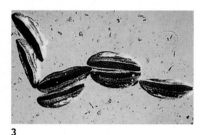

1   2   3

1–3 Mosquito eggs
Culex eggs (**1**, left) are deposited on the water surface in 'rafts'; *Aedes* eggs (**2**, centre) are laid singly and often have a conspicuously sculptured surface. *Anopheles* eggs (**3**, right) have lateral floats and tend to aggregate on the water surface, forming 'Chinese figure' patterns. (**1** × *25;* **2, 3** × *27*)

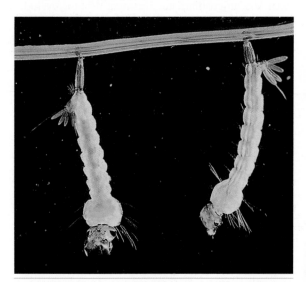

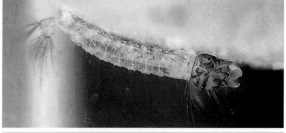

5 Third-stage larva of *Anopheles*
The larvae of *Anopheles* lie parallel to the water surface. (× 9)

4 Third-stage larvae of *Culex* (*Culex*) *quinquefasciatus* and *Aedes* (*Stegomyia*) *aegypti*
The larvae of *Culex* and *Aedes* are suspended under the air–water interface by their siphons. This figure illustrates the differences between the larvae of the two genera, *Culex* (left) with a longer siphon and several tufts of lateral siphon hairs, the *Aedes* (right) with a short siphon and single hair tuft. (× 9)

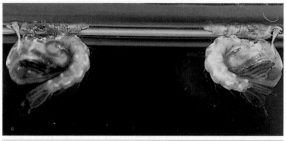

6 Pupae of *Culex*
Pupae of *Culex*, *Aedes* and *Anopheles* are very similar. They obtain air through siphons on the cephalothorax. (× 9)

7 Pupae of *Anopheles*
Compare the shorter siphon of this pupa with that of *Culex* (6). (× 9)

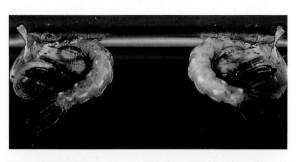

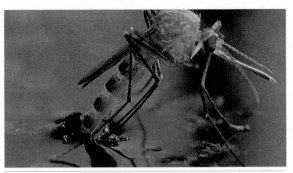

8 Adult *Culex* (*Culex*) *quinquefasciatus* hatching from pupa

The mature pupa, with the siphons penetrating the surface film, splits open and the adult mosquito, in this case a female, emerges, allowing its wings to expand and harden. (× 8)

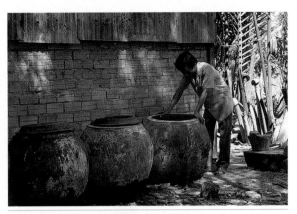

11 Larval breeding in water storage jars

Such containers attract *Aedes* (*Stegomyia*) *aegypti* and *Aedes* (*Stegomyia*) *albopictus*, which readily colonise them even when the jars are covered. Generally, the lids are ill-fitting and do not keep the female mosquitoes out (as seen in this South Vietnam village).

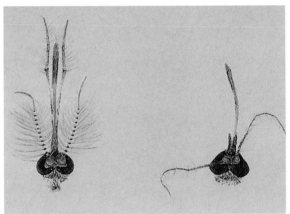

9

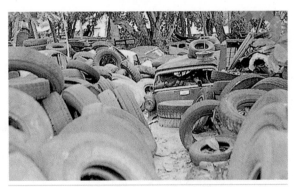

12 Larval breeding in discarded motor tyres

In recent years, the eggs of *A.* (*Stegomyia*) *aegypti* and *A.* (*Stegomyia*) *albopictus* have been carried from continent to continent in motor tyres, which are often sent to central collection areas for recycling. While awaiting transport, the tyres are usually left in dumps exposed to the rain, and such dumps provide ideal sites for egg laying.

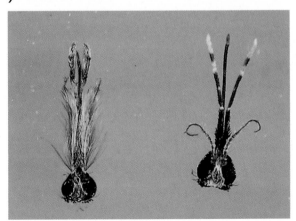

10

9 & 10 Heads of adult culicine and anopheline mosquitoes

The adults are distinguished by the form of the antennae and palps. *Culex* ♂ (left) ♀ (right) (**9**, left); *Anopheles* ♂ (left) ♀ (right) (**10**, right). (× 16). *Aedes* males and females are similar to those of *Culex*. Compare the short palps of the female *Culex* with the long ones of the female *Anopheles*.

Yellow fever

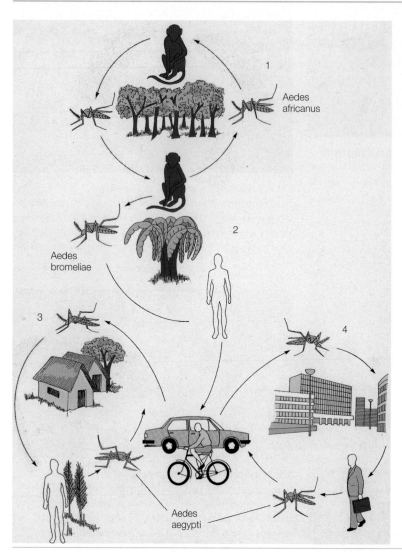

13 Transmission cycles of yellow fever

'Jungle' yellow fever is enzootic among monkeys in the tropical forests of Africa and South America. Although the main reservoirs are now generally believed to be the mosquito vectors, the virus is enzootic in Africa in species of *Cercopithecus* (vervets), *Cercocebus* (mangabeys), *Colobus* and *Papio* (baboons), in which the infections are usually inapparent. Epidemics of yellow fever occur in Africa when the virus is passed by a succession of *Aedes* (*Stegomyia*) species between the monkey reservoirs and humans. The infection is maintained in the forest (1) by several species of mosquito including *Aedes* (*Stegomyia*) *africanus* and *Aedes* (*Stegomyia*) *bromeliae*. The latter may leave the forest to breed in plantations (2), where farmers can become infected. The virus that causes sylvatic yellow fever in east Africa differs from the one that is responsible for urban epidemics in the west of the continent. There, villagers (3) who acquire viraemia serve as a source of infection, which is readily transmitted in more urban areas (3) by *Ae.* (*Stegomyia*) *aegypti* that breeds in domestic and peridomestic sites, thus starting the urban cycle of transmission (4). In South America, epidemics are usually preceded by severe enzootics in which large numbers of forest monkeys may die. (Adapted from Service MW 1980 A guide to medical entomology. Macmillan, London)

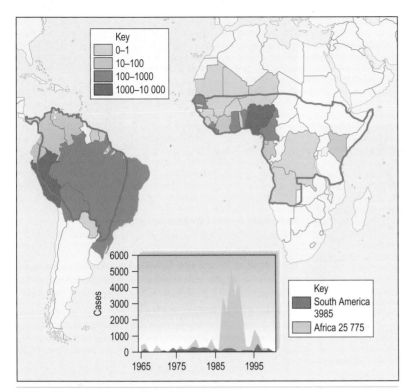

14 Distribution map of yellow fever virus

Focal outbreaks of mosquito-borne yellow fever still occur in South America but are especially a problem in tropical Africa where the disease is endemic in 34 countries with a total population of 468 million. It has been estimated that more than 200 000 cases with up to 30 000 deaths from yellow fever occur annually, the great majority in Africa. Vaccination provides a high level of protection for 10 years and is a legal requirement for travellers entering endemic countries. The virus is transmitted by mosquitoes of the subgenus *Aedes (Stegomyia)*. It is now accepted that the main reservoirs are the susceptible mosquitoes, in which the virus is transmitted from generation to generation by transovarial infection. The map indicates the endemic areas of Africa and South America as indicated by serological surveys and the range of cases reported to the World Health Organization between 1990 and 1999 (upper key). There were no case reports from the areas shown in yellow. The inset shows the incidence of yellow fever in Africa compared to that in South America between 1965 and 2000 (lower key). Nine epidemics occurred in Nigeria between 1986 and 1994. In 2003 and 2004 Colombia experienced outbreaks of yellow fever and the disease extended to the human population of adjacent areas of Ecuador in early 2005, necessitating the institution of a mass vaccination campaign. (Map adapted from Dr T P Monath 2001 Yellow fever: an update. Lancet Infectious Diseases 1: 13.)

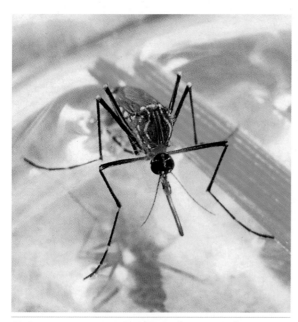

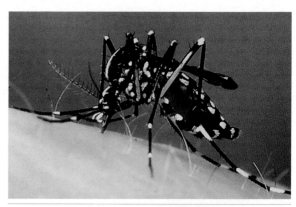

16 Female *Aedes (Stegomyia) albopictus*
Imported in tyres sent from Japan to Houston in the United States in 1985, *Ae. albopictus* (the 'Asian tiger mosquito') has now colonised most states of the USA. *Ae. albopictus* has been shown to be capable of supporting the development of over 24 arboviruses including those causing yellow fever, dengue 1–4 (with which it has been found naturally infected), eastern, western and Venezuelan encephalitis, chikungunya and La Crosse encephalitis. It can truly be considered as the '*Aedes aegypti* of the 1990s', and could readily cause epidemic yellow fever if the virus is reintroduced into the southern parts of the USA. Moreover, this mosquito has genetically adapted to higher temperatures and has already invaded Latin America and parts of west Africa. *Ae. albopictus* may prove to be a far more dangerous vector of arboviruses than *Ae. (Stegomyia) aegypti* because of its ability to thrive in both cold and hot climates. (× 7.5)

15 Newly emerged female *Aedes (Stegomyia) aegypti*
The main vector of yellow fever within village and urban settlements in both the Old and New Worlds is *Ae. (Stegomyia) aegypti*. Over the centuries, its eggs have been transported from Africa in containers made by humans so that this species is now found in most parts of the tropics and subtropics. It breeds readily in all types of domestic and peridomestic collections of fresh water, including flower vases, water drums, tin cans, broken coconut shells, etc. (× 12)

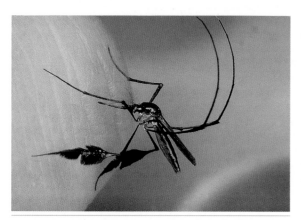

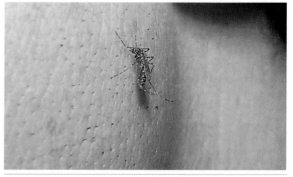

18 *Aedes* biting
Photograph taken at midday in rain forest near Belém, Brazil, at the mouth of the River Amazon. Mosquitoes of the genera *Aedes* and *Haemagogus* transmit yellow fever virus to forest monkeys, in which there is a sylvatic reservoir, from monkeys to humans and subsequently from human to human. Viraemia in monkeys, as in humans, is short-lived. (× 2)

**17 Female *Sabethes (Sabethoides) chloropterus*
probing on a man's hand**
Within the forest, transmission of yellow fever virus between reservoir hosts is also maintained by colourful mosquitoes of the genus *Sabethes*. (× 5)

19 Temperature chart of yellow fever case

The increasing slowness of the pulse relative to the temperature (Faget's sign – also seen in typhoid fever, paratyphoid and brucellosis) is of clinical diagnostic value. P, pulse; T, temperature (°C).

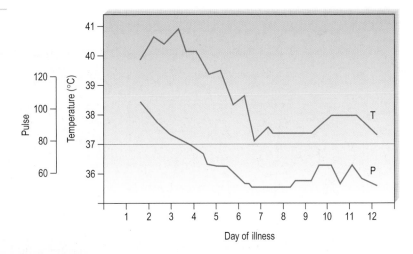

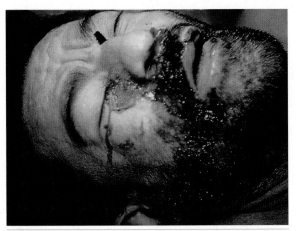

20 'Black vomit' in terminal stage of yellow fever

Despite the name, jaundice is usually not marked in yellow fever. Bleeding from the gut is a grave portent. The Costa Rican patient seen here with severe jaundice vomited material resembling coffee grounds ('black vomit'), as well as fresh blood shortly before dying.

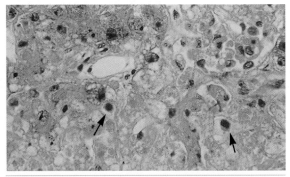

21 Section of liver from fatal yellow fever case

Midzonal necrosis with fatty degeneration and eosinophilic, intranuclear inclusions (Councilman bodies) are characteristic histological features. Here the periportal area contains relatively well preserved cells. (*Giemsa × 800*) (AFIP No. 71-1981)

22 Electron micrograph of yellow fever virus

This RNA virus in the genus *Flavivirus* (Togaviridae) is shown here growing in a Vero cell culture. (× *80 000*) (Courtesy of Mr Bruce Cropp, CDC Fort Collins, CO.)

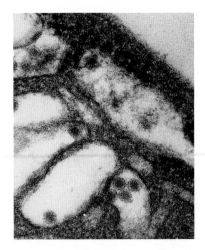

Dengue

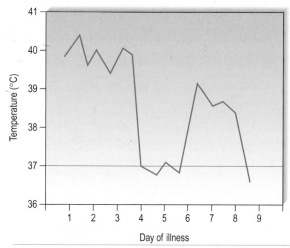

23 Dengue temperature chart

Dengue is an *Aedes* (*Stegomyia*)-borne disease of wide distribution in the tropics and subtropics, and is caused by four serotypes of a species of positive, single-stranded RNA flavivirus. The incubation period is short, on average about 5 days. The illness is often of short duration, with a characteristic 'saddle-back' fever.

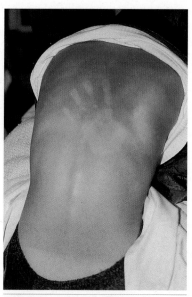

24 Rash of dengue

The figure shows the characteristic blanching rash of dengue fever. The rash is thought to be due to capillary vasodilatation in the skin and occurs shortly after defervescence on about day 5 of the infection. The rash lasts 1–5 days, sparing the palms and soles. It may be followed by a transient morbilliform or scarlatiniform rash that spreads centrally from the extremities during the second bout of fever.

Dengue haemorrhagic fever

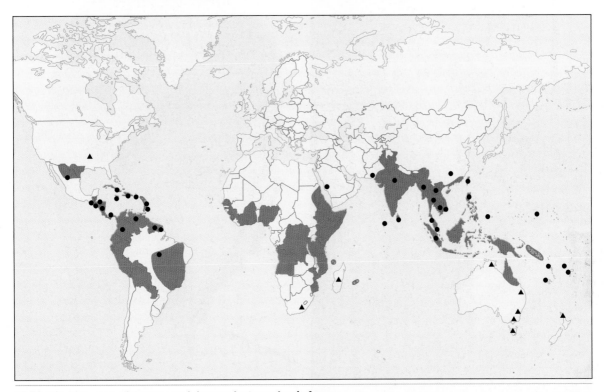

25 Distribution map of dengue and dengue haemorrhagic fever

The distribution of dengue is expanding rapidly. The map indicates the general distribution of the disease (yellow), those countries in which outbreaks of dengue haemorrhagic fever (DHF) were recorded between 1975 and 1996 (●) and localities where imported cases were reported during that period (▲). (During the last two decades, numerous epidemics of DHF have occurred in south-east Asia and Latin America. All four known serotypes of dengue virus have been isolated in almost all of the countries involved, and *Ae.* (*Stegomyia*) *aegypti* has been identified as the main vector. Its peridomestic habits ensure intimate human–vector contact. Strict control of peridomestic breeding sites is the most effective weapon against the spread of infection. In Argentina and Cuba, field trials have shown that the insecticidal fumigant canisters developed for the control of the vectors of Chagas' disease (see **245**) are also extremely effective against *Ae.* (*Stegomyia*) *aegypti* in human dwellings. As several dengue viruses have been proved to pass transovarially also in *Ae.* (*Stegomyia*) *albopictus*, it is likely that epidemics will continue to increase in distribution and number in the future. Monkeys may serve as amplifier hosts in some areas.

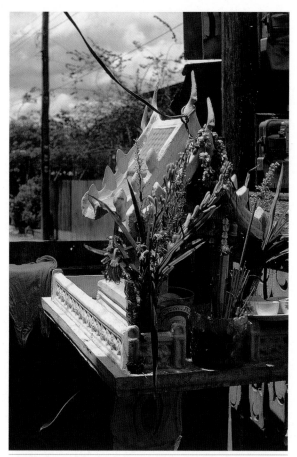

26 Breeding site of *Aedes (Stegomyia) aegypti* in a Thai cemetery
Numerous larvae of this vector were detected in flower pots decorating this altar in a Thai cemetery during an extensive outbreak of dengue.

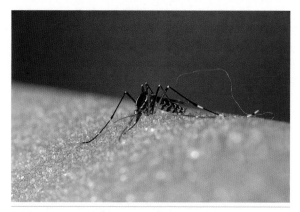

27 Female *Aedes (Stegomyia) polynesiensis*
An important vector of dengue in the Pacific region. (× 4)

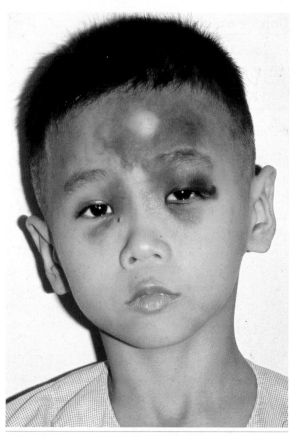

28 Marked ecchymoses in a Chinese boy
Dengue haemorrhagic fever is believed to arise as a result of a second infection, possibly with a different serotype, following an initial attack of uncomplicated dengue via antibody-mediated enhancement. Immune complex formation leads to increased capillary permeability, which may be followed by hypovolaemia and even disseminated intravascular coagulation. Cutaneous haemorrhagic manifestations ranging from petechiae to gross ecchymoses characterise the infection, especially in children. Outbreaks of variable severity occur yearly in south-east Asia. For example, over 200 patients were admitted daily in an outbreak in Vientiane, Laos, in 1987. The peak age specific prevalence was 4–9 years and the severity of cases ranged from grade I (fever and positive tourniquet test) to grade IV (undetectable blood pressure and pulse – dengue shock syndrome). Rapid restoration of plasma volume is mandatory. The case fatality rate can be as high as 15% in the absence of optimal medical management. A tetravalent vaccine is currently undergoing clinical trials but, for the time being, limitation of the infection depends largely on vector control.

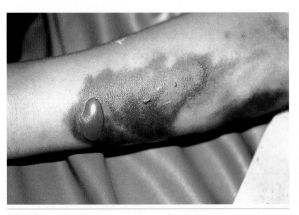

29 Subcutaneous haemorrhage in dengue haemorrhagic fever
This Thai patient had a large haemorrhagic lesion on his upper arm. (Image ID: 9914015, courtesy of Wellcome Trust and WHO, figure WHO/TDR/STI/Hatz.)

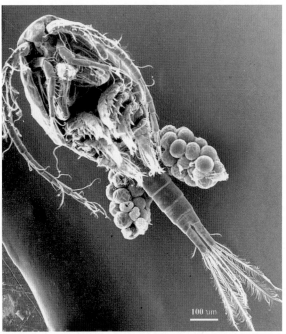

31 Scanning electron micrograph of a copepod used in dengue control
Although the major vector of dengue, Ae. (*Stegomyia*) *aegypti*, breeds in small water containers such as those shown in **11, 12** and **26**, it will also colonise larger containers that are used for storing drinking water where piped water is not available. The deployment of carnivorous copepods, for example the water flea *Mesocyclops thermocyclopoides* shown here, in such larval breeding sites has interrupted the transmission of dengue in parts of Vietnam and Central America. In a programme based on the use of this copepod between 1998 and 2005 in Vietnam, Ae. (*Stegomyia*) *aegypti* was virtually eliminated from 32 of 37 communes occupied by about 310 000 villagers, with a parallel fall in the incidence of dengue. However, constant vigilance has to be observed to ensure that such breeding sites are not further colonised by dengue vectors. (× *75*) (From Hernandez-Chavarria F and Schaper S. Rev Latinamericana de Microbiologica, Mesocyclops thermocyclopoides (Copepoda: Cyclopoida): a scanning electron microscope study. Fig 1, p. 54.)

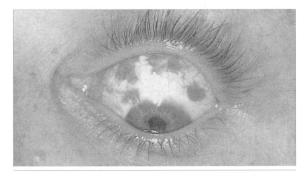

30 Scleral haemorrhage in dengue haemorrhagic fever
Scleral haemorrhages often accompany the skin rash in this condition.

Congo–Crimea haemorrhagic fever

See **1173–1187** for this and other zoonotic viral infections.

West Nile virus

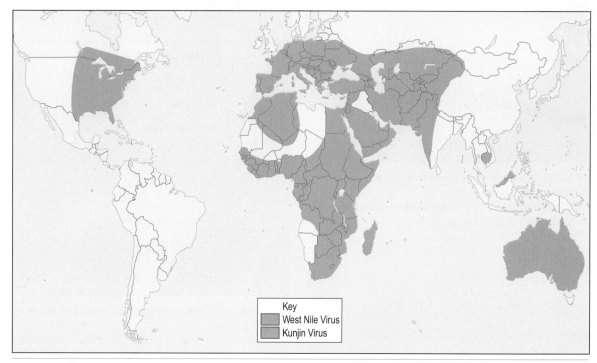

32 Distribution of West Nile virus

Until the end of the 20th century West Nile (WN) virus was endemic in Africa, Asia and Europe, including the far east of Russia. A subtype of this virus, Kunjin virus, is endemic in Australasia. Since 1994 the virus has become established in the New World, where it was responsible for a severe epidemic in New York state associated with meningoencephalitis. The virus is transmitted by species of *Culex* including *C. pipiens*, which maintains a mosquito–bird–mosquito cycle, species especially in the family Corvidae being the main amplifying hosts. WN virus has recently been detected in humans and in dead birds across the entire USA, in parts of Canada and as far south in the New World as Argentina. Moreover, in certain areas of the USA where the American alligator (*Alligator mississippiensis*) is farmed, viral titres of a level sufficient to infect vector culicines have been reported, suggesting that this animal may also serve as an amplifier host. However, the pattern of spread of the virus in the USA would suggest that bird migration is the main route of transport. The figure shows the approximate distribution of WN virus (red) and the closely related *Flavivirus* Kunjin (blue) at the end of 2003. Since that time the virus has been detected over almost the whole of the USA mainland. (Adapted from Campbell G L, Martin A A, Lanciotti R S, Gubler D J 2002 West Nile Virus. Lancet Infectious Diseases 2: 520.)

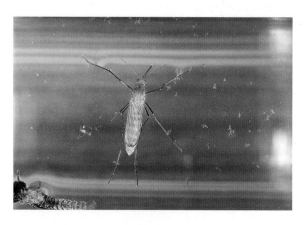

33 Newly emerged female *Culex pipiens*

This common culicine, which is one of the most widely distributed in the world, will feed on both human and avian blood. Some subspecies (e.g. *C. pipiens molestus*) breed in peridomestic collections of polluted water even in total darkness, as well as in cleaner, open sites. *C. pipiens pipiens* feeds primarily on birds and is one of the commonest vectors of West Nile virus. In cold, northern areas this species can hibernate in sheltered sites at temperatures approaching or even below freezing. In the western states of North America *Culex tarsalis* has been shown to be an extremely effective vector that is present mainly in rural areas. (× 3)

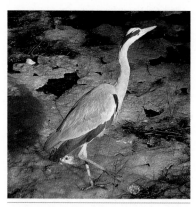

34 Grey heron, a potential carrier of West Nile fever virus

This is one of a number of species of water birds that migrate seasonally from endemic areas and that can carry this and other viruses such as that causing Japanese encephalitis (see **39**).

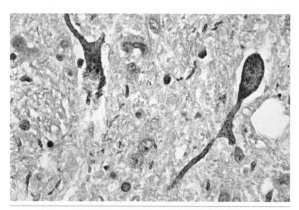

35 A section of human brain from a fatal case of encephalitis caused by West Nile virus

The section was stained to demonstrate viral antigen in neurones and neuronal processes. Most human infections present with mild and nonspecific symptoms, especially in children, but the virus has given rise to meningoencephalitis, especially in older or immunocompromised individuals in the New World. This suggests that vaccination should be directed especially towards older individuals who are at risk. Moreover, infection can induce acute flaccid paralysis resembling that caused by poliomyelitis, with which West Nile infection could be confused. (Methylene blue × *200*.) (Courtesy of Drs W J Shieh and S R Zaki, Centers for Disease Control and Prevention.)

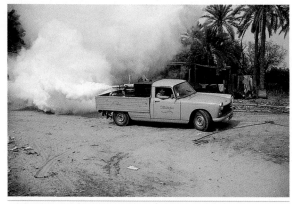

36 Control of culicine vectors of West Nile virus

In urban areas where peridomestic culicine mosquitoes transmit West Nile virus the distribution of insecticides by fogging machines is a valuable method of vector control.

Japanese encephalitis

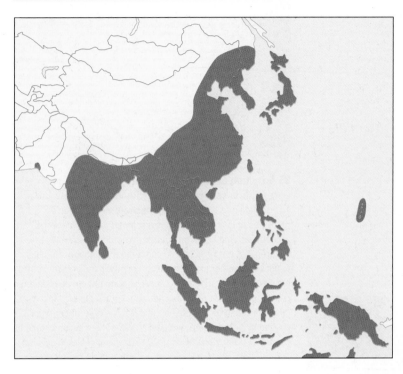

37 The distribution of Japanese encephalitis

This disease is caused by a flavivirus which is spread through birds and transmitted by various species of *Culex* and *Anopheles* mosquitoes. These are commonly found breeding in surface water such as flooded paddy fields. Birds form a reservoir for the virus which is amplified in infected pigs. It is believed that only 1 in 200 people who are infected develop the full-blown disease but, among these the mortality may range between 5 and 35%. Of the survivors 75% may develop neurological sequelae. Although between 30 000 and 50 000 cases are reported yearly the actual total number is probably much greater. The map shows the distribution of Japanese encephalitis in Asia between 1970 and 1998. (Adapted from Division of Vector-borne Diseases, CDC, Atlanta (2003) Japanese encephalitis. http://www.cdc.gov/ncidod/dvbid/jencephalitis/map.htm.)

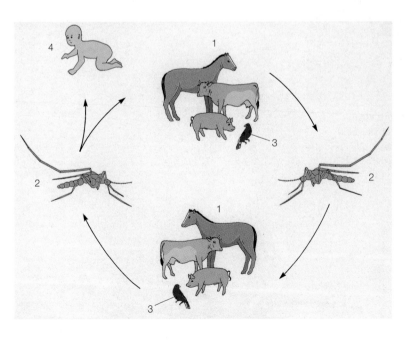

38 Cycle of transmission of Japanese encephalitis

The virus is passed between the amplifier hosts (equines, sheep and, mainly, pigs) (1) and humans (4) by culicine mosquitoes. The amplifier hosts are infected by mosquitoes (2) that have fed on migratory water birds (herons and egrets) (3). The human (4) is a dead-end host.

Scrub typhus

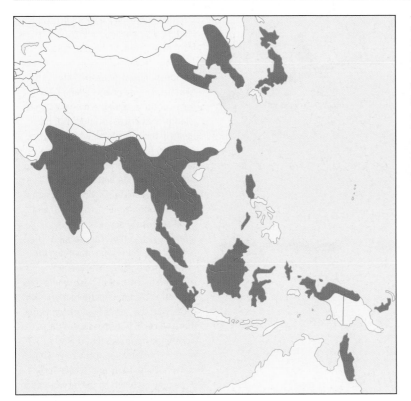

47 Distribution map of scrub typhus
Scrub typhus, or tsutsugamushi disease (from a Japanese word meaning 'noxious bug'), is caused by infection with *Orientia tsutsugamushi* and is transmitted by larval trombiculid mites of the genus *Leptotrombidium* (see **Table 23**). The disease occurs in the Indian subcontinent, south-east Asia, the far east and islands of the south-west Pacific including the Republic of Palau.

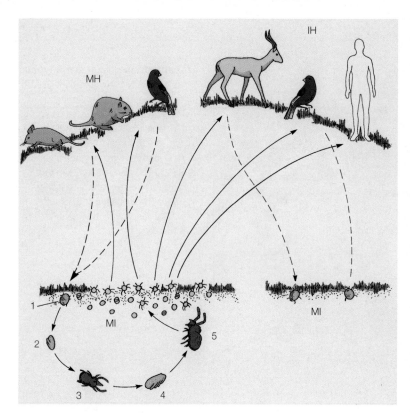

48 Epidemiological cycle of scrub typhus

O. tsutsugamushi is present in trombiculid-infested rodents. Not far from Kuala Lumpur, for example, *Leptotrombidium deliensis* is found in the forest, and *Leptotrombidium akamushi* in the grass ('lalang'). The mites occur in colonies known as 'mite islands' that are associated with the nests of the rodents on which they normally feed. They pass through a cycle that includes a parasitic, blood-feeding, hexapod larva (1A and 1B), a nymphochrysalis (2), followed by eight-legged, nonparasitic nymphal (3) and adult stages (5) between which is interposed an imagochrysalis (4). The cycle of infection is maintained in the focus, since engorged larvae are returned to the rodent nest, where they drop off and complete the rest of their cycle, with the adults finally laying eggs there. Vertical transmission of the rickettsiae occurs so that the true reservoir of infection is the mite. Other mammals, humans and occasionally birds may be bitten by the larvae, which cause severe irritation. Thus, scrub typhus, although a zoonosis, can occur in small outbreaks if groups of people (e.g. soldiers in the jungle) rest in the vicinity of a mite island. (IH, incidental hosts; MH, maintenance hosts; MI, mite island; adapted from Audy JR 1968 Red mites and typhus. Athlone Press, London.)

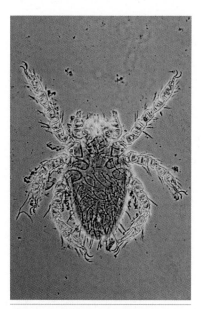

49 Larva of Leptotrombidium

Larval mites transmit the infection from rodent to humans when they come into accidental association with mite-infested terrain. The mites act as reservoirs since transovarial transmission of the *Rickettsia* occurs. (× *80*)

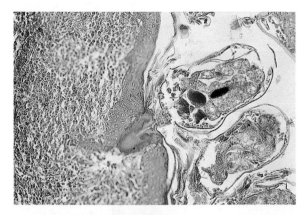

50 Longitudinal section through a feeding trombiculid larva to show the 'stylostome'

When the larvae feed they penetrate the upper dermis of the host with their chelicerae, then inject a histiolytic salivary secretion that dissolves the underlying tissue which appears to harden to form an attachment to the chelicerae. In this 'stylostome' a central tubular cavity develops through which more saliva is passed. This contains digestive enzymes that render the host tissue liquid enough to be taken up through the stylostome, the larva thus feeding not on blood but on partially digested host tissues. (*Haematoxylin and eosin (H&E) × 100*)

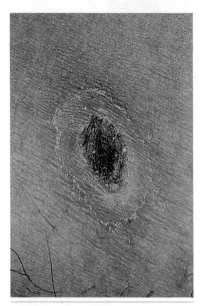

51 Eschar of mite bite

A typical 'eschar' forms at the site of the trombiculid bite and precedes the fever. That seen here on the lower abdomen of a Thai patient appeared 7 days before the photograph was taken. (© D A Warrell)

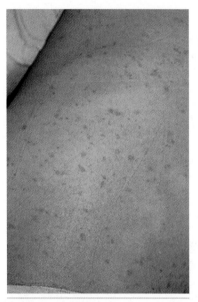

52 Scrub typhus rash

The maculopapular eruption which appears on about the sixth or seventh day of the illness, lasts for 3 or 4 days. While mainly seen on the trunk, upper arms and thighs, it may also appear on the face, hands and feet. The diagnosis of scrub typhus can be made by an immunofluorescent antibody method or by a more sensitive polymerase chain reaction (PCR) technique such as a nested PCR procedure to detect specific DNA fractions in blood. The PCR can confirm the prolonged persistence of *O. tsusugamushi* DNA in blood for several weeks following clinical recovery.

Spotted fevers (tick typhus)

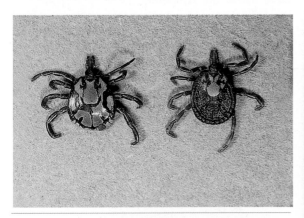

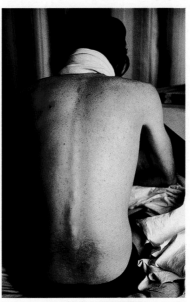

53 Adult male and female *Amblyomma hebraeum*, a vector of African tick-borne spotted fever
Various species of hard ticks transmit a variety of *Rickettsia* species, e.g. *Rickettsia africae* in sub-Saharan Africa and parts of the French West Indies. In the latter region the vector is *Amblyomma variegatum*, the main vector in west, central and east Africa, from where this arthropod was probably transported at the time of the slave trade. Compare the characteristic markings of the scutal shield of *A. hebraeum*, the main vector in South Africa, with those of *A. variegatum* (**60**). The immature stages of both tick species readily feed on humans. (× *1.8*) (♂ left, ♀ right.)

54 Eschar at site of tick bite
As with mite-borne typhus, 'eschar' forms at the site of the infective tick bite. The distribution of the rash is also seen clearly on the back of this individual infected in South Africa.

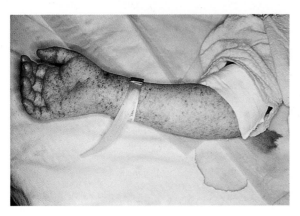

55 Petechial rash of Rocky Mountain spotted fever
Rickettsia rickettsii causes three types of tick-borne infection in the USA. The western type is transmitted by *Dermacentor andersoni*, the eastern type by *Dermacentor variabilis* and the southern type by *Amblyomma americanum* and *Rhipicephalus sanguineum*. Various small rodents, gophers and woodchucks serve as mammalian hosts. This 4-year old child, seen here comatose on the eighth day of the illness, recovered fully. An eschar marked the site of the bite. The application of a tourniquet, as seen here, accentuates the haemorrhagic nature of the rash distal to the site of the pressure (Hess test).

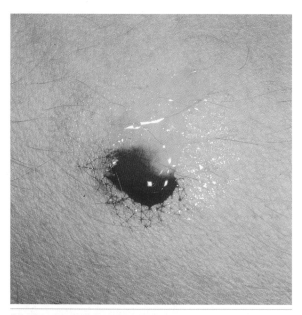

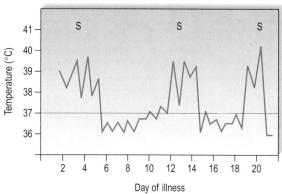

86 Temperature chart of tick-borne relapsing fever
The infection acquires its name from the typical relapsing nature of the fever. *B. duttoni* appears in the blood only during the febrile episodes, which are numerous and of short duration. S, spirochaetes in blood.

85 Site of the bite of *O. moubata*
Note the reddening of the skin proximal to the point of attachment immediately after the fully engorged tick has released itself, the continual bleeding caused by the anticoagulant component of the tick's saliva and the coxal fluid. Infection occurs both from the injection of blood containing the organisms and when the *Borrelia* that are shed with the coxal fluid enter the wound.

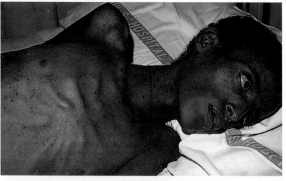

87 Louse-borne relapsing fever in an Ethiopian
B. recurrentis transmitted by body lice occurs in epidemic form in Ethiopia and Eritrea. The febrile periods recur usually on one or two occasions only (up to five in some cases, however). This patient, who presented with fever, jaundice and large petechial haemorrhages on the trunk, was severely emaciated. Mortality in untreated patients may be as high as 40% during epidemics. (© D A Warrell)

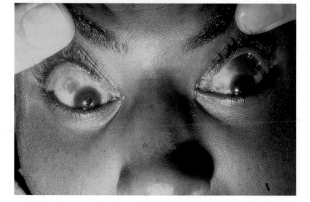

88 Conjunctival haemorrhages in a patient with *B. recurrentis* infection
This sign is common associated with severe louse-borne relapsing fever. (© D A Warrell)

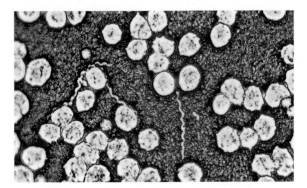

89 Borrelia recurrentis in blood film
Infection is acquired from the body fluids of lice crushed on the skin while scratching. The spirochaetal organisms are readily seen in this Indian ink preparation. (× *800*)

Lyme disease

Lyme disease is a zoonosis of rodents caused by several species of *Borrelia*, which are spread by the bites of infected ixodid ticks. Human infection is caused by *Borrelia burgdorferi sensu stricto*, *Borrelia afzelii* and *Borrelia garinii*. It is now recognised to be cosmopolitan in distribution. In humans, three stages are recognised: (I) an acute phase often associated with a rash, (II) early disseminated infection involving the circulatory, nervous and skeletal systems, and (III) a chronic stage of multiple organ involvement that may only become apparent months or years after the initial infection.

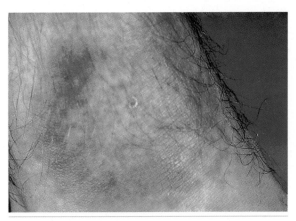

90 Erythema chronicum migrans
This unusual type of chronic rash is associated with the early stage of Lyme disease. It spreads centrifugally in 1–2 weeks following infection and usually resolves spontaneously within a month or two. The best diagnostic procedure at present is the examination for serum IgG and IgM antibodies using an enzyme-linked immunosorbent assay (ELISA) test with recombinant proteins as antigens. This is claimed to yield a 20% detection rate in stage I, 50% in stage II and nearly 100% in stage III infection.

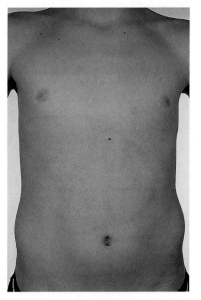

91 Later stage of erythema chronicum migrans
A very extensive centrifugal extension of the rash can be seen on this man's abdomen.

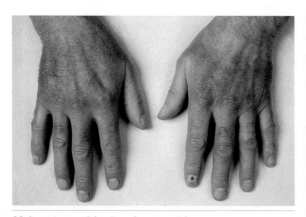

92 Acrodermatitis chronica atrophicans
In some patients, acrodermatitis chronica atrophicans can develop in the chronic stage III. The typical bluish-red inflammatory lesions are usually found on the acral portions of the extremities. (Courtesy of Dr. Eva Asbrink. From Sivadas R, Rahn DW and Luft BJ. Lyme Disease. In: Cohen J and Powderly W, eds. Infectious Diseases, 2nd edn. Edinburgh: Mosby 2004; 591–604.)

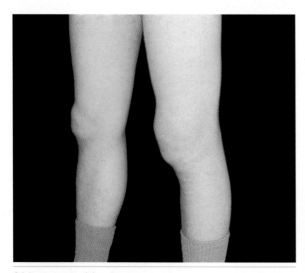

94 Lyme arthritis of knees
Severe deformity of both knees is seen in this man with chronic Lyme disease. (Courtesy of Dr A C Steere).

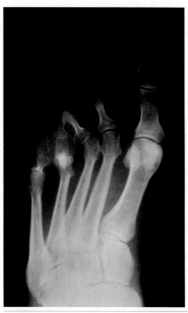

93 Arthritis caused by *B. burgdorferi* infection
Acute arthritis and chronic, disabling arthritic lesions (both usually associated with skin lesions) are late sequelae of Lyme disease. Neurological changes such as meningoencephalitis (sometimes with cranial or peripheral radiculopathy) are being increasingly reported. The severity of lesions associated with *B. burgdorferi* may be related to host genetic factors. The infection, in fact, appears to produce protean manifestations and the diagnosis is probably missed in many cases. If the diagnosis – which may be confirmed by culturing the organisms from skin or other tissues and by serology – is made sufficiently early, the disease is usually cured rapidly by chemotherapy.

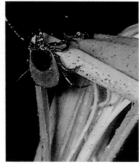

95 Adult female *Ixodes dammini*
The larvae and nymphs feed mainly on rodents but occasionally on humans, to whom they pass the spirochaetes from the rodent reservoirs. This species is responsible for the transmission of Lyme disease in the northeast of Canada and the USA, where it is also the vector of *Theileria microti*. The organisms are transmitted trans-stadially. (× 2.5)

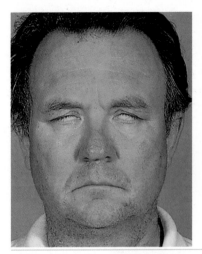

96 Bilateral Bell's palsy lesion in Lyme disease

Meningoradiculitis leading to bilateral, peripheral, facial palsy (Bannwarth's syndrome), was caused by Lyme borreliosis (confirmed serologically) in this 50-year-old German patient. The majority of neurological lesions improve spontaneously with time. In this case, the right facial palsy recovered completely after chemotherapy but the left only partially.

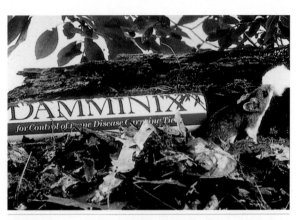

97 *Peromyscus leucopus*: the white-footed mouse – permethrin-impregnated acaricide for control of *Ixodes dammini*

P. leucopus is the most important maintenance host for *B. burgdorferi* on the eastern seaboard of the USA. Other rodent species harbour the organisms in other countries – e.g. species of *Apodemus* and *Clethrionomys* in Europe, where *Ixodes ricinus* is an important vector. Careful ecological observations revealed that this rodent likes to line its nest with soft materials such as cotton wool. When the wild rodents are provided with a ready source of this material in the form of cotton wool balls impregnated with a synthetic pyrethroid, they convey the acaricide into their nests, where it kills the rodents' ticks, thus interrupting the cycle of transmission both of Lyme disease and *Babesia microti* (see **101**) – a prime example of the importance of good fieldwork and its practical application.

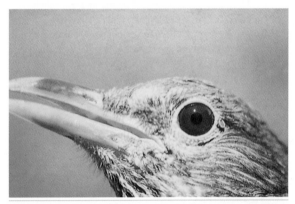

98 Female blackbird (*Turdus merula*) infested with larvae and lymphs of *I. ricinus*

Two-thirds of the ticks found on birds in surveys in Switzerland were larvae and one-third nymphs, among which 25% were infected with *B. burgdorferi*.

Rat-bite fever ('sodoku')

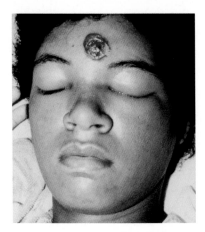

99 A patient with 'sodoku' following a rat bite

Infection with *Spirillum minus* in this young Brazilian woman following a rat bite resulted in a local ulcerative lesion associated with high fever and cervical lymphadenopathy. The spirochaete-like organisms were detected by dark field examination of material from the ulcer. This patient's infection responded to antibiotic therapy, but untreated infections may cause death in over 10% of cases. *Streptobacillus moniliformis* is another rare infection associated with rat bites or accidental contamination with rat excreta. This pathogen can induce systemic infection leading to fulminant septicaemia and death but is more commonly associated with a relatively mild fever and sometimes a maculopapular rash of the extremities.

PROTOZOAL INFECTIONS See Table 5.

Piroplasmosis in humans

Babesiosis and theileriosis are apicomplexan infections that are of considerable economic importance in domestic cattle, as well as in horses, smaller domestic animals and a wide range of wild mammals. The causative organisms belong to at least two genera, *Babesia* and *Theileria*, which are commonly referred to as 'piroplasms', their exact systematic status remaining a subject for debate. The first genus belongs to the family Babesiidae and the second to the family Theileriidae. A common feature of these families is that the organisms are transmitted to their vertebrate hosts by different species of ixodiid tick (in rare exceptions argasiid ticks are involved), in the tissues of which they undergo a complex life cycle. Its terminal phase involves the development of an infective sporozoite stage. When sporozoites of *Babesia* are injected by the tick, they enter circulating erythrocytes, in which they multiply by repeated cycles of binary fission to form large numbers of asexual stages and, at some stage, gametocytes that are infective to feeding ticks. Infection in the acarine host is both trans-stadial and transovarian. In the mammalian host, *Theileria* first undergoes a cycle of development within lymphocytes, producing a leukaemia-like, generalised lymphatic infection before entering circulating red blood cells. The destruction of the latter results in severe anaemia and this, together with severe damage to the host's immune system, may lead to the loss of a high proportion of the infected animals. The ticks become infected when they take up the intraerythrocytic gametocytes of either genus.

Until about 30 years ago infection of humans with piroplasms (which was first reported as recently as 1957) was considered to be an extremely rare event and was limited to individuals who, usually by virtue of a prior loss of their spleen, were severely immunodeficient. The outcome was generally fatal and the parasites in question were invariably identified as species that normally infect cattle. The discovery of mild piroplasm infections, mainly self-limiting even without chemotherapy, on the eastern seaboard of the USA, revealed that ixodiid ticks in that area not uncommonly transmit a rodent piroplasm to humans. This organism, which is enzootic in a high proportion of wild rodents, has been found also to infect rodents and humans in the Gulf of Mexico and has, on a few occasions, been identified in forest workers in Germany and other parts of Europe.

Table 5 The protozoa (phylum Apicomplexa) of medical importance

Phylum	Subclass	Order	Family	Genus and Species
Sarcomastigophora (see **Tables 17** and **18**) *Ciliophora* (see **Table 17**) *Microspora* (see **Table 19**) Apicomplexa				
	Piroplasmasina		Babesiidae[1]	*Babesia bovis* *B. divergens* *B. microti* *Babesia* sp. Near *odocoilei*
	Coccidiasina			
		Eucoccidiorida Suborder Haemospororina		
			Plasmodiidae	*Plasmodium (Plasmodium) vivax* *P. (P.) ovale* *P. (P.) malariae* *P. (P.) knowlesi*[2] *P. (Laverania) falciparum*
		Suborder Eimeriorina		
			Sarcocystidae	*Toxoplasma gondii* *Sarcocystis hominis*[3] *S. suihominis*[4] *Sarcocystis* spp.[5]
			Eimeriidae	*Isospora belli* *Cyclospora cayetanensis*
			Cryptosporidiidae	*Cryptosporidium hominis* *C. parvum* *Cryptosporidium* sp. near *parvum*[6]

[1] All rare in man. Genus names are still under review.
[2] A common zoonotic infection in parts of Southeast Asia, especially the island of Borneo
[3] Man definitive, cattle intermediate host
[4] Man definitive, pig intermediate host
[5] 'Sarcocystis lindemanni' consists of a number of unidentified species for which humans are the intermediate hosts.
[6] Rare in humans.

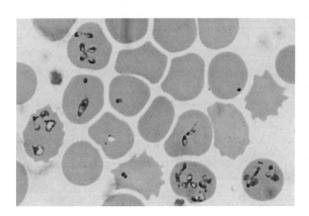

100 *Babesia divergens* in human blood
Human infection with species of piroplasm transmitted by the bite of the tick *Ixodes ricinus* infected from cattle is a rare occurrence. Infection in normal people with this piroplasm may give rise to a self-limiting fever and parasitaemia, as in the case of infection with the rodent parasite *Babesia microti* on the north-eastern seaboard of the USA via the tick *Ixodes scapularis*. Heavy red-cell infection may develop, however, in splenectomised patients, leading to fatal haemolytic anaemia. This patient died from an infection acquired from the cattle parasite *B. divergens* in Scotland. Other species of *Babesia* that occasionally infect humans, e.g. the WA1, CA1 and MO1 isolates from the USA are now being recognised by molecular characterisation. (*Giemsa* × *700*)

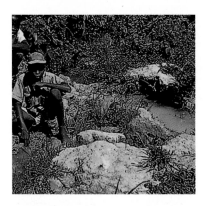

105 Breeding site of *Anopheles gambiae* in west Africa
A. gambiae and closely related species are the most dangerous malaria vectors in tropical Africa. *A. gambiae* breeds in small temporary collections of fresh surface water exposed to sunlight and in such sites as residual pools in drying river beds. The majority of important vectors in other parts of the world are also surface-water breeders. Malaria control operations since the early 1950s were based mainly on the destruction of house-haunting anopheline vectors by DDT or other insecticides sprayed on the interior walls where mosquitoes usually rest before and/or after feeding; larviciding played a relatively minor role (see **190, 191**).

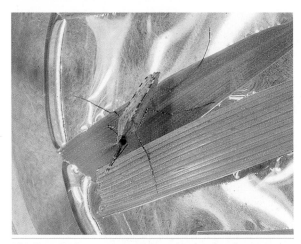

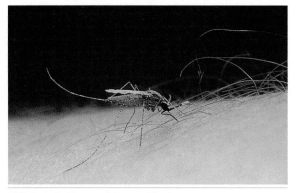

107 *Anopheles gambiae* probing
Malaria is transmitted by numerous species of female *Anopheles* mosquito (see **Table 6**). Most species bite indoors at night but some are outdoor-feeding. The adults are distinguished from culicine mosquitoes by the structures of the antennae and palps. (See also **5** and **7**.) (× 4)

106 Female *Anopheles stephensi* emerging from pupa
This is a peridomestic mosquito that is responsible for the transmission of malaria in urban areas over a wide geographical range from the east of the Arabian peninsula, through central Asia to Pakistan and India and as far east as Burma. It breeds mainly in water cisterns, domestic water tanks, wells and other collections of fresh water. In rural areas it breeds in fresh, clean water in ground pools but will also tolerate brackish water. *A. stephensi* is largely endophilic in western India but less so in such areas as Calcutta in the east. Although zoophilic by choice, *A. stephensi* is a very efficient malaria vector, particularly in urban areas. (× 4)

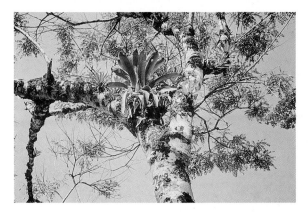

108 A bromeliad in the Amazonian rain forest
Bromeliads provide breeding sites for *Anopheles* (*Kerteszia*) *bellator* and *Anopheles* (*Kerteszia*) *cruzi*. These species are found from the Caribbean islands south to Brazil. The females feed mainly before or just after dusk, in shaded woody areas or in houses, but they are generally exophagic. Up to 1% of *A. bellator* have been found to be naturally infected with sporozoites in the hills above Rio de Janeiro, Brazil, where this species is considered to be a secondary vector. Some South American vectors of this subgenus breed in the axils of bromeliads, the destruction of which is only possible on a very limited scale in most endemic areas. The adults bite outdoors rather than inside houses. Consequently, the control of these vectors by insecticides is often extremely difficult.

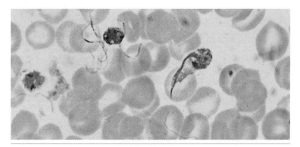

109 Development of male gametes

Male gametes develop by a process of flagellar extrusion, known as exflagellation, from microgametocytes contained in the bloodmeal in the midgut of the female anopheline. (× *950*)

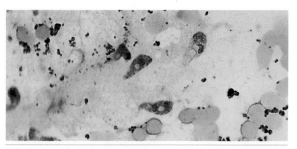

110 Ookinetes in midgut

Male and female gametes fuse to produce motile ookinetes, which enter midgut epithelial cells. (× *950*)

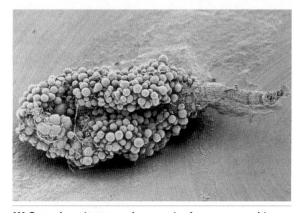

111 Scanning electron micrograph of oocysts outside anopheline midgut

Infective stages (sporozoites) develop in oocysts that lie on the outside of the mosquito midgut. (× *65*)

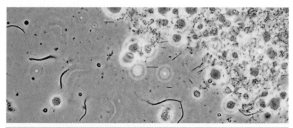

112 Living infective sporozoites

Bow-shaped sporozoites emerge from the oocysts and enter the insect's salivary glands. They are passed into the small vessels of the skin with saliva when the mosquito next takes a blood meal. (× *370*)

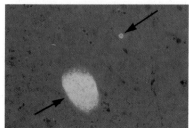

114 Hypnozoite and preerythrocytic schizont in liver biopsy

The unicellular, dormant hypnozoite (arrowed, right) stands in sharp contrast to the maturing PE schizont (left) in this fluorescent-antibody-stained section of Rhesus monkey liver containing *Plasmodium cynomolgi* – a relapsing species with the same life cycle as *P. vivax*. (× *270*)

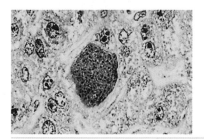

113 Exoerythrocytic schizont of *Plasmodium malariae* in liver

Within 30 minutes, the sporozoites enter the parenchymal cells of the host's liver where they may form large pre-erythrocytic (PE) 'tissue' schizonts or, in *P. vivax* and *P. ovale*, hypnozoites (see **114** and **115**). The PE schizonts mature in 6–14 days according to the species, before liberating daughter cells ('merozoites') into the hepatic circulation.
(*Giemsa–colophonium technique* × *350*)

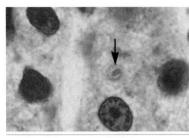

115 Hypnozoite of *Plasmodium cynomolgi*

Enlarged view of a single hypnozoite. (*Giemsa – colophonium technique × 2000*).

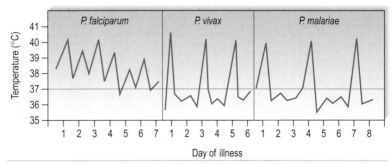

116 Tertian and quartan fever patterns

The asexual blood stages of *P. falciparum*, *P. vivax* and *P. ovale* require 48 hours to complete their schizogony. Fever is produced when the schizonts mature, i.e. at 48-hour intervals. This gives the classical tertian periodicity, which is, however, uncommon in a primary attack of *P. falciparum* malaria. *P. malariae* requires 72 hours and is associated with quartan fever, i.e. 72 hours between paroxysms.

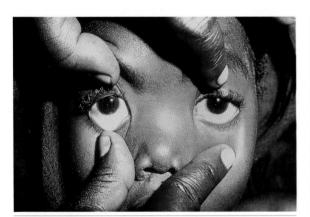

117 Malarial anaemia

The pathogenesis of malarial anaemia is multifactorial, involving destruction of parasitised cells, haemolysis of uninfected cells, dyserythropoiesis and iron sequestration. In parts of Africa, malarial anaemia is an important cause of death in children under 2 years of age. This young Kenyan boy with *P. falciparum* parasitaemia had profound anaemia with a haemoglobin of 12 g/l. (See also **1208**.) (© D A Warrell)

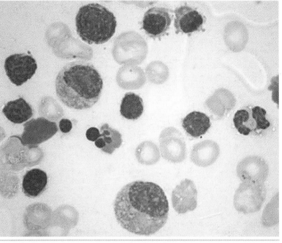

118 Spleen smear showing association of dyserythropoiesis with malaria

Although erythropoiesis is usually normoblastic in individuals with acute or chronic malaria, the examination of bone marrow frequently shows changes reflecting dyserythropoiesis such as the irregular nuclei and cytoplasmic bridges in erythroblasts seen in this figure. Two young rings of *P. falciparum* can be seen in an erythrocyte. (*Giemsa stain × 900*). (Courtesy of Dr Saad H Abdalla).

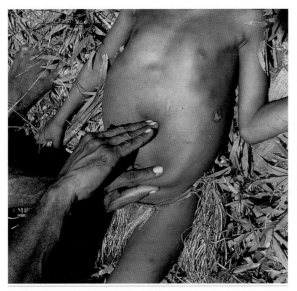

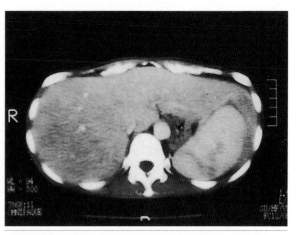

120 Massive hepatosplenomegaly in a patient with severe malarial anaemia
Computed tomography scan of the abdomen of a traveller from west Africa who presented with a haemoglobin less than 50 g/l. The scan shows a massively enlarged liver, the left lobe of which is encircling an enlarged spleen.

119 New Guinea child with grossly enlarged liver and spleen
Haemolysed red cells and parasite debris are phagocytosed by macrophages, particularly of the spleen and liver, which become enlarged. This child was seen on a field survey in a holoendemic area of northern Papua New Guinea.

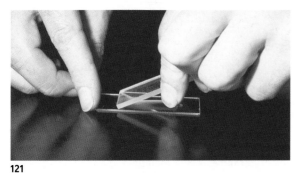

121   122

121 & 122 Preparation of thick and thin blood films
Although a number of rapid diagnostic tests such as those shown in **123** and **124**, as well as polymerase chain reaction (PCR) are becoming widely available, the 'gold standard' diagnosis of malaria is still based primarily on the recognition of parasites in well-prepared thick and thin blood films stained with a Romanowsky stain (Giemsa, Leishman, Field, etc.) at pH 7.2–7.4. A small drop of blood from a finger or ear is placed on a clean slide. The thin film is made by pulling a second slide away from the drop (**121**, left). A thick film is made by spreading two or three larger drops on a slide, then spreading them out with the corner of a second slide. The thick smear should still be sufficiently transparent to see print through it, as shown here (**122**, right). Sophisticated diagnostic tools such as *Plasmodium*-specific DNA probes are of value mainly for epidemiological surveys but are of little value in diagnosing malaria in individual patients.

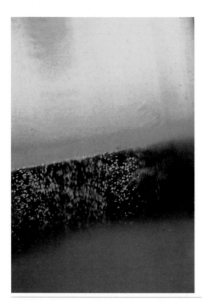

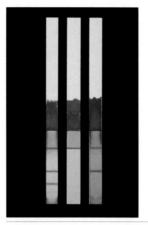

124 Immunochromatographic assay for *P. falciparum* and *P. vivax*

To aid the rapid diagnosis of falciparum and other species of malaria in individual patients and for ease and speed of diagnosis as an alternative to microscopy in field surveys, a number of simple immunochromatographic assays have been devised based on the use of monoclonal antibodies to detect parasite histodine-rich protein (HRP-2) or parasite-specific lactate dehydrogenase (pLDH). The paper-like dipstick shown here, based on the recognition of pLDH, is impregnated with antibodies and dye-containing microcapsules and is reported to detect as few as 100–200 parasites/μl of blood, i.e. a parasitaemia of 0.002%. In this figure the left-hand strip shows a positive reaction for *P. falciparum* and the right-hand strip for *P. vivax*, *P. ovale* or *P. malariae*. The centre strip is a negative control. Such rapid diagnostic tests (RDAs) should be used with caution for self-diagnosis by, for example, travellers as false-negative results may occur. (Figure of OptiMAL® Rapid Malaria Test courtesy of Dr D Bashforth DiaMed, Cressier, Switzerland.)

123 Diagnostic test based on fluorescent staining of centrifuged blood

In this technique, a fluorescent stain (green in this case) is used to stain malaria parasites in blood containing anticoagulant, which is centrifuged in a special capillary tube containing a float. With ultraviolet epi-illumination, the parasites can readily be seen just beneath the buffy coat and in a thinned-out layer of red cells. The procedure can also be used to detect other parasites such as trypanosomes (see also **223**) and microfilariae. (Figure of QBC Test® courtesy of Becton Dickinson, Tropical Diseases Diagnostics, Sparks, MD.) (× *40*)

Plasmodium falciparum

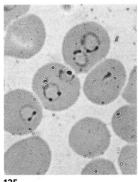

125

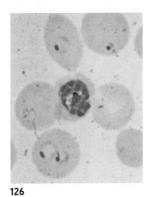

126

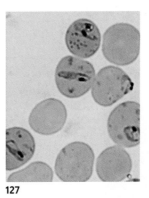

127

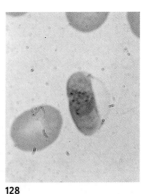

128

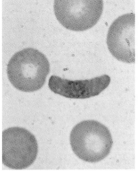

129

125–129 Life cycle of the blood stages (thin blood films)

Fine rings (**125**) predominate, with mature trophozoites and schizonts (**126**) appearing uncommonly in the peripheral circulation because parasites bind (cytoadhere) to the post capillary venules of the internal organs. Host cells are not enlarged. Basophilic clefts and spots of irregular shape and size (Maurer's clefts and dots) may be seen in erythrocytes containing more mature parasites. They are thought to be aggregates of parasite proteins which are being exported from the parasite to the surface of the red cell (**127**). Crescent-shaped male (**128**) and female gametocytes (**129**) are diagnostic. Infection with *P. falciparum* gives rise to 'malignant tertian malaria', so-called because severe, often lethal complications such as those figured below can develop; such cases must be treated as medical emergencies. (*Giemsa × 1500*)

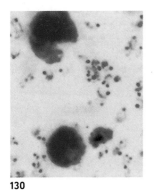

130

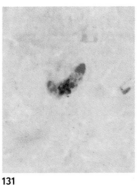

131

130 & 131 Thick blood films

Usually only young rings (**130**, left) are seen in acute infections, although sometimes in very large numbers. Heavy parasitaemia leads to severe haemolytic anaemia. Gametocytes (**131**, right) appear about a week after the onset of the illness. (*Field × 1500*)

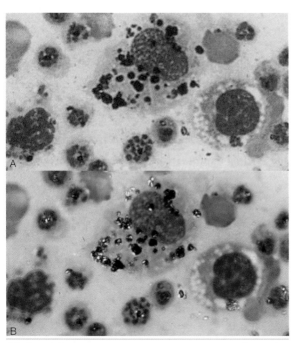

A

B

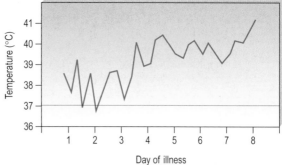

134 Temperature chart in falciparum malaria

In first infections, the fever is usually irregular rather than tertian. Thrombocytopenia is commonly found. Relapses do not occur after adequate treatment with blood schizontocides since there are no hypnozoites and hence no secondary tissue schizogony (cf *P. vivax* and *P. ovale*). Recrudescences, as opposed to relapses, occur when treatment is inadequate and asexual parasites are not cleared from the blood.

132 A & B Macrophage from the spleen of a patient with acute falciparum malaria

Parasitised erythrocytes are removed from the peripheral circulation by macrophages in the reticuloendothelial tissues. **A** shows a large monocyte/macrophage, which contains large quantities of malaria pigment (haemozoin), the residue from the digestion of infected red cells. The use of a polarising filter (**B**) clearly reveals the haemozoin, which is birefringent, a technique particularly useful in material that contains only scarce parasites. (*Giemsa* × *1500*).

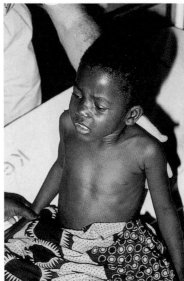

135 Prostration in malaria

A common manifestation of severe malaria in children is the inability to sit up and take fluid by mouth. Here a child with falciparum malaria, while fully conscious, is being supported to take water.

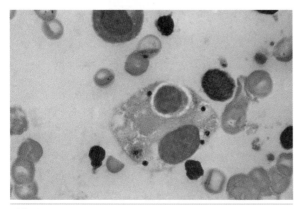

133 Macrophage from the bone marrow in acute falciparum malaria

Macrophage activation can be profound in acute malaria. Here a macrophage contains an uninfected red cell, a schizont, clumps of haemozoin and even a lymphocyte. (Leishman × *900*)

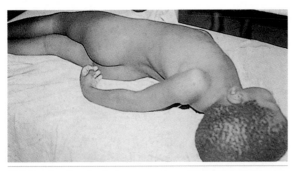

136 Cerebral malaria in a comatose Malawian child with opisthotonus

In holoendemic areas of Africa, cerebral malaria commonly occurs in children between 6 months and 3 years of age – often older than those with severe malarial anaemia. Cerebrospinal fluid opening pressures are often raised in children when measured at lumbar puncture. About 10% of children who survive cerebral malaria have neurological sequelae. These include hemiparesis, cerebellar ataxia, cortical blindness, severe hypotonia, mental retardation, generalised spasticity and aphasia.

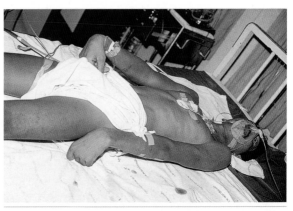

137 Decerebrate rigidity in cerebral malaria

The Thai man shown here had unrousable coma and peripheral parasitaemia. Other causes of encephalopathy were excluded, mainly on clinical grounds. He therefore fulfilled the World Health Organization definition of cerebral malaria. (See also **135** showing a less advanced stage of cerebral malaria.) Decerebrate rigidity may also be associated with hypoglycaemia, which may be quinine-induced. This is more common in pregnant women, in whom the warning signs are fits, abnormal behaviour and a change in the level of consciousness.

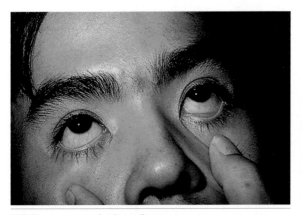

138 Severe malarial jaundice

Deep jaundice, which is clearly seen in this Vietnamese man who had severe falciparum malaria, is much commoner in adults than in children. Liver failure, however, occurs only in individuals in whom a concurrent viral hepatitis is present. (© D A Warrell)

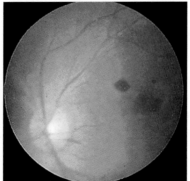

139 Retinal haemorrhage in severe falciparum malaria

Examination of the fundus is an important part of the physical examination of a patient. In this Thai with cerebral malaria, the haemorrhage is near the macula. Such haemorrhages have been found in as many as 18–30% of patients with cerebral malaria and are an indication for parenteral therapy. In children, papilloedema and extramacular retinal oedema predict a poor prognosis. (© D A Warrell)

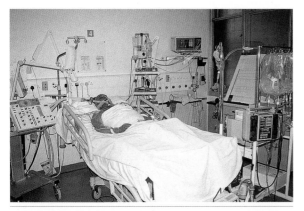

140 Multiorgan failure in severe falciparum malaria
Patients with severe malaria should be cared for at the highest level of clinical care, in this case in an intensive therapy unit. This patient presented with renal failure and is being haemodiafiltered. In addition he developed Gram-negative septicaemia with hypotension and metabolic acidosis ('algid malaria'). These complications developed in the absence of cerebral malaria.

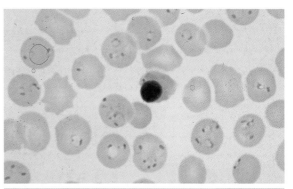

141 Blood film from a patient with hyperparasitaemia in acute falciparum malaria
This patient presented with jaundice and was initially mistakenly thought to have hepatitis. The blood films show 80% parasitaemia. Included is a late erythroblast, which has emerged from the bone marrow and is also interestingly infected with a ring form of *P. falciparum*. Within half an hour of this blood film being made the patient died. (*Leishman* × *900*)

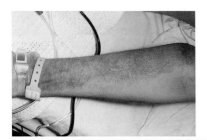

142 Disseminated intravascular coagulation in falciparum malaria
Bleeding into the skin seen in a patient who demonstrated disseminated intravascular coagulation with thrombocytopenia, a prolonged prothrombin time, increased fibrinogen degradation products and hypofibrinogenaemia. He had no signs of cerebral malaria.

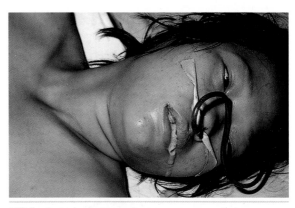

143 Acute pulmonary oedema
Two types of pulmonary oedema occur in severe falciparum malaria. The first, due to overhydration, is preventable with good patient management of the patient. The second, acute respiratory distress syndrome (ARDS) occurs during the fourth or fifth day of the illness when the patient appears to be improving; its causation is not clearly understood. This Vietnamese woman, in addition, had cerebral malaria complicated by hypoglycaemia. (© D A Warrell)

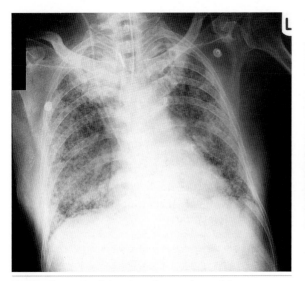

144 Radiograph of the chest in a patient with acute respiratory distress syndrome
The radiograph shows new, bilateral, diffuse, homogeneous pulmonary infiltrates without evidence of cardiac failure, fluid overload or chronic lung disease in an adult with severe falciparum malaria. This condition is rare in children.

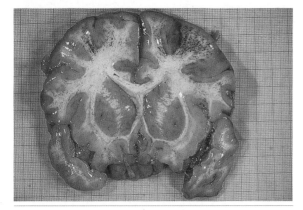

146 Gross section of brain in cerebral malaria
Cerebral malaria results when cerebral capillaries are blocked by erythrocytes containing developing falciparum schizonts (see also **147**). The blockages lead to petechial haemorrhages round many of the capillaries, as seen in this section. Cerebral malaria is a medical emergency that demands immediate treatment by intravenous administration of suitable antimalarials. Rehydration is also often required but careful attention must be paid to avoiding overhydration, which may result in pulmonary oedema. It is now recognised that other factors, such as the over-production of certain cytokines (e.g. tumour necrosis factor, TNF), are involved in the pathogenesis of cerebral malaria.

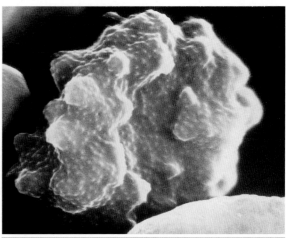

145 Scanning electron micrograph of a mature *P. falciparum* schizont in a red cell
The merozoites form asexual parasites, which grow inside erythrocytes to form the trophozoites. These ingest haemoglobin, producing insoluble pigment (haemozoin) as a waste product. When growth is complete, the parasites undergo cell division (schizogony) and the daughter cells (merozoites), after rupture of the host erythrocyte membrane, invade new red cells. The biconcave shape of the red cell is lost as the parasite develops and the infected red cell becomes more spherical in shape. Moreover it develops tiny but regularly arrayed knobs on its surface, which are the sites at which schizont-infected red cells bind to endothelial surfaces in the deep tissues in organs such as the brain, liver, heart and spleen. There is loss of red cell deformity, which appears to be correlated with the clinical outcome. ($\times$ *11 000*)

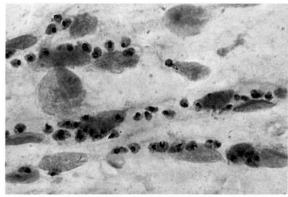

147 Brain smear from a fatal case of cerebral malaria
The capillaries are seen to be full of erythrocytes containing maturing trophozoites and schizonts of *P. falciparum*. (*Giemsa* $\times$ *350*)

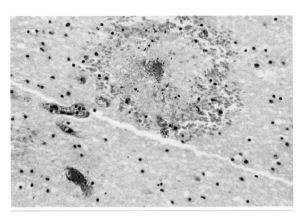

148 Microhaemorrhage around a disrupted cerebral capillary

A clear ring of erythrocytes forms a halo, at the centre of which can be seen a disrupted cerebral capillary. Other capillaries contain mature schizonts of *P. falciparum*. Dürck's granulomas are probably the sequelae of what, at the time of acute malaria, would appear as such microhaemorrhages (*H&E × 125*)

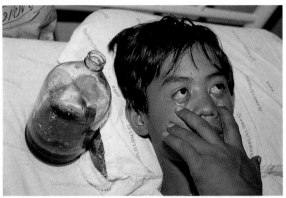

149 Malarial haemoglobinuria, 'blackwater fever'

This condition may be due to severe intravascular haemolysis and is mainly seen in semi-immune patients. More commonly, however, haemoglobinuria is due to haemolysis developing in patients deficient in the enzyme glucose-6-phosphate dehydrogenase (G6PD), in response to oxidant antimalarials, e.g. primaquine, quinine or other drugs. Note the small quantity of very dark urine passed by this Thai patient and the pale conjunctivae. (© D A Warrell)

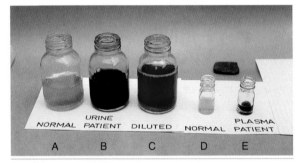

150 Urine and serum in blackwater fever

The figure shows normal urine (**A**) compared with a specimen of urine from a patient with blackwater fever undiluted (**B**) and diluted (**C**). Also shown are a normal serum sample (**D**) compared with that from a patient with blackwater fever (**E**).

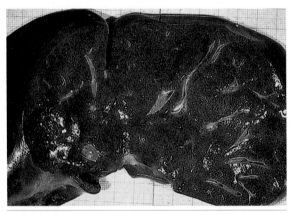

151 Liver in chronic malaria

In chronic infection, accumulation of malaria pigment (haemozoin) in the macrophages produces a dark brown coloration of liver and spleen.

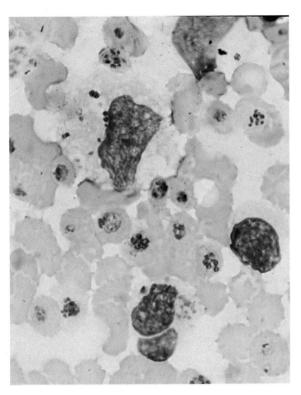

152 Placental smear with falciparum schizonts and macrophage

The accumulation of falciparum schizonts in the maternal side of the placental circulation may result in the delivery of underweight infants, especially in primigravidae. True congenital malaria is very rare. Note the presence of haemozoin granules in the macrophage. Pigment-loaded macrophages and neutrophils in the peripheral circulation usually indicate that the blood infection has been present for some days. (*Giemsa × 900*)

Plasmodium vivax

153–157 Life cycle of the blood stages (thin films)

All stages of asexual parasites – from young trophozoites (**153**) to schizonts – appear in the peripheral circulation in vivax malaria together with gametocytes. The parasites are large and amoeboid (**154**), and produce schizonts with about 16 daughter cells (merozoites) (**155**). Pigment is well developed. Host red cells are enlarged and uniformly covered with fine eosinophilic stippling (Schüffner's dots). Gametocytes are round, with the male (microgametocytes; **156**) being about 7 μm, and the female (macrogametocytes; **157**) being 10 μm or more in diameter. (*Giemsa × 1500*) (See also **104**.)

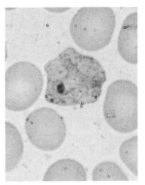

153

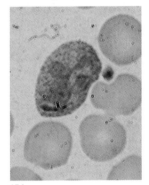

154

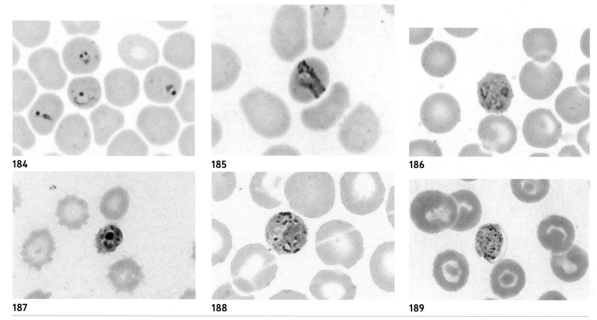

184   185   186

187   188   189

184–189 Life cycle of the blood stages (thin films)

The host erythrocytes are usually of a normal size. Young rings (**184**) strongly resemble the young ring stages of *P. falciparum*. Band forms (**185**) similar to those of *P. malariae* are commonly seen, as well as more rounded young trophozoites (**186**), in which dark pigment granules are prominent, often forming a halo around the periphery of the parasites. The host erythrocyte may contain light stippling and be coloured a light mauve with Romanowsky stains. Some older trophozoites are in rather ovoid, fimbriated erythrocytes in which the cytoplasm has a granular, mauvish colour with Romanowsky staining, somewhat resembling *P. ovale*. (This is seen also in *P. knowlesi* infections in Rhesus monkeys.) Maturing and mature schizonts (**187**) commonly contain up to 12 or 16 merozoites and the pigment forms a large more or less central clump as in those of *P. malariae*. In erythrocytes containing macro- (**188**) or microgametocytes (**189**), the cytoplasm stains a distinctly mauve colour and the edges are often lightly fimbriated. Macro- and especially microgametocytes are smaller than the host cells, the former containing a heavily staining, solid nucleus and small number of large, dark pigment granules and the latter, larger numbers of smaller granules and a more diffuse nucleus. (*Giemsa × 1500*) (Blood films provided courtesy of Professor Balbir Singh and Dr David LK Sung. Photography by Dr David LK Sung, J Williams, LB Stewart and W Peters.)

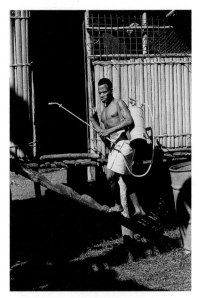

190 Indoor house spraying in malaria control
The ambitious global programme that started in the 1950s to eradicate malaria by spraying the inside of all dwellings in endemic areas with long-lasting insecticides such as DDT failed to meet its objective in all but a few areas. Residual spraying still retains a place, however, as one of the effective means of controlling transmission in some areas, in spite of popular fears over the possible ecological hazards of deploying such organochlorines widely. Here a malaria worker is seen entering a village house in the north of Papua New Guinea to apply a DDT suspension to the inside walls. Although at the time that the photograph was taken house spraying radically reduced transmission in this holoendemic area, the project did not produce a lasting effect and the area remains highly endemic. Insecticide resistance has been, unfortunately, an all too frequent consequence of the mass use of DDT and other residual chemicals.

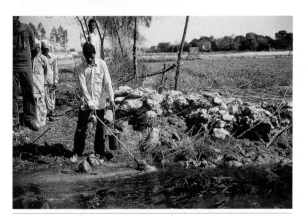

191 Larviciding of anopheline breeding site near New Delhi
The management of larval breeding sites has been a traditional means of limiting malaria transmission and is still of value in specific circumstances. This figure illustrates the spraying with oil of a stream in which several species of anopheline vectors were breeding.

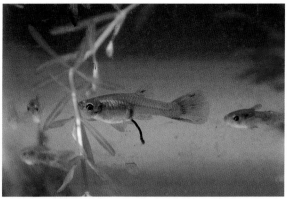

192 Larvivorous fish
Small freshwater fish such as species of *Gambusia* and *Poecilia reticulata* (seen here), which feed on mosquito larvae, still retain a minor but useful place in the control of vector breeding in peridomestic containers such as that harbouring the Indian malaria vector *Anopheles stephensi*.

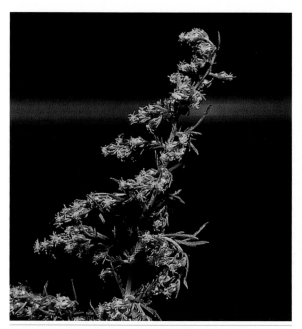

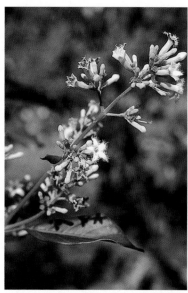

194 Flowers of *Cinchona ledgeriana*, the source of quinine
A young plant growing in a plantation in Madagascar. Quinine and related alkaloids are harvested from the bark of the *Cinchona* tree. (*Natural size*)

193 Qinghao: the oldest antimalarial

Resistance of parasites, especially *P. falciparum*, to antimalarial drugs is currently one of the biggest problems in the management of malaria. In the search for new drugs with which to combat drug-resistant malaria, attention has moved away from synthetic chemistry to a search for natural products, some of them used from time immemorial in traditional therapy. Among such remedies is qinghao (the Chinese wormwood, *Artemisia annua*), which has yielded one of the most potent compounds available currently: qinghaosu (artemisinin). Qinghao has been recorded as an anti-fever plant in traditional Chinese medicine for over 2000 years, considerably longer than the Peruvian plant that yields quinine (see **194**), the beneficial effects of which were first recorded a mere 400 years ago. A number of semisynthetic derivatives and others based on the active pharmacore of artemisinin are now under development or clinical trial. (*Natural size*)

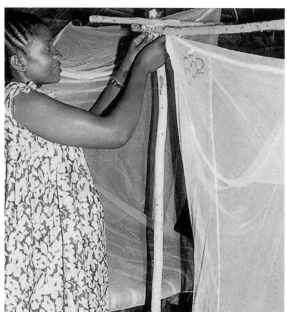

195 The mosquito net: an emerging method for malaria control!

In addition to the widespread problem of multiple drug resistance in *P. falciparum*, vector control has failed in many countries because of insecticide resistance or other factors, some of them socioeconomic. Protection of the populations of endemic countries remains an elusive target. These obstacles have necessitated a vigorous search for additional, sustainable ways of preventing malaria. Field trials of mosquito nets impregnated with synthetic pyrethroids have given promising results in terms of lowering the rate of infected bites in the community, but are still far from eliminating transmission in most places. The situation is especially challenging in tropical Africa, where transmission is very intense.

TRYPANOSOMIASIS See **Tables 7** and **18**.

Table 7 Trypanosomes of medical and veterinary importance

Section	Genus (Subgenus)	Species	Host Species	Disease
Africa				
Salivaria	*Trypanosoma (Duttonella)*	*vivax*	Antelopes, ruminants, equines, dogs	Souma
		uniforme	Antelopes, ruminants	(Pathogenic)
	Trypanosoma (Nannomonas)	*congolense*	Antelopes, ruminants, equines, pigs, dogs	(Pathogenic)
		simiae	Pigs, warthogs, camels	(Pathogenic)
	Trypanosoma (Trypanozoon)	*brucei brucei*	Antelopes, domestic mammals	Nagana
		brucei rhodesiense	Antelopes, humans	Sleeping sickness (acute form)
		brucei gambiense	Humans, pigs	Sleeping sickness (chronic form)
		*evansi**	Bovines, equines, camels, dogs, etc.	Surra
		equiperdum[†]	Equines	Dourine
	Trypanosoma (Pycnomonas)	*suis*	Domestic and wild pigs	(Pathogenic)
South America				
Salivaria	*Trypanosoma (Duttonella)*	*vivax*[‡]	Bovines	(Pathogenic)
	Trypanosoma (Herpetosoma)	*rangeli*[§]	Many wild animals, humans	(Nonpathogenic)
Stercoraria	*Trypanosoma (Schizotrypanum)*	*cruzi*[§]	Humans, armadillos, opossums, dogs, etc.	Chagas' disease

See Table 5 for general systematic position in protozoa (Sarcomastigophora).
All species transmitted by tsetse flies except: * by tabanid flies; † by coitus; ‡ by various biting flies; § by reduviid bugs.

African trypanosomiasis

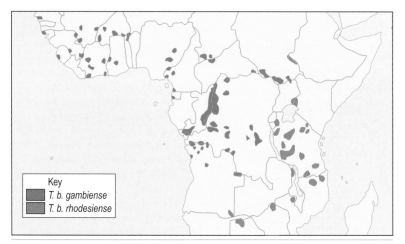

Key
T. b. gambiense
T. b. rhodesiense

196 Distribution of infection in humans

African trypanosomiasis is confined to equatorial Africa, with a patchy distribution depending upon detailed topographical conditions. It is caused by two subspecies of *Trypanosoma brucei*: *T. b. gambiense* infection is widespread in West and Central Africa, mainly by riverine species of tsetse fly (*Glossina*), but *T. b. rhodesiense*, transmitted mostly by savannah species, is restricted to the east and east central areas, with some overlaps between the two. While domestic pigs form an important reservoir for *T. b. gambiense* infection, various wild ruminants are the major sources for *T. b. rhodesiense*. The epidemic re-emergence of African trypanosomiasis in recent years is exemplified by the death of at least 96 people in Angola in 2003 when 3115 cases were confirmed among a suspected 270 000 new cases in that country. In the same year it was estimated that some 500 000 people across Africa were suffering from trypanosomiasis, which was likely to have a mortality rate of about 80%. Recent reports indicate a spread of transmission from the northern towards the southern parts of Angola. (Adapted from WHO Map No. 98005)

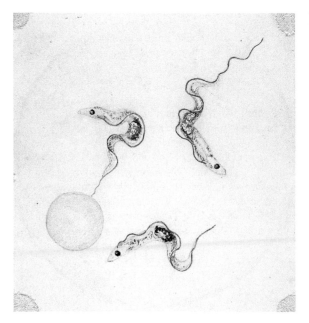

197 Original illustration of *Trypanosoma* (*Trypanozoon*) *brucei gambiense* in human blood by J. Everett Dutton

Polymorphic trypanosomes were first discovered a century ago, in 1895, by Bruce in the blood of domestic cattle suffering from the wasting disease nagana in South Africa. The first observation of these protozoa in humans was by R. M. Forde, who noted, in 1902, 'small worm-like, extremely active bodies' in the blood of a sick European seaman in the Gambia. The parasites seen here in a Romanowsky-stained, thin blood film, which were described and named by Dutton in the same year, are responsible for sleeping sickness in west Africa. (Reproduced by kind permission of the Director, Liverpool School of Tropical Medicine.)

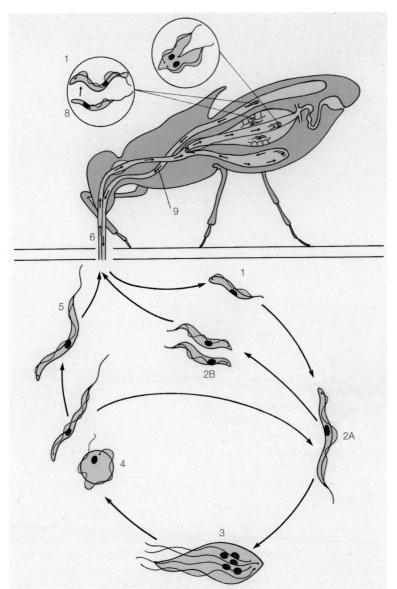

198 Life cycle of African trypanosomes in humans and reservoir hosts

There are three phases in the life cycle of African trypanosomes: (A) – in the reservoir host; (B) – in the tsetse fly; (C) – in humans. Metacyclic trypomastigotes (1) pass from the fly's proboscis into the mammalian host's skin. There, the parasites reproduce, forming long, flat trypomastigotes (2A) and (in humans) a chancre develops. The trypomastigotes enter the blood and circulate to the tissues. Some, in the liver, appear to form multinucleate giant forms (3), from which arise sphaeromastigotes (4) and further long, flat forms (2A) or very long, slender trypomastigotes (5). Some of the long, flat forms develop into short stumpy forms (2B) but these degenerate trypomastigotes, although taken up by the tsetse fly (6), are not infective. The slender forms, directly or via the crop, enter the midgut, in which they reproduce by binary fission (7). Most of the progeny exit via the terminal part of the peritrophic membrane and pass back from the ectoperitrophic space, through the hypopharynx, to reach the salivary ducts and thence, in reverse direction to the salivary flow, to the glands themselves, where they become attached and reproduce further as epimastigotes (8). These convert back to metacyclic trypomastigotes (1), which pass back down the salivary ducts to enter a new mammalian host when the fly bites again. (See also **199, 201, 202** and **211**.)

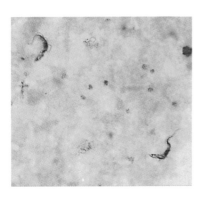

199 *Trypanosoma brucei rhodesiense* in human blood

T. b. brucei parasitises wild and domestic animals but does not infect humans. The different subspecies can be distinguished with certainty only by biochemical techniques, such as electrophoretic typing of their isoenzymes (see also **249** and **658**) or by the use of DNA probes. *T. b. gambiense*, *T. b. rhodesiense* (and *T. b. brucei* of animals) are virtually indistinguishable in blood films. Note the small kinetoplast and free flagellum. Both subspecies from humans will infect guinea pigs, but only *T. b. rhodesiense* is infective to rats, in which the parasites are polymorphic, i.e. long, thin, intermediate and short, stumpy forms of trypomastigotes may coincide. (*Giemsa* × 900)

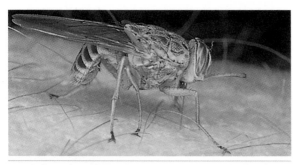

200 Tsetse fly feeding
The common vectors of *T. b. gambiense* in west Africa are *Glossina palpalis* and *Glossina tachinoides*. *T. b. rhodesiense* is associated with *Glossina morsitans*, *Glossina swynnertoni* and *Glossina pallidipes*. Other, secondary, vectors have more localised distributions. (× *5.5*)

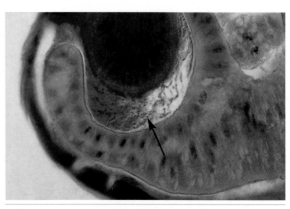

201 Trypanosomes in section of tsetse fly
After ingestion by the tsetse fly, the trypomastigotes pass to the midgut. After asexual reproduction, the parasites migrate forward between the peritrophic membrane and gut wall to re-enter the pharynx and proboscis. They migrate back into the salivary glands, where they transform first into epimastigotes (see also **198**), then to the infective stage (metacyclic trypomastigotes; **202**). The section shows trypomastigotes massed at the entrance to the midgut ready to enter the proventriculus. (× *90*)

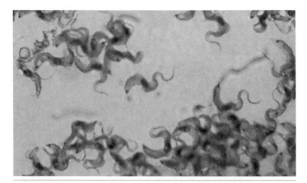

202 Metacyclic trypanosomes in salivary 'probe'
The infective stages are passed into the bite together with the saliva when the fly next feeds. They may be observed in saliva expressed from the proboscis of the fly on to a microscope slide. (× *900*)

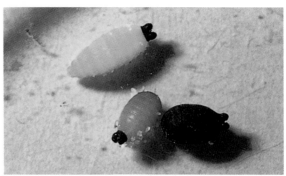

203 Larva, pre-pupa and pupa of *Glossina morsitans*
A single larva develops inside the female tsetse fly and is deposited when mature in dry soil. Here it pupates, and metamorphoses to the adult. (× *3.2*)

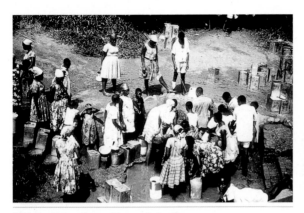

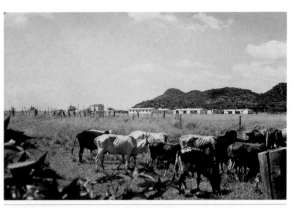

204 Ecology of gambiense infection

Gambiense trypanosomiasis is transmitted by riverine species of *Glossina*, requiring optimum shade and humidity – shady trees near lakes, rivers and pools of water are ideal habitats. The figure shows a typical site for transmission by *G. tachinoides*, one of the *G. palpalis* group that transmit human trypanosomiasis over a wide geographical area. Human–fly contact is intimate when villagers congregate around pools for collecting water or washing, as at this riverside near Kampala in Uganda. Domestic pigs are an important reservoir of infection with *T. b. gambiense* in west African villages. *G. tachinoides* is second in importance to *G. palpalis* as a vector of this parasite. In contrast to gambiense trypanosomiasis, the rhodesiense form is transmitted by *G. morsitans* and its subspecies, whose habitat is scrubby savannah woodland. These flies are less dependent on moisture. Moreover, in such terrain, wild animals and domestic cattle provide alternative feeding opportunities for the fly. Trypanosomiasis due to other species is a serious disease of domestic animals, causing great economic loss and depriving human populations of much needed protein. *T. b. brucei*, *Trypanosoma vivax* and *Trypanosoma congolense* are the commonest parasites involved. Pigs may also be decimated by other species such as *Trypanosoma suis* or *Trypanosoma simiae*.

205 Domestic cattle infected with *Trypanosoma brucei rhodesiense*

Chronic infection with trypanosomes of the *T. brucei* complex, resulting in progressive emaciation, as seen in these cattle on a central African farm, poses a serious burden on the rural economy and increases the problem of protein malnutrition in many communities.

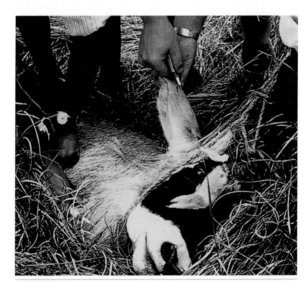

206 Blood sample being taken from a roan antelope

The reservoir of *T. b. rhodesiense* was long suspected to be wild animals; the first species found infected with this trypanosome was the bushbuck (*Tragelaphus scriptus*) but other species of game animals have since been found to harbour these parasites. This antelope was immobilised with an anaesthetic dart for a blood sample to be collected.

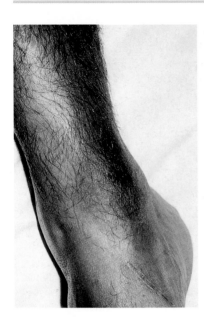

207 Trypanosomal chancre

The bite reaction, the earliest clinical lesion, is known as a 'trypanosomal chancre'. It resembles a boil but is usually painless. Fluid aspirated from the nodule contains actively dividing trypanosomes. This reaction is seen more commonly in rhodesiense than in gambiense infection.

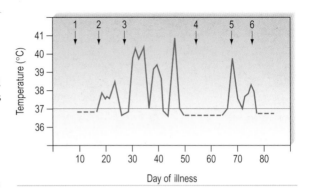

208 Temperature chart in a patient with trypanosomiasis

Episodes of pyrexia that occur irregularly are often associated with the rash. Trypanosomes appear in the blood 1–3 weeks after infection. They may be scanty in gambiense but are commonly numerous in rhodesiense infection, which is usually a more fulminating disease. 1, headache; 2, trypanosomal chancre; 3, oedema of left eyelid; 4, 5, 6, rash.

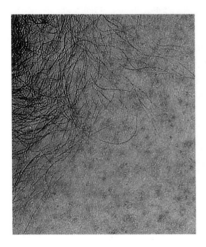

209 Trypanosomal rash

In fair-skinned individuals, each peak of fever may be accompanied by a remarkable skin eruption in the form of annular patches of erythema. In other cases, the rash may be more generalised, as seen here on the sixth day of an infection with *T. b. rhodesiense*.

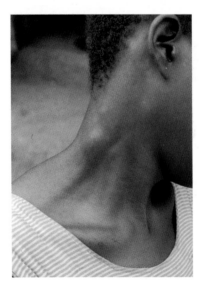

210 Cervical lymphadenopathy

Enlargement of lymphatic glands, especially in the posterior triangle of the neck ('Winterbottom's sign'), is an important clinical feature of *T. b. gambiense* infection and calls for diagnostic gland puncture. Examination of a needle aspirate from the glands is a valuable and simple means of providing an early diagnosis, especially in Gambian trypanosomiasis.

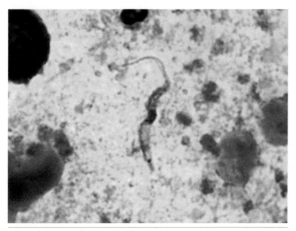

211 Trypanosome in gland fluid

The trypanosomes are easily identified as actively motile organisms in the wet preparation of aspirated gland juice. Their identity can be confirmed by staining. (*Giemsa* × *1650*)

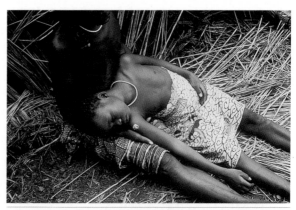

212 Nigerian child with early sleeping sickness due to *Trypanosoma brucei gambiense*

Involvement of the central nervous system (CNS) is first manifested by nonspecific neurological symptoms, partly due to meningeal irritation, followed by a classical reversal of the sleep rhythm and daytime somnolence, as seen in this child.

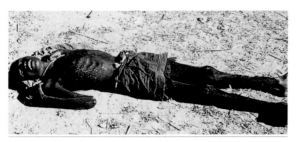

213 Sleeping sickness

In the absence of treatment, the patient with gambiense infection becomes progressively more wasted and comatose, finally showing the classical picture of sleeping sickness as the CNS becomes further involved. Although infection with *T. b. rhodesiense* often leads to death from toxic manifestations before CNS changes are evident, this man, who was infected in Juba, southern Sudan, displayed early cerebral manifestations.

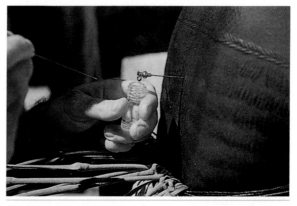

214 Lumbar puncture

This procedure should be carried out to determine whether the CNS has been invaded. In such instances, the cerebrospinal fluid (CSF) will reveal a lymphocytic pleocytosis, an increased protein content, and trypanosomes may be found in stained films of the centrifuge deposit. In *T. b. rhodesiense* infection, invasion of the CNS may occur very early, whereas several months or years usually elapse before meningoencephalitis develops in gambiense disease. (Note: this procedure should be carried out with full sterile and other precautions that are not shown in this figure.)

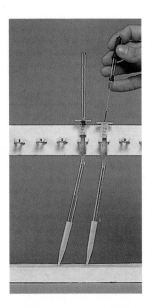

215 'Minicolumn' separation of trypanosomes

The Sephadex 'minicolumn', which permits the detection of very small numbers of trypanosomes in specimens of blood or CSF, can be an invaluable diagnostic aid in individual patients and has been employed in field surveys. Once eluted from the base of the column, even a single parasite is readily identified under the microscope.

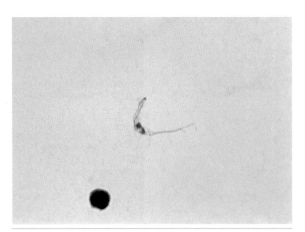

216 Trypomastigote of *Trypanosoma brucei brucei* in cerebrospinal fluid

A single organism is seen in this sample taken from cerebrospinal fluid filtered in a 'minicolumn'. (*Giemsa × 1200*)

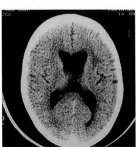

217 Cerebral changes in *T. b. rhodesiense* infection

Computed tomography may show evidence of cerebral involvement prior to treatment. Atrophic changes with hydrocephalus are seen in the scan of this young child 9 months after clinical cure.

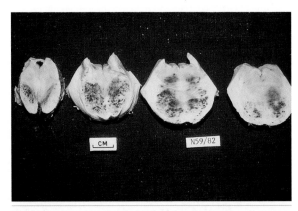

218 Acute haemorrhagic leucoencephalopathy

Numerous small haemorrhagic foci, some of them confluent, are seen in these sections of the brain-stem from a fatal case of African trypanosomiasis. (Original figure from the Department of Neuropathology, Southern General Hospital, Glasgow, reproduced by courtesy of WHO. ID: 9204178, WHO/TDR.)

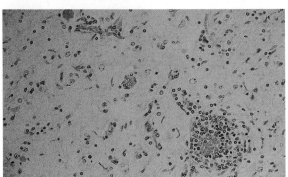

219 Microscopic changes in brain

The leptomeninges are congested, there may be oedema, and small haemorrhages are commonly present. The basic pathological change is a meningoencephalitis in which perivascular cuffing with round cells is often pronounced. (*H&E × 200*)

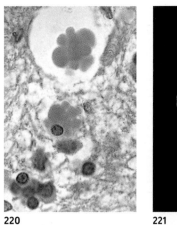
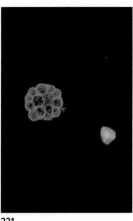

220

221

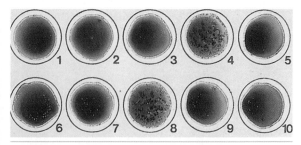

220 & 221 Morula cells in brain

Scattered irregularly through the brain substance, there occur large eosinophilic mononuclear cells (**220**, left) with eccentric nuclei, known as morula cells of Mott (*H&E × 1500*). These are IgM-producing plasma cells as shown in this preparation (**221**, right) treated with anti-IgM antibody. (× *1500*)

222 Card agglutination test for (gambiense) trypanosomiasis (CATT)

Anti-trypanosomal IgM, which is raised both in the blood and the CSF in trypanosomiasis, can be detected by this simple test, which is invaluable for rapid diagnosis, especially in field surveys. Other useful serological aids are the complement-fixation test, quantitative IgM radial immunodiffusion assay and fluorescent antibody (FAT) staining. In the CATT test card shown here, the presence of blue granular deposits in wells 4 and 8 is indicative of infection.

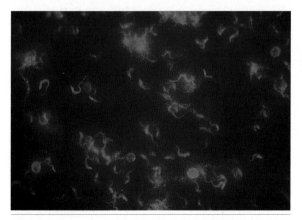

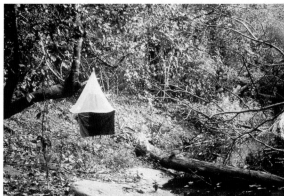

223 Acridine-orange-stained *T. b. rhodesiense* in centrifuged blood

The examination of centrifuged blood to detect trypanosomes is facilitated by the use of the QBC^R technique with fluorescent staining, as seen here. The method is highly sensitive and simple to use. (*See also* **123**.) (× *200*)

224 Vavoua trap in use at a *G. palpalis*-infested riverine site in west Africa

This is a cheap and simplified version of the Lancien trap. Note the alternating black and blue cloth, which provides a colour attractant for this species of tsetse. The trap contains a liquid bait at the apex of the cone. It is used extensively in west Africa. Impregnating the material from which it is constructed with a synthetic pyrethroid such as deltamethrin improves its performance.

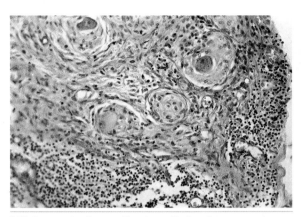

240 Sympathetic ganglion in wall of atrium
Degenerative changes in neuronal cells from a ganglion in the heart of a patient with Chagas' disease who died of sudden cardiac failure. Mononuclear cellular infiltration is conspicuous, especially round the capsule of the ganglion. CNS involvement may present as diffuse meningoencephalitis with necrosis in individuals who develop AIDS. The recent finding in a number of patients with chronic disease that sequences of *T. cruzi* DNA may be integrated into the hosts' genome has led to the hypothesis that this phenomenon may be one of the factors that underlie the evolution of the disease to the chronic phase. (*H&E* × *130*)

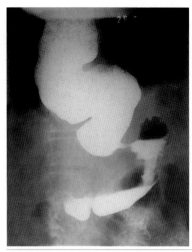

241 Radiograph of megaoesophagus
Muscular degeneration and denervation of segments of the alimentary tract through destruction of the cells of Auerbach's plexus cause megaoesophagus, megastomach and megacolon, etc., which can be detected radiologically.

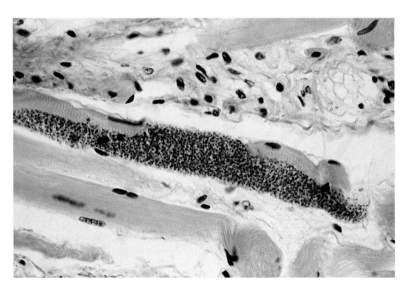

242 Amastigotes in oesophageal muscle
Pseudocysts containing amastigotes of *T. cruzi* can rarely be demonstrated in ganglion cells of the intestinal tract, although the smooth muscle is often invaded. (× *480*)

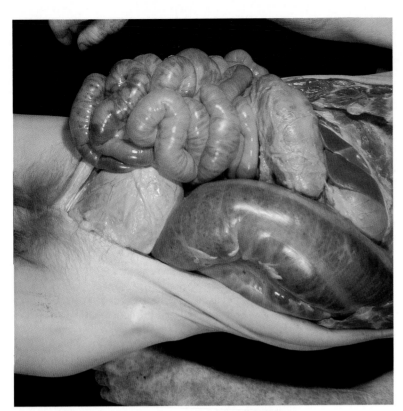

243 Post-mortem of patient with megacolon

Gross megacolon is shown here in a man who died of chronic Chagas' disease.

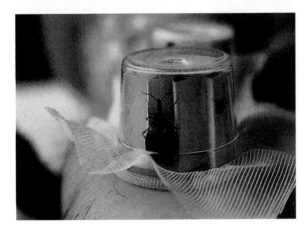

244 Xenodiagnosis

Various serological tests are of value in confirming a diagnosis of Chagas' disease. An ELISA test employing antigen from epimastigotes of *T. cruzi* cultivated in vitro is widely used, and is one of the most sensitive means of diagnosis, especially if the antigen is derived from an autochthonous strain. It can indicate past or present infection but does not necessarily imply the presence of parasites. Fluorescent antibody tests may also be employed, using whole cultured epimastigotes as the antigen. The exquisitely sensitive PCR technique, which is capable of detecting the DNA from a single parasite, is invaluable in the control of blood for transfusion in endemic countries, as well as for the diagnosis and follow-up of individual patients in whom few parasites may be accessible for detection by other methods. However, absolute confirmation of active infection is obtained by demonstrating that the patient can infect the vector (xenodiagnosis). Laboratory-bred, clean reduviid bugs are fed on patients suspected of having trypanosomiasis. Two weeks later the hindgut is dissected out and is examined for metacyclic trypanosomes. The screening of all blood donors to reduce transmission is an integral part of the 'Southern Cone Initiative' since chemotherapy of established infection remains unsatisfactory.

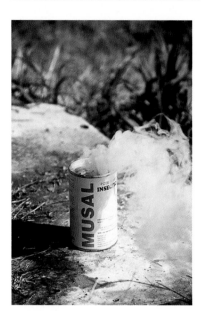

245 Fumigant canister releasing insecticide
This type of canister was especially designed to kill domestic insects. When lit, it releases a cloud of insecticide that is very effective in killing the triatomine vectors of Chagas' disease, as well as other insect pests. The large scale deployment of such canisters has made a major contribution to the reduction or arrest of transmission of Chagas' disease in a major part of the endemic areas. (Figure by courtesy of WHO, ID: 9905250, WHO/TDR/Crump.)

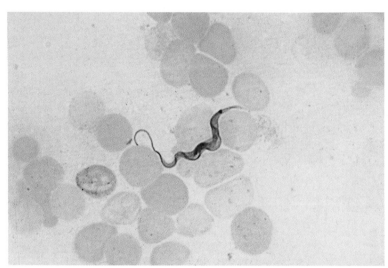

246 *Trypanosoma rangeli*
T. rangeli is a long, slender trypanosome also transmitted by reduviid bugs from wild animals to humans. It is readily distinguished by its shape from *T. cruzi* in blood films, and appears to be nonpathogenic to humans. (*Giemsa × 1200*)

LEISHMANIASIS See **Tables 8** and **9**.

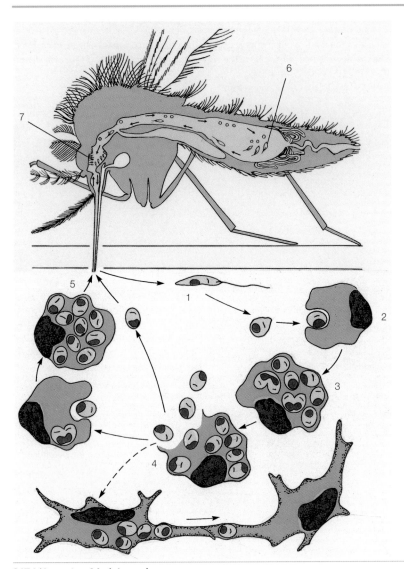

247 Life cycle of *Leishmania*

(1) Infective, flagellated promastigotes pass from the proboscis with the saliva into the subcutaneous tissues when a sandfly feeds. (2) The promastigotes penetrate local tissue macrophages, becoming rounded amastigotes (also known as Leishman–Donovan bodies) as the flagellae degenerate. (3) The amastigotes multiply by asexual binary fission to form 'cell nests', which rupture the host cells – the progeny are taken up by other local or circulating macrophages. (4) Depending on the species of parasite, some amastigotes remain in the superficial tissues, where the reproductive cycle continues, whereas others settle in macrophages in the deep organs of the reticuloendothelial system such as lymph glands, bone marrow, spleen and liver. (5) When another sandfly takes a blood meal, some amastigotes in macrophages (either in the skin or in the peripheral circulation) are taken into the midgut, where they convert to promastigotes within the peritrophic membrane. (6) The promastigotes reproduce further, mainly by binary fission, and escape into the midgut when the peritrophic membrane breaks down; some possibly undergo a form of sexual conjugation. (7) Promastigotes of *Leishmania* (*Leishmania*) move forward to the oesophagus and proboscis, attaching for some time en route to the stomodeal valve (situated between the thoracic midgut and oesophagus), where some species continue to divide. Species of *Leishmania* (*Viannia*) move posteriorly to the pylorus and ileum of the hindgut, where they reproduce further before once again moving anteriorly to the proboscis. (See also **248,250,257,270,275,276,294** and **313**.)

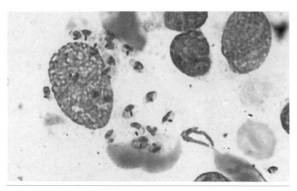

248 Amastigotes of *Leishmania infantum* in a macrophage from dog skin

The amastigotes of different species are very similar on light microscopy (apart from their sizes), and can be distinguished – even by experts – to a limited degree only. (*Giemsa × 1250*)

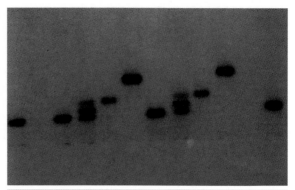

249 Isoenzyme electrophoresis: a tool for biochemical taxonomy

A widely used method for identifying species of *Leishmania* (which is also of considerable value for other parasites, e.g. trypanosomes, amoebas, schistosomes and their molluscan hosts) is the characterisation of isoenzymes by electrophoresis on starch gel or other bases. This figure of duplicate specimens of five *Leishmania* isolates illustrates banding of glucose phosphate isomerase in four distinct patterns, each of which indicates a different species; two of the pairs are identical. This technique has now largely been superseded by the use of specific DNA probes and PCR to identify isolates from vertebrate or invertebrate sources (see also **271, 298**).

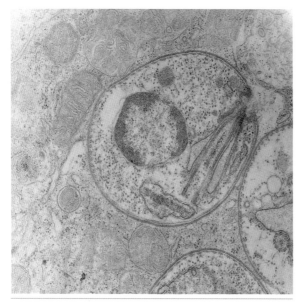

250 Ultrastructure of amastigotes

Leishmanial amastigotes are seen within a parasitophorous vacuole in the host cell. The short flagellum (or mastigote) does not extend beyond the outer cell membrane in this stage. (*× 23 500*)

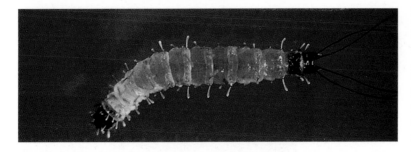

251 Third instar larva of *Phlebotomus perfiliewi*
Leishmania are transmitted by sandflies of the genus *Phlebotomus* in the Old World and far east, and by *Lutzomyia* in the New World. The photograph shows the larva of *P. perfiliewi*, which is a vector of leishmaniasis in southern Europe. In dry areas, the larvae occupy cracks and crevices, which provide a humid, cool microclimate; forest species possibly prefer leaf mould on the forest floor. ($\times$ 9)

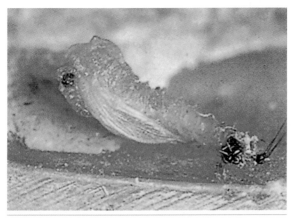

252 Pupa of *Lutzomyia longipalpis*
L. longipalpis transmits visceral leishmaniasis in Brazil. ($\times$ 20)

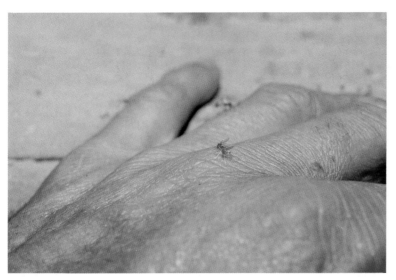

253 Adult female *Lutzomyia longipalpis* biting
This figure gives an impression of the small size of these flies. ($\times$ 2)

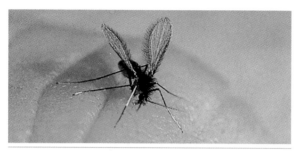

254 Close-up view of *Lutzomyia longipalpis*
The female has a 'blunt' end on the abdomen (× 10)

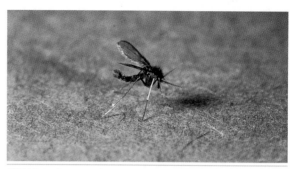

255 Male *Lutzomyia longipalpis*
The claspers of the male genitalia as seen in this figure readily distinguish the male from the female. (× 10)

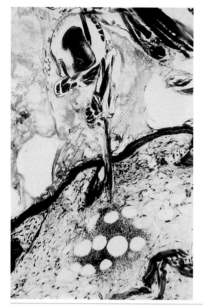

256 Cross-section through *Phlebotomus argentipes* in the process of feeding
The female feeds from the pool of capillary blood that accumulates at the tip of the proboscis. (*Haematoxylin* × 100) (Photographed from a specimen prepared by the late Colonel H. E. Shortt FRS.)

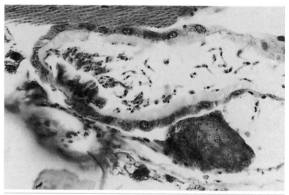

257 Promastigotes in vector midgut
In the midgut of the poikilothermic vector, amastigotes transform to promastigotes, which then divide asexually. (*Giemsa* × 1150)

258 Reaction to sandfly bites
A persistent macule appears at the site of each bite, even from an uninfected fly; this may be the starting point of the lesion in simple cutaneous leishmaniasis. Multiple primary lesions occur when the sandfly probes repeatedly in the course of feeding.

Visceral leishmaniasis (kala-azar, dum-dum fever, black sickness)

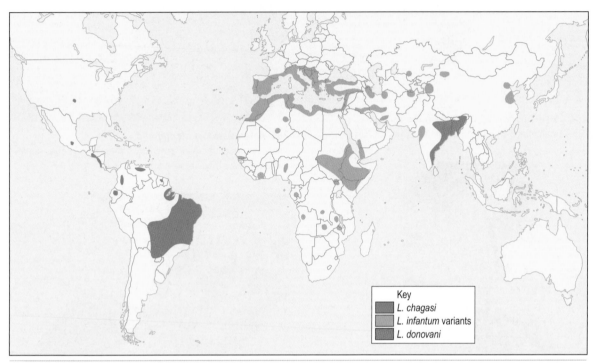

259 Distribution

Visceral leishmaniasis caused by parasites of the *L. donovani–L. infantum* complex occurs in the Mediterranean littorals, the Middle East and adjacent parts of the former Soviet Union, the Sudan, east Africa, the Indian subcontinent and China, and South America ('*Leishmania chagasi*') (Table 8). An arid, warm environment provides ideal ecological conditions for the breeding of many species of sandfly. Zoonotic kala-azar due to *L. infantum* and *L. chagasi* is commonly associated with dry, rocky, hill country where cases are typically scattered. In India, *L. donovani* is essentially an anthroponosis. This type of kala-azar may occur in severe epidemic fashion, as can kala-azar in the Sudan.

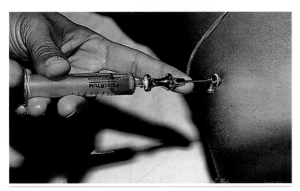

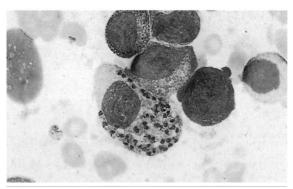

274 Iliac crest puncture of bone marrow
This procedure is less commonly used than splenic aspiration. In general the newer serological techniques shown above avoid the necessity for these more invasive procedures, which are not always necessary.

275 *Leishmania infantum* in macrophage from bone marrow
While typically found in macrophages as shown here, isolated extracellular amastigotes from disrupted host cells are commonly seen in such preparations. (*Giemsa* × *810*)

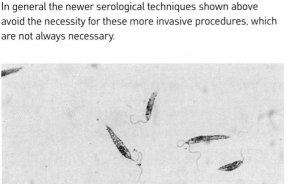

276 Promastigotes in NNN culture
After inoculation of aspirated material into appropriate media such as blood agar (NNN – Novy–Nicolle–MacNeal – medium) and incubation at 28°C for 1–4 weeks, promastigotes may appear in the fluid overlay. *L. donovani* is more readily isolated in culture than *L. infantum*, which sometimes grows better in Schneider's insect tissue culture medium than in NNN. The parasites may also be isolated by intrasplenic inoculation into hamsters; after 4–6 weeks, characteristic visceral lesions are seen macroscopically and amastigotes are found in large numbers in smears of the liver and spleen. (*Giemsa* × *950*)

Old World cutaneous leishmaniasis (zoonotic cutaneous leishmaniasis)

Table 9 The genus *Leishmania* and the leishmaniases – cutaneous and mucocutaneous disease

Type of disease	Species	Localities	Main vectors	Main reservoirs
Cutaneous leishmaniasis (Old World)				
Oriental sore and recidiva	Leishmania (Leishmania) tropica	India	Phlebotomus sergenti	Dog
		Former Soviet Union (urban)*	P. sergenti	Humans
		Iran	Phlebotomus ansarii	Dog
		Mediterranean basin	P. sergenti	Humans
			Phlebotomus perfiliewi	
		Saudi Arabia	P. sergenti	?
Oriental sore and oronasal	Leishmania (Leishmania) major	Former Soviet Union (rural)	Phlebotomus papatasi	Gerbils
		Saudi Arabia, Central Asia	P. papatasi	Gerbils, merions
		Mediterranean basin	P. papatasi	Gerbils, merions
		Sudan	? P. papatasi	Rodents
		Senegal	Phlebotomus duboscqi	Rodents
		India	Phlebotomus saheli	Rodents
	L. (L.) tropica complex	Namibia	Phlebotomus rossi	Hyrax
		Kenya	Phlebotomus guggisbergi	?

continued

Table 9 The genus *Leishmania* and the leishmaniases – cutaneous and mucocutaneous disease—*cont'd*

Type of diseases	Species	Localities	Main vectors	Main reservoirs
Oriental sore	Leishmania (Leishmania) infantum	Mediterranean basin, Italy	?	Dog, ? Rattus rattus
	Leishmania (Leishmania) donovani	Kenya	?	?
Single sore and diffusa	Leishmania (Leishmania) aethiopica	Ethiopia Kenya	Phlebotomus longipes Phlebotomus pedifer	Hyrax Hyrax, Cricetomys
New World cutaneous and mucocutaneous leishmaniasis				
Simple cutaneous and diffusa	Leishmania (Leishmania) mexicana L. (L.) mexicana complex	Mexico, Guatemala, Belize Belize Trinidad São Paulo State Dominican Republic Texas	Lutzomyia olmeca ? Lutzomyia flaviscutellata ? ? ? Lutzomyia anthropophora	Forest rodents ? Forest rodents ? ? Neotoma micropis
	Leishmania (Leishmania) pifanoi	Venezuela	? Lu. flaviscutellata	?
	Leishmania (Leishmania) amazonensis	Brazil (Amazon basin)	Lu. flaviscutellata	Forest rodents
	Leishmania (Leishmania) venezuelensis	Venezuela	? Lu. olmeca bicolor	?
	Leishmania (Leishmania) garnhami	Venezuela	? Lutzomyia townsendi	Opossum
	Leishmania (Viannia) naiffi	Brazil (Pará)	? Lutzomyia paraensis, Lu. anduzei	Armadillo
	Leishmania (Viannia) lainsoni	Brazil (Pará), Peru	Lutzomyia ubiquitalis	Paca
	Leishmania (Viannia) spp.	Belize Central America	? Lutzomyia ovallesi ? Lutzomyia crucians	? ?
Espundia	Leishmania (Viannia) braziliensis	Brazil† Brazilian Amazon Bolivian lowlands Venezuela, Peru Paraguay, Ecuador Colombia	Lutzomyia wellcomei Lu. wellcomei Lutzomyia squamiventris Lutzomyia complexus Lutzomyia carrerai ? ? ?	Forest rodents ? ? ? ?
Pian bois	Leishmania (Viannia) guyanensis	Guyanas Northern Brazil	Lutzomyia umbratilis Lutzomyia whitmani Lu. anduzei	Sloths, ant-eaters ? Rodents
Simple sore or pian bois	Leishmania (Viannia) panamensis	Panama Costa Rica Colombia	Lutzomyia trapidoi Lutzomyia ylephiletor ? Lutzomyia gomezi ? Lutzomyia panamensis	Sloths monkeys kinkajou olingo
	Leishmania (Viannia) colombiensis	Colombia	Lutzomyia hartmanni	Sloths
	Leishmania (Viannia) shawi	Brazil (Pará)	Lu. whitmani	Sloths, monkeys, coatimundi
Uta	Leishmania (Viannia) peruviana	Peru (west of Andes), Peru (southwest Andes) Peru (central Andes) Argentina	Lutzomyia verrucarum Lu. ayacuchensis Lu. tejadai Lu. peruensis	Dog ? ? ?

The genus *Leishmania* has been divided into *Leishmania (Leishmania)*, type species *L. donovani*, and *Leishmania (Viannia)*, type species *L. (V.) braziliensis*.
* Soviet Union = Turkmenia, Uzbekistan of former Soviet Union. † Forested areas east of the Andean chain.

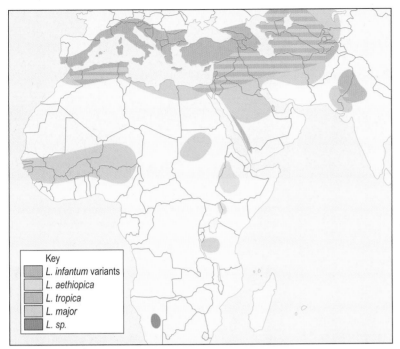

277 Distribution

Cutaneous leishmaniasis in the Old World is caused by *L. major*, *L. tropica*, *L. aethiopica* and certain zymodemes of the *L. infantum* complex (see **Table 8**). With the possible exception in some localities of *L. tropica*, these infections are essentially zoonoses that occur in scattered foci throughout the tropical and subtropical belts. Depending upon the area, cutaneous leishmaniasis is known as Oriental sore, Aleppo button, bouton de Biskra, Baghdad boil, Delhi sore, etc.

Key
- *L. infantum* variants
- *L. aethiopica*
- *L. tropica*
- *L. major*
- *L. sp.*

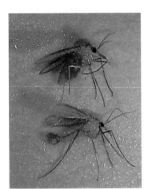

278 Male and female *Phlebotomus papatasi*

This is the most important vector of *L. major* from north Africa, through the Middle East to Mongolia. The female (upper figure) has a fully engorged midgut. Note the contrast between the terminal abdominal segments of the two sexes of this pale sandfly. (× 9)

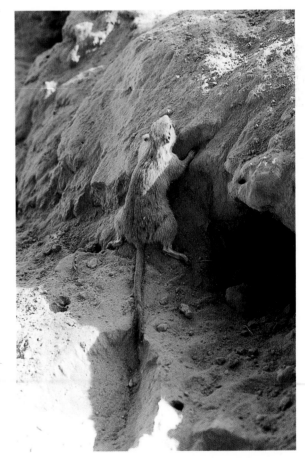

279 Animal reservoirs of *Leishmania major*

Various rodent species such as this 'great gerbil', *Rhombomys opimus*, of eastern Iran and neighbouring parts of the former Soviet Union, and the 'fat-tailed sand rat', *Psammomys obesus* (see **280**), in Libya, Israel and Saudi Arabia, are important reservoirs of *L. major*.

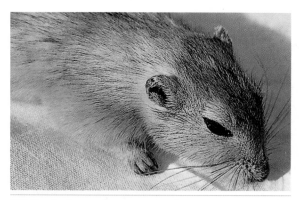

280 Ear lesion on *Psammomys obesus*

These rodents and the sandflies that rest in their burrows are responsible for outbreaks of zoonotic cutaneous leishmaniasis (ZCL) in newly urbanised areas that intrude on their normal habitat – arid or even semidesert terrain. The burrows provide ideal breeding and resting sites for sandfly vectors such as *Phlebotomus papatasi* that transmit *L. major*, the species causing ZCL. Sandflies also rest during the day in cool deep crevices in the ground, between rocks, in caves, cellars, house walls, etc. Although the eroded ear seen here is typical of *L. major* in its natural host, many infected animals have no obvious skin lesions.

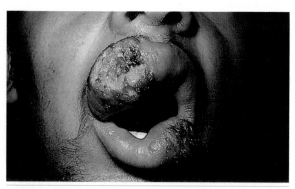

281 'Wet' lesion of mouth

L. major occurs most commonly in rural areas, causing moist, ulcerative lesions that may be extensive and sometimes involve the epithelium of lips and nose.

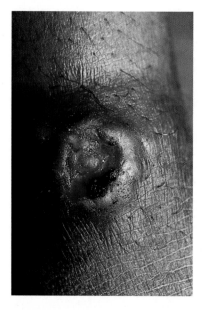

282 Nodulo-ulcerative lesion of *Leishmania major*

These are the commonest types of lesion caused by *L. major*. The prominent 'rolled' edge of the lesions is the best area in which to demonstrate the parasites, which are present in macrophages or are free in surrounding tissue, often in small numbers.

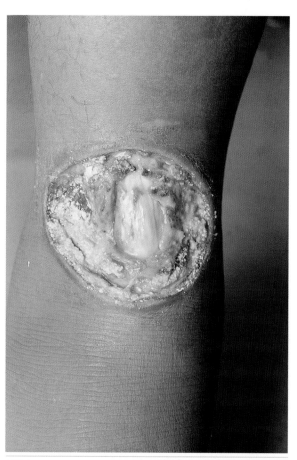

283 Invasive ulcerative lesion of *Leishmania major*

The extensive lesion on the lower leg of this Sudanese woman near Khartoum has exposed deep tissues, including a tendon sheath. (Courtesy of Dr S El-Safi.)

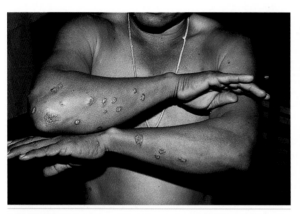

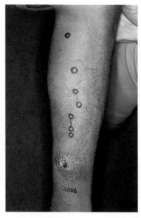

285 Lymphatic spread of *Leishmania major*
The ink marks indicate a line of subcutaneous nodules along the lymphatic, passing proximally from the lesion on the lower part of this man's arm. Readily palpated, the lymphatic is sometimes referred to as a 'beaded cord'. The nodules usually resolve without complications when the primary lesion heals with or without specific therapy.

284 Multiple lesions of *Leishmania major* in a non-immune man
This Thai builder received multiple bites by infected *P. papatasi* through sleeping outdoors without protection in a highly endemic area of eastern Saudi Arabia.

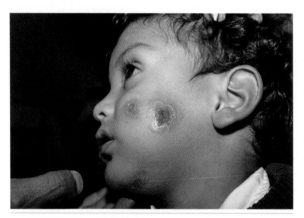

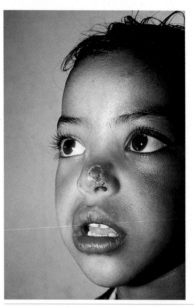

286 Simple 'dry' lesion of *Leishmania tropica*
This parasite often produces dry, usually self-healing lesions, which, unlike the infection seen here, are generally single. This form is commonly seen in and around towns from north Africa and the Middle East to the former Soviet Union, Afghanistan and western states of India, especially in mountainous areas. The lesions frequently contain very large numbers of parasites. Following 20 years of war it was shown in 2004 that about 67 500 residents of Kabul were suffering from anthroponotic infection with *L. tropica*, and that this number was only about one-third of the total Afghans infected, who represented 4% of the entire population of that country.

287 Cutaneous leishmaniasis due to *Leishmania tropica* transmitted by *Phlebotomus sergenti* in an Arabian child
The lesions caused by this parasite are commonly found on the head or neck and may become chronic, leading to the condition known as leishmaniasis recidivans.

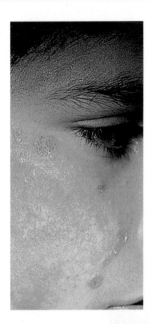

288 Leishmaniasis recidivans

Infection with *L. tropica* may become very chronic, with a hyperallergic reaction leading to lupus-like lesions such as seen in this child in Israel. Amastigotes may be very difficult to find in the lesions.

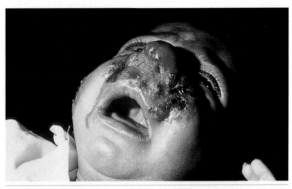

289 Infant with mucocutaneous lesions caused by *Leishmania major*

In some cases, especially in young infants or older individuals whose cellular immune responses are impaired, ZCL may proceed to involve mucous tissue, much as occurs in the New World disease known as espundia (see **307**). This infant was seen in eastern Saudi Arabia but the condition is also reported from the Sudan and Ethiopia (see **290**), where it may also be associated with *L. major*.

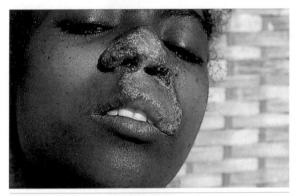

290 Mucocutaneous leishmaniasis in Ethiopia

In addition to simple cutaneous lesions due to infection with *L. aethiopica*, other forms are seen in the Ethiopian highlands where rock hyraxes are the reservoirs. It has not yet been ascertained whether the mucocutaneous condition seen here is due to this or another species of *Leishmania* (*see also* **281, 289**). Mucocutaneous lesions in Sudanese patients are probably associated with *L. major*.

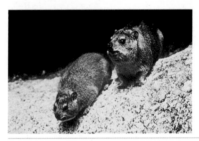

291 *Procavia capensis*

Widely distributed in Africa and Arabia, this hyrax is the reservoir of cutaneous leishmaniasis in Namibia. An unnamed species of *Leishmania* similar to *L. major* causes cutaneous leishmaniasis in parts of Namibia where *Phlebotomus* (*Synphlebotomus*) *rossi* is the probable vector.

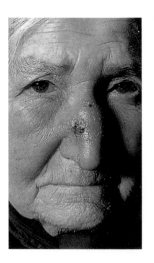

292 Dry lesion on nose of woman in Southern France

This lesion proved to be due to a zymodeme of the *L. infantum* complex.

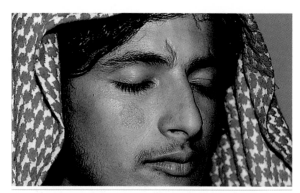

293 Typical healed cutaneous lesion

An atrophic, papery, slightly depressed scar results when healing occurs. This man was probably infected with *L. tropica* which healed spontaneously.

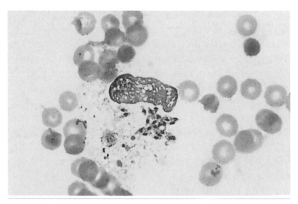

294 Amastigotes in macrophages from skin

The diagnosis is confirmed by demonstrating amastigotes in smears made from the cutaneous lesions (see captions for **286** and **287**). Various simple techniques such as biopsy by dental broach or skin-slit and scrape can be used. (*Giemsa* × *950*)

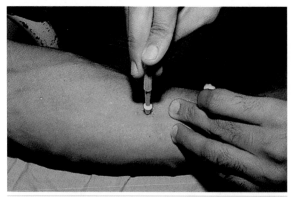

295 Punch biopsy

A piece of tissue may be removed under local anaesthetic with a disposable skin punch for histology, culture and the direct demonstration of amastigotes. For the isolation of parasites for identification a microculture method using microcapillary tubes is simpler, more rapid and more sensitive than the classical use of NNN medium.

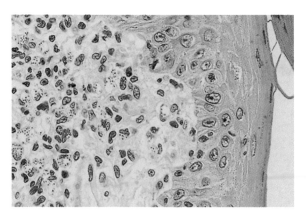

296 Parasitised macrophages in skin section

Many parasitised macrophages can be seen in this section from an acute lesion caused by *L. major*. (*H&E* × *220*)

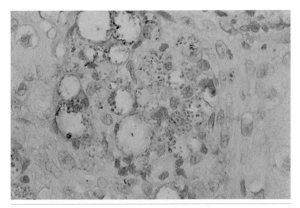

297 Immunoperoxidase staining of *Leishmania*
This procedure is very useful to demonstrate small numbers of amastigotes in tissue sections in which H&E staining is often unsatisfactory. The section shown here has many brown staining amastigotes in parasitophorous vacuoles within mauve-staining macrophages. (× 260)

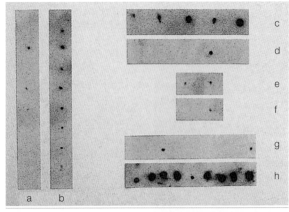

298 DNA probe for the identification of *Leishmania major* in *Phlebotomus papatasi*
Highly specific DNA probes have been developed not only for *Leishmania* but also for sandflies; their combined application can be invaluable in epidemiological studies. Sandflies collected in the field are squashed on to special papers and are then hybridised sequentially with probes against the parasite and suspected vector species. This permits both the numbers of the vector in the collection and the proportion of those vectors that are infected to be determined in parallel in a short time, thus avoiding the need for laborious and time-consuming dissections and subsequent cultivation and identification of the parasites. The figure shows autoradiographs of *P. papatasi*, some of which are infected with *L. major* (**a**, positive hybridisation to an *L. major* probe in 3/8 flies found positive on dissection; **b**, positive responses to a *Ph. papatasi* probe in 8/8 flies; **d**, **e**, **f**, **g**, positive responses to *L. major*; **c**, **h**, positive responses to both probes.)

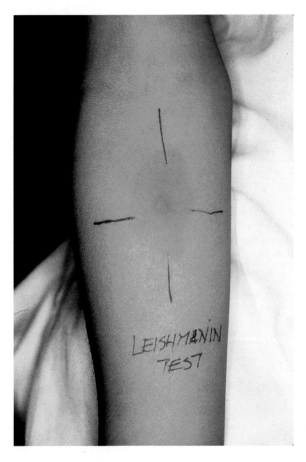

299 Leishmanin (Montenegro) test
The diagnosis may be assisted by the injection of an intradermal antigen prepared from cultured promastigotes of *L. major* or other species. This produces a typical cell-mediated, delayed hypersensitivity response in most cases of active cutaneous disease within 1–2 months of its onset; the test usually remains positive for life. It is negative in the active stages of kala-azar but may become faintly positive during the course of treatment, especially in east African patients. The reaction shown in the antigen site is maximal after 48 hours; it should be measured by first feeling and marking the limits of the induration as shown. The size is then compared with that of a control injection (not shown here).

New World cutaneous leishmaniasis

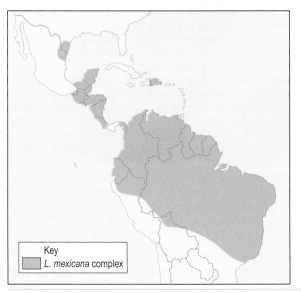

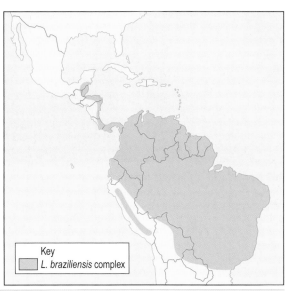

300 Distribution (including espundia)

New World cutaneous and mucocutaneous leishmaniasis ('espundia') occurs focally from Texas (USA) and Mexico southwards throughout Central America and South America as far south as São Paulo State in Brazil. The disease is limited by the Andean chain to the west except in Peru where a special form of cutaneous disease, 'uta', is found on the western slopes of the Andes. (See **Table 8**.)

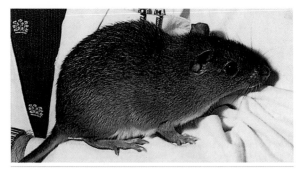

301 Rodent reservoir of *Leishmania amazonensis* in the Brazilian rain forest

Most cutaneous leishmaniases in the New World are zoonoses associated with rodents of the rain forest. *L. amazonensis* has been isolated from this species, *Proechimys guyanensis*, in the Amazon basin of Brazil. Recent surveys using PCR confirmed that a variety of ground-loving mammals such as rodents are the primary reservoirs also of *L. (V.) braziliensis*.

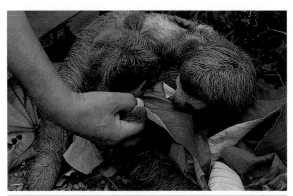

302 Arboreal animals as reservoirs

In other areas, e.g. Panama, Brazil and the Guyanas, a wide variety of arboreal animals serve as reservoirs for *L. panamensis* and *L. guyanensis*. The hosts include species of monkeys, marmosets, ant-eaters, and such bizarre animals as the three-toed sloth (*Bradypus variegatus*) shown here in Panama.

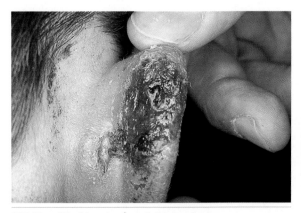

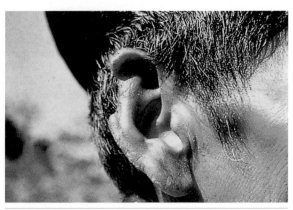

303 New World cutaneous leishmaniasis

The early stage of a lesion caused by *L. mexicana* is seen on the back of the ear of a man infected in the jungle near Belize.

304 Chiclero's ulcer

Forest workers collecting gum from wild chicle trees commonly sleep near the forest floor and are bitten on exposed parts of the head by vectors that normally maintain transmission of *L. mexicana* among the forest rodents. Ulcers leading to erosion of the auricular cartilage are known as 'chiclero's ulcers'.

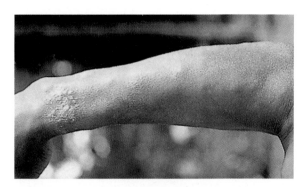

305 'Sporotrichoid' dissemination

As noted for *L. major* (see **250**), lymphatic spread may also occur with New World species. This patient was infected with *L. guyanensis*, the agent of 'pian bois'. In such infections the lymphatic nodules may ulcerate, resulting in chains of 'sporotrichoid' lesions. *L. guyanensis* has also been identified as the cause of disseminated cutaneous leishmaniasis in an HIV-negative woman in Cayenne who developed over 400 lesions. Unlike cases of anergic, diffuse cutaneous leishmaniasis (DCL), her infection responded rapidly to chemotherapy.

Mucocutaneous leishmaniasis

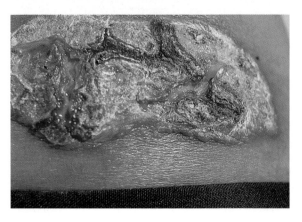

306 Cutaneous lesion caused by *Leishmania braziliensis*

Chronic cutaneous ulceration as seen on the lower abdomen of this man living in the town of Coarí along the river Amazon frequently precedes the development of the nasopharyngeal lesions of espundia.

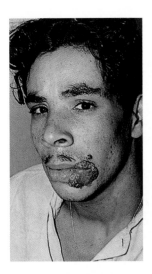

307 Early lesion of espundia

The lesions of mucocutaneous leishmaniasis due to infection with *L. braziliensis* may first become evident as ulcers involving the mucocutaneous junctions of the mouth and nose. This condition frequently follows a primary cutaneous lesion, which may have healed with or without specific therapy some years earlier.

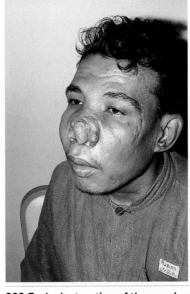

309 Early destruction of the nasal septum

The progress of the disease in this man, seen in Belo Horizonte, Brazil, was arrested by intensive chemotherapy, leaving him with the need for reconstructive surgery.

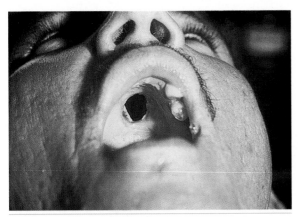

308 Pharyngeal involvement

Ulceration often extends to the pharynx and soft palate, and the first symptoms may be related to tissue destruction in this area. This man from Pará, Brazil, had a large, destructive lesion of the hard palate.

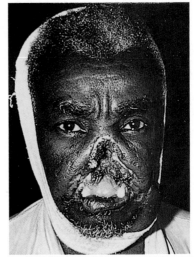

310 Destructive espundia

Gross destruction of the nose, including the septum and palate, may follow inadequate treatment of *L. braziliensis* infection. Many patients with this disease respond very poorly if at all to any form of chemotherapy and reconstructive plastic surgery is called for. The tissue destruction is probably due to cytotoxic immune complexes formed in this hyperallergic response.

Diffuse cutaneous leishmaniasis

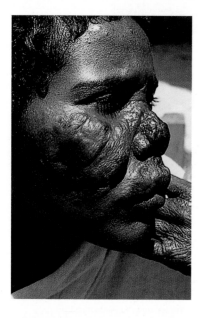

311 Diffuse cutaneous leishmaniasis in the Old World
The diffuse form of leishmaniasis was first described from Ethiopia. This patient, who was infected with *L. aethiopica*, was treated for years in a leprosarium with no improvement in the mistaken belief that he was suffering from lepromatous leprosy (cf **268**).

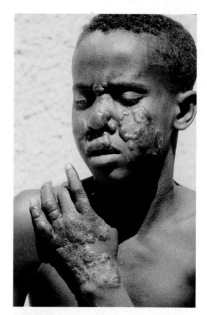

312 Diffuse cutaneous leishmaniasis of face and hand
The diffuse lesions in this Ethiopian are also advanced on the patient's hands.

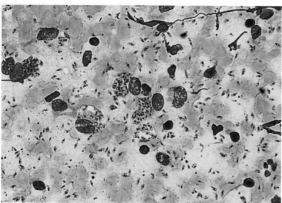

313 Skin smear in diffuse cutaneous leishmaniasis
This smear from a skin biopsy from another Ethiopian patient with DCL shows large numbers of amastigotes. Parasites are rarely so numerous in biopsies from patients with other forms of cutaneous leishmaniasis. (*Giemsa* × *390*)

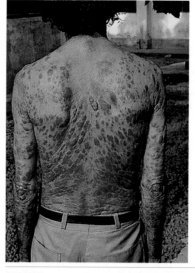

314 Diffuse cutaneous leishmaniasis in the New World
In rare individuals, a failure of specific cell-mediated immunity may result in the development of chronic disseminated disease, 'leishmaniasis diffusa', resembling lepromatous leprosy, following infection with parasites of the *L. mexicana* complex. In such cases chemotherapy produces only a temporary remission at best and complete cure is unknown to date. This Brazilian patient first developed lesions due to *L. amazonensis* more than 20 years before this picture was taken. A similar syndrome occurs in Ethiopia and western Kenya in patients infected with *L. aethiopica*. DCL never affects the mucosae and is thus readily distinguished from PKDL or espundia (*cf* **268**, **310**).

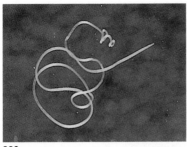

332

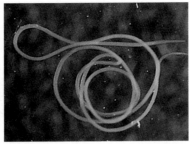

333

332 & 333 Male and female *Wuchereria bancrofti* adults

On maturation, the infective larvae copulate and the adult filariae become localised in lymph glands (e.g. in the groin). Adult male *W. bancrofti* (**332**, left) are about 4 cm long; females (**333**, right) are about 8–10 cm long. (× 9)

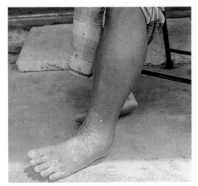

334 Lymphangitis

Acute involvement of lymphatic vessels is common, especially in the extremities. In association with lymphangitis, there is almost always some local lymphadenitis and fever.

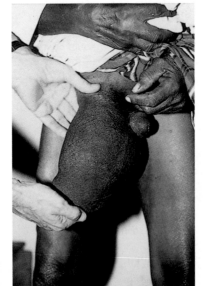

335 Hydrocele

Orchitis may occur in the acute stages; it is commonly associated with hydrocele, and microfilariae may be found in the hydrocele fluid. This is a relatively late lesion seen in a Tanzanian patient.

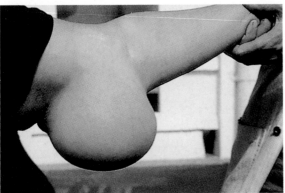

336 Elephantiasis of right epitrochlear gland in a Fijian

A feature that is unusually frequent in the South Pacific and is also due to *W. bancrofti* is gross enlargement of the epitrochlear lymph node.

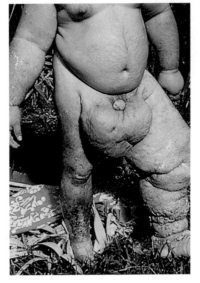

337 Elephantiasis of the leg and scrotum due to *Wuchereria bancrofti* in Tahiti

Gross elephantiasis of the scrotum may produce gross and incapacitating deformity that requires radical surgery to remove the surplus tissue.

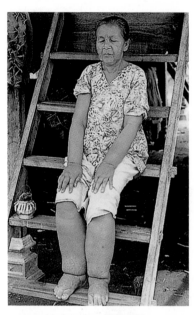

338 Early elephantiasis due to *Brugia malayi*
Lymphatic obstruction (especially in the leg) progressing in chronic cases to elephantiasis may occur in regions of high endemicity. This may also arise in the arm, breast or scrotum. By this late stage, microfilariae are rarely found in blood films.

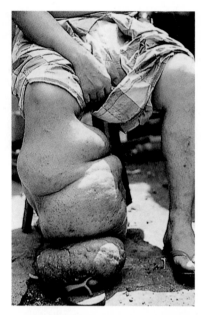

339 Massive elephantiasis due to *Brugia malayi*
As in elephantiasis caused by *W. bancrofti* (see **337**), the enlargement is commonly unilateral.

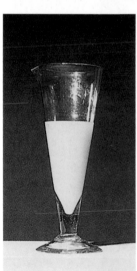

340 Urine containing lymph
The dilated lymph vessels rupture and discharge chyle into the urinary tract, thus producing the milky appearance known as chyluria.

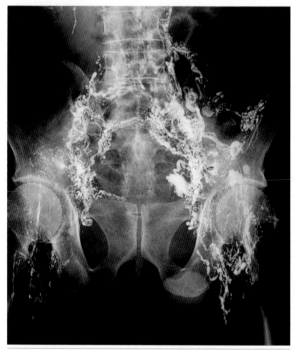

341 Lymphogram in patient with chyluria
Obstruction of the cisterna chyli or its tributaries may occur, giving rise to chyluria.

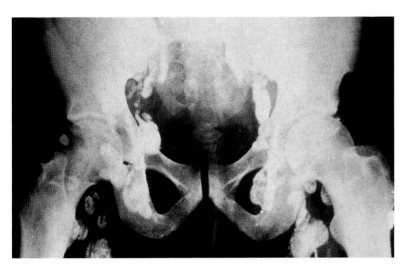

342 Calcified lymph nodes
Numerous calcified inguinal lymph nodes and ducts are seen in this X-ray of a patient with chronic *W. bancrofti* infection.

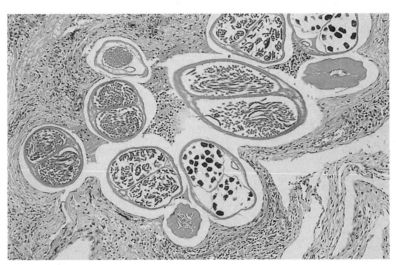

343 *Wuchereria bancrofti* in an occluded lymphatic vessel
Note the marked cellular reaction surrounding the microfilaria-containing female worms, seen here in cross-section. (*H&E* × *20*)

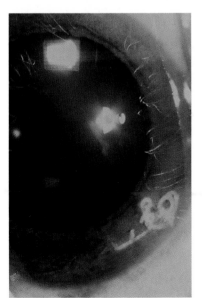

344 Male *Wuchereria bancrofti* in the anterior chamber of the eye
A motile nematode was removed from the anterior chamber of the eye of this 20-year-old Indian man who had soreness of the eye and diminished vision of 1 week's duration. The worm, which measured about 20 × 0.1 mm was identified as a male *W. bancrofti*. The patient made a complete recovery following surgery, which is the treatment of choice for this rare condition.

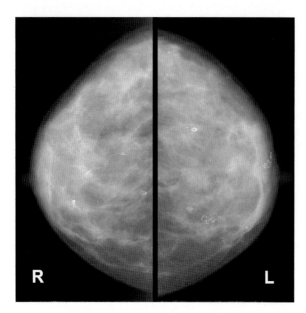

345 Calcified adult filaria in a mammogram

Adult filaria such as those of *W. bancrofti* can develop from infective larvae that enter and settle in the lymphatic vessels of the mammary gland. The adults seen here in the mammogram of a young Cameroonian woman have become calcified, forming palpable nodules appearing here as serpiginous shadows that are readily distinguished from neoplastic changes. (Courtesy of Drs H Alkadhi and E Garzoli. © Massachusetts Medical Society.)

346–352 Microfilariae in blood films

Identification of microfilariae and parasite counts per unit quantity of blood are necessary for the epidemiological evaluation of filariasis (although not for individual diagnosis). 20 ml pipettes are commonly used to make a thick blood film of specific size. If microfilariae are present in the peripheral circulation, they can usually be found by examining a fresh preparation of blood that has been taken between 10 pm and midnight. The worms may be seen in a wet preparation but morphological differentiation is only possible after suitable staining with a Romanowsky stain (Leishman or Giemsa) or haematoxylin. *W. bancrofti* (**346**); *B. malayi* (**347** and **348**); *Loa loa* (**349** and **350**); *Mansonella ozzardi* (**351**); *Mansonella perstans* (**352**). (× 920) (See **Table 10, 382** and **383** for skin-snip technique for other species.)

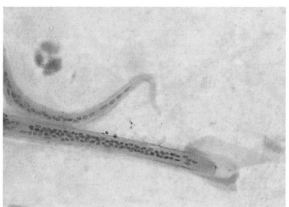

346

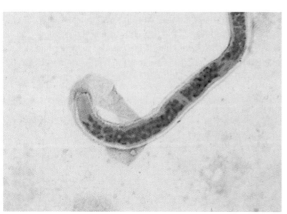

347

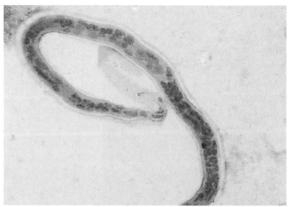

348

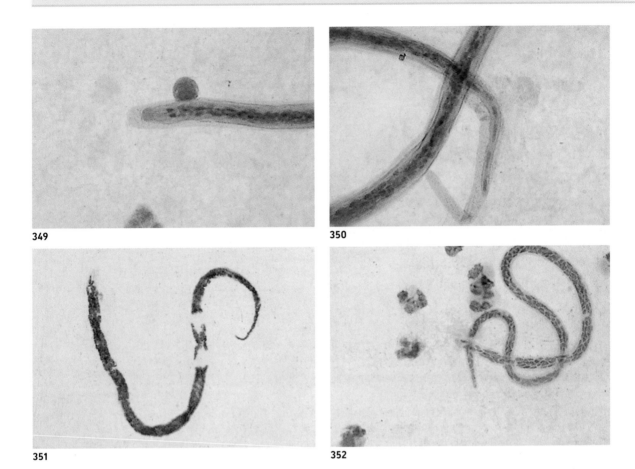

349

350

351

352

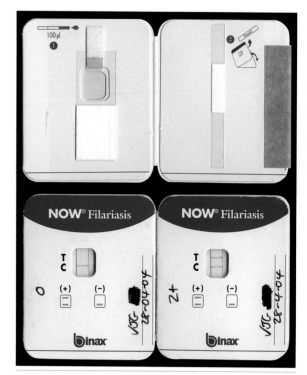

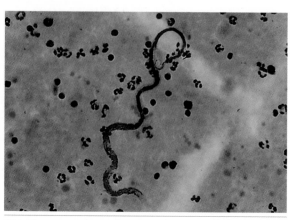

354 Giemsa-stained microfilariae
The sheathed microfilaria of *B. timori* is easily distinguished from that of *B. malayi* and *W. bancrofti* by its large size, the lack of staining of the sheath of *B. timori* in Giemsa stain, and the distribution of the nuclei in the posterior end. *B. timori*, like *B. malayi*, has two distinct nuclei in the tail (cf **346** and **348**). In *B. timori*, as in *B. malayi* or typical *W. bancrofti*, infection–parasite counts reveal a marked nocturnal periodicity. (In the diurnal, subperiodic type of *W. bancrofti*, microfilariae are readily seen in blood taken during the day.) ($\times$ *310*)

353 Rapid serological diagnosis of filariasis
A global programme for the elimination of lymphatic filariasis by 2020 based primarily on mass drug administration was initiated in 2000 by the Global Programme for Elimination of Lymphatic Filariasis, a broad partnership of organisations coordinated by the World Health Organization. An essential component of this programme is the mapping of the distribution and prevalence of infection with the responsible nematodes. The diagnosis of infection with *W. bancrofti* in individuals and especially for field surveys is facilitated by the use of affordable immunochromatographic test cards that detect antigen released by the adult nematodes. The example shown here of the Binax Filariasis Now® card demonstrates a negative test (bottom left) and a positive test (bottom right) in samples from two people who live in a filariasis-endemic area in Papua New Guinea. This test is usually positive in persons with microfilaraemia and in 'antigen-positive endemic normal' subjects with amicrofilaremic infections. Antigen tests are negative in old cases with, for example, lymphoedema or elephantiasis in whom the adult worms are no longer viable. This test is highly sensitive and species-specific. To date there is no sensitive antigen test available for diagnosis of filariasis caused by *B. malayi* or *B. timori*. Antibody tests (ELISA or dipstick tests that detect IgG4 antibodies to native or recombinant filarial antigens) are useful for verifying infection (or heavy exposure) for these parasites. (Courtesy of Professor G J Weil.)

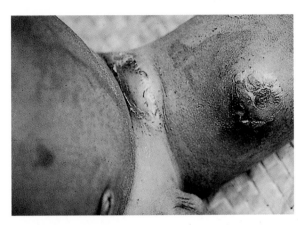

355 Abcesses in groin and thigh due to *Brugia timori*
Both this species and *W. bancrofti* are found in some Indonesian islands (see **315**) where up to 25% of village populations have been found to be infected with *B. timori*. The clinical disease resembles that caused by *B. malayi*, except that abcess formation is fairly common in the early stages along the line of the great saphenous vein in the upper thigh (as seen here), while chronic lymphoedema is commoner than frank elephantiasis in later cases. This parasite is transmitted by *Anopheles barbirostris*. The apparent absence of an animal reservoir increases the chances of eradicating this parasite by a combination of mass chemotherapy and anopheline vector reduction, the latter being facilitated by malaria control activities. Tests based on the detection of *B. malayi* antigens in blood have also proved valuable in assessing the levels of exposure of infection with *B. timori* in individuals and communities.

Mansonella perstans and *Mansonella streptocerca*

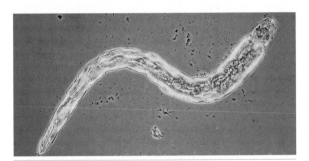

356 Larva of *Culicoides*
M. perstans is found in tropical Africa and in coastal regions of Central and South America. The vectors of *M. perstans* are small, speckled-wing flies of the genus *Culicoides*, of which *C. austeni* and *C. grahami* appear to be the main vectors in west Africa. The aquatic stages are commonly found in tree holes, leaf axils and other small natural water containers. (× 16)

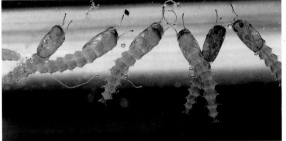

357 Pupae of *Culicoides*
Like mosquito pupae, the pupae of *Culicoides* obtain air by piercing the surface water film with their respiratory trumpets. (× 10)

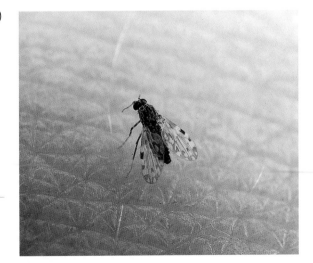

358 Adult *Culicoides* female
Although these flies are very small, their bites can cause severe irritation. The distinctive type of wing pattern is well shown in this figure. (× 15)

359 Breeding sites of *Culicoides* in an African village
The leaf axils of banana, such as this in a Liberian rain forest village plantation, the 'travellers' palm' and *Strelitzia* species are excellent breeding sites for *Culicoides* species in tropical areas.

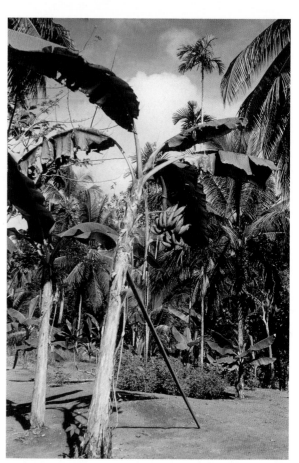

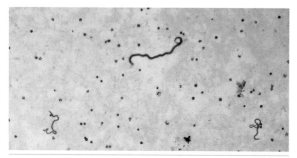

360 Mansonella perstans and Loa loa in blood film
The unsheathed microfilaria of *M. perstans* is readily distinguished (even at a fairly low magnification) from the sheathed microfilaria of *Loa loa* (or that of *W. bancrofti*) in blood films by its smaller size. Multiple infections with several species of blood-dwelling microfilariae are common.
M. perstans infection is usually asymptomatic and may last for many years. Males measure about 45 mm in length, and females about 70–80 mm. (*Giemsa × 100*)

Loaiasis

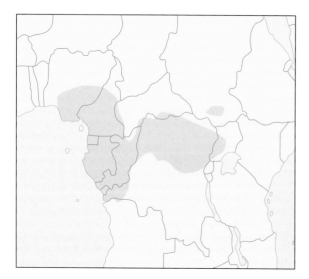

361 Distribution of loaiasis
Loaiasis is confined to Africa, extending from the Gulf of Guinea in the west to the Great Lakes in the east. Infection with an almost identical parasite is common in these areas in certain monkeys (such as the mandrill), and some infections may be zoonotic.

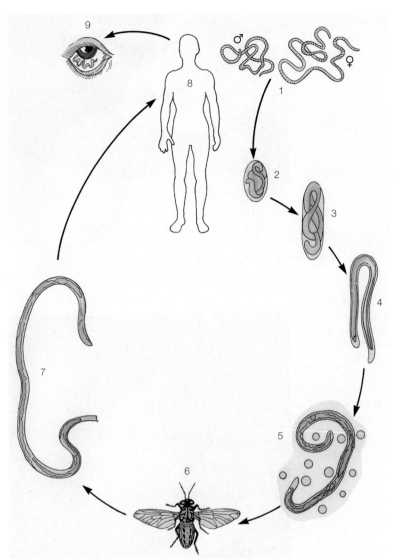

362 Life cycle of *Loa loa*

The adult worms (1) live in humans for 4–12 years. The females (which are about 7 cm long) migrate through the subcutaneous tissues and may cross the front of the eye under the conjunctiva (9). Microfilariae (5) develop from larvae (2–4) in the female and circulate in the blood, in which they are picked up by a *Chrysops* (6). In the gut of the fly, the microfilariae exsheath and enter the fat bodies in which they mature first to 'sausage-like' forms, then to infective third-stage larvae (7). These larvae infect a new host (8) when the *Chrysops* takes another blood meal, and mature to adult worms within about 1 year.

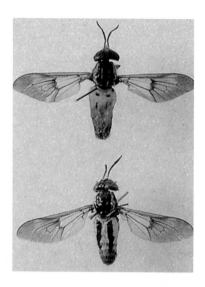

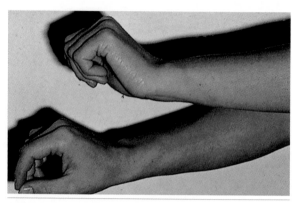

363 Female *Chrysops silacea* (top) and *Chrysops dimidiata* (bottom)
Tabanid flies of the genus *Chrysops* transmit loaiasis. *C. silacea* and *C. dimidiata* are the most important vectors in Nigeria, the Cameroons and the Congo highlands. (× 2.5)

364 Calabar swelling in left forearm
Recurrent large swellings lasting about 3 days are characteristic and indicate the tracks of the migrating adults in the connective tissue. They are most frequently seen in the hand, wrists and forearm. A marked eosinophilia (60–90%) accompanies this phase of the infection.

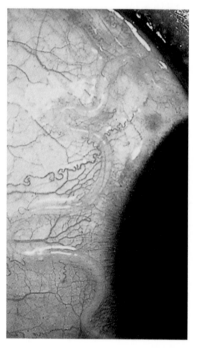

365 Adult *Loa loa* in the eye
The movement of the adult worm under the conjunctiva gives rise to considerable irritation and congestion.

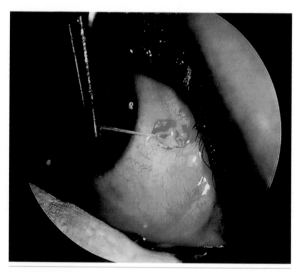

366 Extraction of worm
The adult worm can be extracted with fine forceps after anaesthetising the conjunctiva.

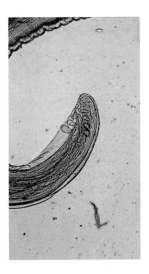

367 Tail of male *Loa loa*
The spicules at the posterior
end of the male worm are
typical of this species. (× *90*)

Onchocerciasis

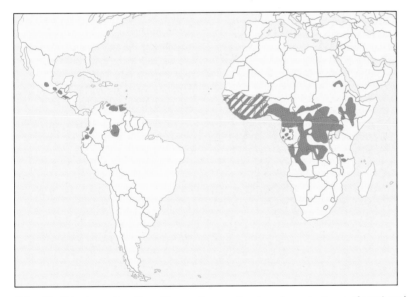

368 Former areas of distribution of onchocerciasis

Onchocerca volvulus is a tissue-dwelling nematode, the microfilariae of which are found predominantly in the skin and eye. Onchocerciasis had a focal distribution in Africa as well as parts of Central and South America. In Africa, onchocerciasis is mainly a disease of riverine country – e.g. of the extensive ramifications of the Niger and Volta in west Africa, and of mountainous regions in Zaire, Ethiopia and east Africa. In addition, small foci of transmission exist in the mountainous country of Yemen and possibly south-west Saudi Arabia. In the New World, onchocerciasis, once believed to be restricted to Central America, is now known to be endemic in large foci in Colombia, Ecuador and northern Venezuela as well as in an important area of southern Venezuela bordering Amazonian Brazil. Transmission in west Africa has been almost eliminated in the past three decades thanks to a mass campaign to destroy the larvae of the vectors with insecticides and the infective pool of filariae in the human hosts with chemotherapy. The shaded area in west Africa indicates the region in which the Onchocerciasis Control Programme was operative from 1974 (see **391**). In east Africa, where foci were limited mainly to small hill streams, larviciding with DDT largely interrupted transmission in the 1950s. In Central and South America, where vectors also breed in hill streams, chemotherapy has been the main basic weapon in onchocerciasis control. (Adapted from WHO Maps Nos. 94910 and 94911.)

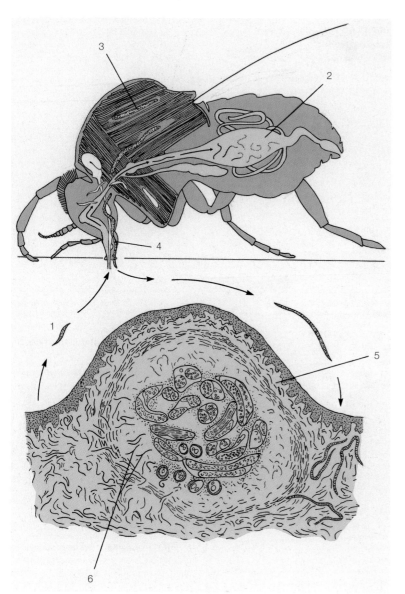

369 Life cycle of *Onchocerca volvulus*

(1) Microfilariae in the subepidermis are taken up with blood when the *Simulium* bites. From the midgut (2), the larvae pass into the haemocoele, then enter the thoracic muscles, where they grow and undergo two moults. In the process, they pass through an L2 'sausage' stage (3), then become long, thin, infective L3 larvae (4); the whole process takes from 6–12 days depending upon the ambient temperature. The infective larvae make their way to the proboscis, through which they enter the skin when the fly again feeds. Infective larvae mature into adults as they migrate through the subcutaneous tissues, with males and females mating and becoming encapsulated by fibrous tissue in prominent subcutaneous nodules (5). Within the nodules, the females produce larvae and these microfilariae (6) migrate into the nearby subepidermal tissues, with those in the head region reaching the tissues of the eye. (Adapted from Geigy and Herbig, 1955) (See also **335, 377, 378** and **383–386**.)

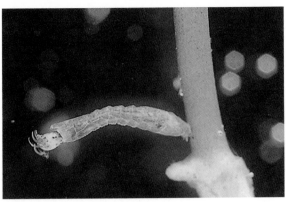

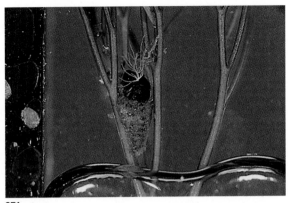

370

371

370 & 371 Aquatic stages of the vectors
The filarial worm is transmitted by biting flies of the genus *Simulium*. The larvae (**370**, left) and the pupae (**371**, right) of *Simulium* are attached to submerged objects in fast-running water from which they extract oxygen through head filaments. ($\times$ 5) (See also **374**.)

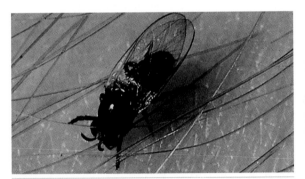

372 Adult *Simulium damnosum*
Because of their hump-backed stance, these insects are commonly known as 'buffalo flies' in some areas. *S. damnosum* is now recognised to be a large complex of sibling species of which at least 10 are proven vectors in different parts of Africa. In east Africa, the *Simulium neavei* complex used to be an important vector in some highland areas. *Simulium ochraceum* and *Simulium metallicum* are important vectors in Central and South America. ($\times$ 10)

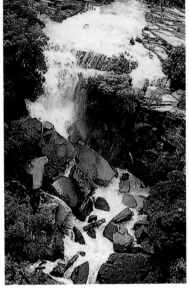

373 Typical locality of *Simulium* in west Africa
Fast-moving, highly oxygenated water in streams, rivers, waterfalls, etc. provides the essential ecological environment. The figure shows a branch of the Upper Volta river. In some hyperendemic villages in west Africa, a third of all adults may be blinded by onchocerciasis.

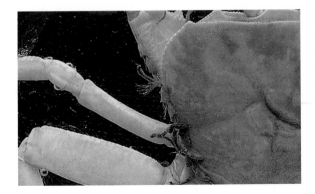

374 *Simulium* larvae and pupae on a crab
In east Africa, larvae and pupae of the *S. neavei* complex are attached to fresh-water crabs. Several of each stage of *S. nyasalandicum* can be seen on this preserved specimen of *Potamonautes pseudoperlatus*, which inhabits small hill streams in Tanzania.

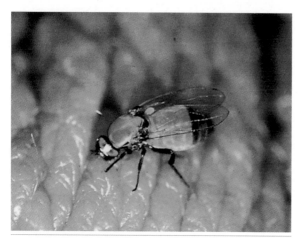

375 *Simulium ochraceum*
This simuliid fly and *S. metallicum* are two of the most
important vectors of onchocerciasis in Central America. (× *12*)

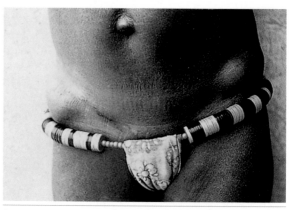

376 *Onchocerca* nodules on iliac crests of an African
The adult filariae become encapsulated in fibrous material,
which forms nodules in the subcutaneous tissues. They are
found predominantly in the lower part of the body in Africa,
while in South and Central America they are more commonly
found on the head and upper trunk.

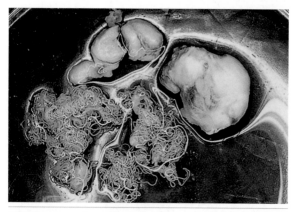

377 Macroscopic section of nodule
In this gross section of a nodule, the adult worms are seen
entwined. They lie in a matrix of inflammatory cells and
fibrinoid material in which microfilariae released by the female
worms become embedded. (× *2*)

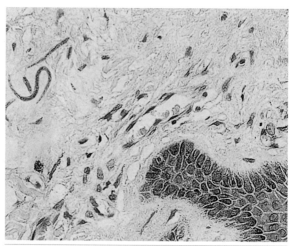

378 Microfilaria in skin biopsy
After discharge from the female uterus, the microfilariae
migrate to the skin and the eye. Treatment even with a single
dose of a microfilaricide such as diethylcarbamazine can
trigger a severe allergic response, the 'Mazzotti reaction', due
to the rapid killing of the skin-dwelling microfilariae. (A similar
reaction can also result if skin-dwelling microfilarial larvae of
Mansonella streptocerca are present.) (*H&E* × *350*)

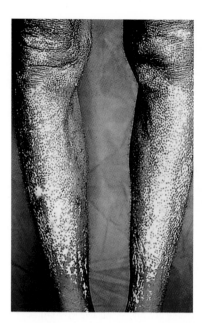

379
Depigmentation
Pretibial atrophy and depigmentation in a patient with late (burnt-out) onchocerciasis. This condition is sometimes called 'leopard skin'. Atrophy of the skin can occur, resulting in a 'tissue paper' appearance.

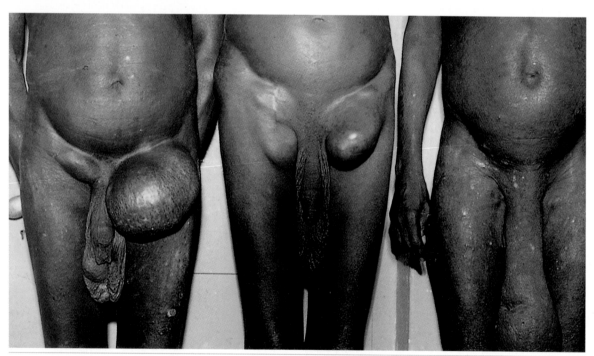

380 'Hanging groin' and scrotal elephantiasis
Involvement of the inguinocrural glands can result in an appearance described as 'hanging groin'. These three African patients show particularly severe anatomical changes due to onchocerciasis.

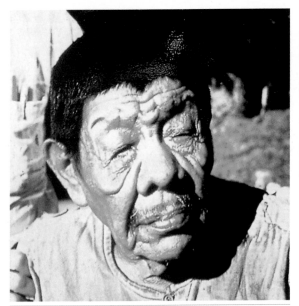

381 'Leonine facies' due to onchocerciasis in Guatemala
Estimates of the number of people infected in the New World are inaccurate but, for example, at least 2 million people inhabit the endemic areas of Venezuela. In Central America, onchocerciasis (*erisipela de la costa*) is characterised by an erythematous appearance of the face or upper trunk. It occurs in heavily infected young people, usually under 20 years of age. Purplish-tinged plaques or papules may be observed in Central America, usually in patients of an older age group. This condition, which is known as *mal morado*, sometimes gives the leonine appearance seen here.

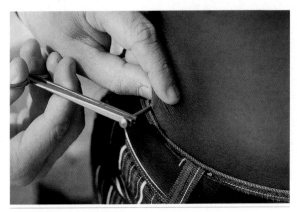

382 Skin-snip technique
A tiny piece of skin, often from the back of the shoulders, iliac regions or calf, is snipped off and placed in a drop of saline on a microscope slide under a cover slip, where it is left for several minutes at room temperature. The use of a scleral puncture as seen here permits the removal of a standard-sized sample to be taken for quantitative assessment of the microfilarial load. A simpler method is to raise the skin with a needle tip, then remove a piece of skin with a scalpel blade.

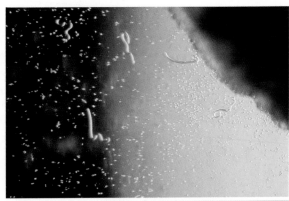

383 Living microfilariae of *Onchocerca volvulus*
After some time, actively moving microfilariae emerge from the skin into the surrounding saline where they can be counted. An ELISA test that is currently being evaluated uses a 'cocktail' of recombinant antigens as the basis of diagnosis and has shown some promise as a replacement for skin snips in diagnosis. However, the use of a nonradioactive PCR procedure on skin snips has proved more sensitive than visual examination and, unlike serological tests, can distinguish between past and current infections. It is likely to gain in importance for the monitoring of the progress of control programmes, rather than for individual diagnosis. (× *350*)

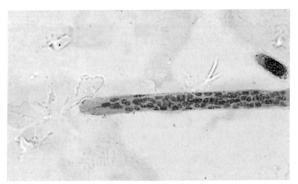

384

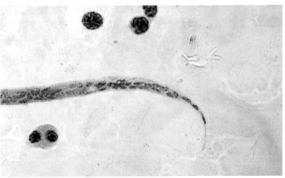

385

384 & 385 Microfilariae in skin-snips
O. volvulus head (**384**) and tail (**385**) (× *930*). (cf **346–352, 392, 393**.)

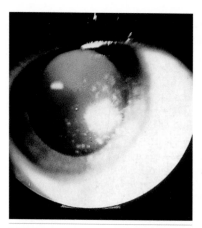

386 Early corneal involvement
The tissue reaction associated with dead microfilariae in the cornea gives rise to a number of 'snowflake-like' opacities as seen in the figure. This punctate keratitis may clear with time. Heavy microfilarial infection can lead to the development of progressive, sclerosing keratitis that commonly produces blindness.

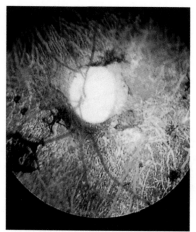

387 Optic atrophy
A variety of choroidoretinal lesions may follow damage by microfilariae to the anterior segments of the eye; optic atrophy may develop finally, as seen in this eye.

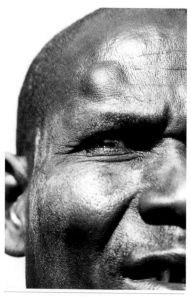

388 River blindness
From the female worm in the nodule of *O. volvulus* on the head of this blind African in Burkina Faso, large numbers of microfilariae will have penetrated the tissues of the eyes, eventually leading to blindness.

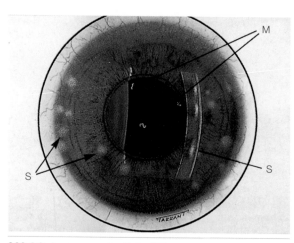

389 Slit-lamp examination of the eye
Slit-lamp examination often reveals numerous microfilariae (M) in the anterior chamber of the eye. They are best sought in the inferior medial quadrant. Note the 'snowflake-like opacities' (S) in the cornea.

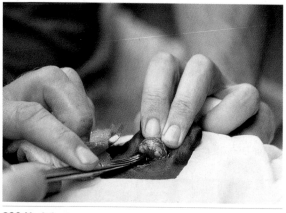

390 Nodulectomy
Serious eye changes can be prevented in some early cases by excising the nodules that contain the adult worms, thus preventing the continuing production of the microfilarae that are the actual pathogenic agents in this disease. Nodulectomy has been widely employed in Central and South America. Control (by larviciding) in the New World has only been successful so far in Mexico and, to a lesser degree, in Guatemala.

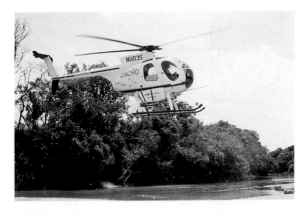

391 Helicopter spraying BTI over a breeding site of *Simulium damnosum* on the River Milo, Republic of Guinea

Fixed wing aircraft and helicopters were used widely in the international Onchocerciasis Control Programme. Following the emergence of insecticide resistance to the organophosphate insecticide, temephos (Abate®), extensive use was also made of the biological agent *Bacillus thuringiensis israelensis* H14 (BTI) to destroy the aquatic stages of *S. damnosum* in a 30-year campaign that dramatically reduced the transmission of *O. volvulus* in much of the endemic area of west and central Africa. However, the risk of reinvasion of infected areas by flies infected outside the controlled area continues to pose a threat.

Other filariases

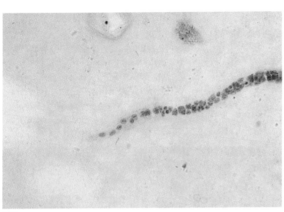

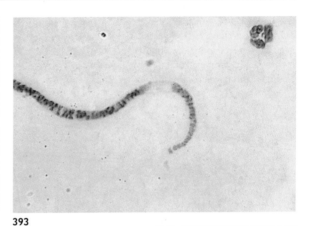

392

393

392 & 393 Microfilariae of *Mansonella streptocerca*

This skin-dwelling, unsheathed microfilaria must be distinguished from that of *O. volvulus* (**384** *and* **385**) in African patients. For this, a stained preparation should be examined (e.g. with haematoxylin). *M. streptocerca* produces few pathogenic effects; it is transmitted by *Culicoides grahami*, also infects chimpanzees, and is known only in Africa. Head (**392**, left), tail (**393**, right). (× *700*) (cf **346–352, 384** and **385**).

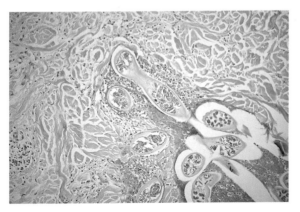

394 *Mansonella streptocerca* adult females in section of human skin

The females which measure approximately 27 × 0.08 mm live tightly coiled in the subcutaneous tissues where they release the unsheathed microfilariae. Sections of these can be seen within the adult worms in this section. (*H&E × 200*)

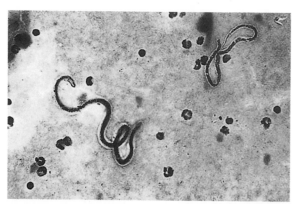

395 Microfilaria of *Mansonella ozzardi*

This unsheathed microfilaria (right) is found in the blood in parts of South America and the Caribbean. The microfilaria is readily distinguished from the larger and sheathed microfilaria of *W. bancrofti* (left) which also occurs in parts of South America. Vague symptoms of various types have been attributed to infection with the parasite, which is also transmitted by *Culicoides* spp. (× *340*)

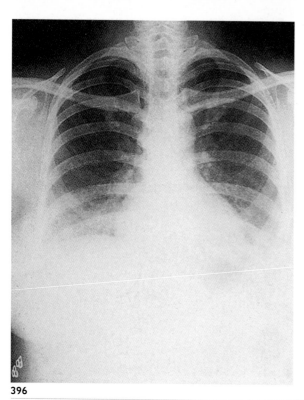

396

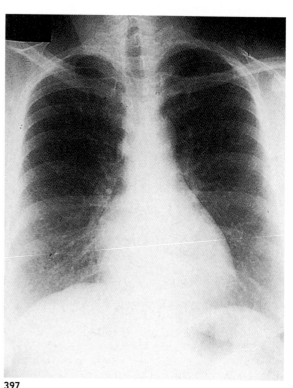

397

396 & 397 Tropical pulmonary eosinophilia (Löffler's syndrome)

This is a peculiar allergic reaction to filarial infections that may be of human or animal origin. It occurs principally in south Asia and affects Indians particularly. The condition is characterised by nocturnal cough and bronchospasm, with transient shadows in the lungs. Eosinophilia may be very marked. Pulmonary nodules caused, for example, by encapsulated *Dirofilaria immitis* may be mistaken for malignant tumours. These radiographs are of the chest of a patient who returned from Sri Lanka with a severe wheeze and eosinophilia and who was found to have an extremely high antibody to filaria (no microfilaria were found on thick blood films). The condition responds well to specific filaricides. **396** before treatment; **397** 10 days after treatment with diethylcarbamazine.

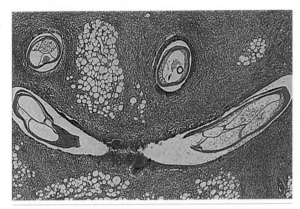

398 *Dirofilaria repens* in retrobulbar tissues

In the human this parasite is found mainly in dermal and subcutaneous tissues. It has been recorded from the eyelids and retrobulbar tissues of the eye of patients in Europe as in this case. *D. repens* is normally a parasite of dogs. (*H&E × 10*)

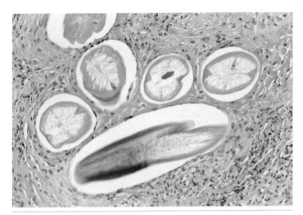

400 Cross sections of a *Dirofilaria* in subcutaneous nodule

This adult *Dirofilaria* (probably *D. repens*) was observed in a biopsy of a subcutaneous nodule occurring in a patient in northern Italy. The muscular layer, lateral nerve cord and uteri can be seen. (*H&E × 10*) (Courtesy of Drs M Lisci and G Cera.)

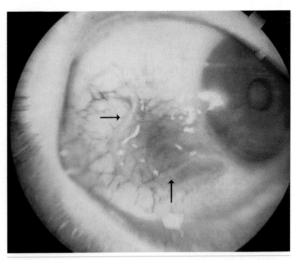

399 Adult female *Dirofilaria repens* in a human eye

The figure shows a mass situated under the bulbar conjunctiva of a 51-year-old Italian farmer. Excision and microscopic examination of the mass revealed an adult female of this nematode measuring 95 mm in length with a diameter of 0.45 mm. (Courtesy of Professor A E Bianco, Dr A Biglino and Dr A Casabianca.)

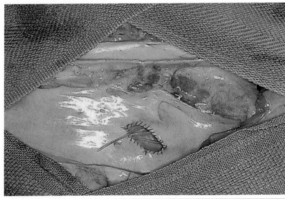

401 *Dirofilaria immitis* in humans

Several cases of infection with the common dog heartworm have been recorded in humans. This figure shows a 25 cm long, adult female *D. immitis* sited within the prosthetic portocaval shunt of a 32-year-old African-American woman in the southern USA who died of hepatic failure from chronic alcoholism. The nematode was first detected at autopsy.

Other arthropod-borne nematodes

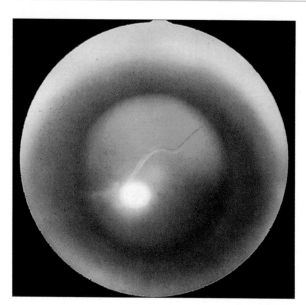

402 *Thelazia callipaeda* in the human eye

The adult worms of this spirurid nematode (see **Table 11**), which are 1–2 cm long, normally inhabit the lachrymal ducts and conjunctival sacs of dogs and rabbits. The females are viviparous and the L1 larvae in the lachrymal secretions may be picked up by eye-haunting flies such as *Musca* and *Fannia*. The flies may then transfer the larvae to fresh hosts, including humans, in whom the worms develop to adults within 3–6 weeks. The two species that have been found in humans are *T. callipaeda* which is common in people living in poor socioeconomic conditions in many Asian countries and *Thelazia californiensis*, which occurs in North America. Seen here is an adult *T. callipaeda* in the eye of a Malaysian man. The natural vector species of the 16 known species in this genus remain uncertain.

2. Soil-mediated helminthiases

Soil-transmitted helminthic infections are of two types: the hookworms, which undergo a cycle of development in the soil (the larvae being infective), and a group of nematodes that survive in the soil merely as eggs that have to be ingested in order for the cycle to continue.

The geographical distribution of the hookworms is limited by the requirements of the developing larvae for warmth and humidity. Generally speaking, the second type can occur not only in the tropics and subtropics but also in temperate regions. All of these helminthiases provide an index of the level of personal hygiene and sanitation in a community, since they depend for their dispersal, among other factors, on the indiscriminate deposition of faecal material on the ground and the use of untreated night soil as an agricultural fertiliser. In temperate regions, as in other areas, those infections that are spread directly (i.e. through the ingestion of eggs) are common in microenvironments that favour such spread (e.g. homes for mentally subnormal people, refugee camps, orphanages). The provision of adequate sewage disposal facilities virtually excludes these diseases.

Faecal contaminated soil in the neighbourhood of human habitations or on farmland is the source of hookworm infection for the barefooted inhabitants. Conversely, the use of footwear greatly reduces the prevalence of *Necator americanus* infection but not necessarily that of *Ancylostoma duodenale* infection, which may also be acquired by the oral route (see **426**). Such people as rubber tappers in Malaysia and farmers planting rice paddies commonly acquire infection from contaminated soil. Larvae of a number of animal hookworm species do not mature in humans but the invasive larvae produce a transitory skin

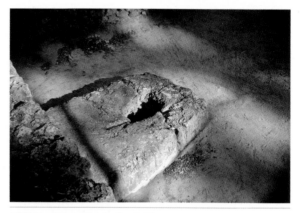

403 A public toilet in Gedi, Kenya
This pit-latrine-type public toilet was constructed in the 14th century Afro-Arab city of Gedi near Malindi on the Swahili coast of Kenya. The value of such a basic public health measure was apparent even earlier to physicians in the days of the Roman Empire when elaborate, water-carriage, public toilets were popular meeting and debating sites for its citizens. The use of this type of latrine in east Africa was a significant contribution to the limitation of infection by the helminthiases described here, as well as by pathogenic viruses, bacteria and protozoa acquired through the gastrointestinal tract (see Ch. 4).

eruption as they migrate (cutaneous larva migrans). Visceral larva migrans may be due to infections with eggs of the dog or cat roundworm (*Toxocara canis*, *Toxocara cati*). The larvae of these worms also do not mature in humans but may set up inflammatory reactions in the viscera (especially the liver), or in the eye.

Generally speaking, the degree of harm done to the host is related to the worm burden in these helminthiases. Hookworm disease results when large numbers of adult worms are present and the loss of blood due to the worms cannot be balanced because the host's diet is deficient in iron and other essential components. Moreover, multiple intestinal helminthic infection is the rule in many areas.

Heavy infections with *Ascaris* may result in intestinal obstruction, particularly in children. Severe *Trichuris* infection of the large bowel can lead to anaemia and rectal prolapse in infants. The prevalence of human infection with the individual nematodes is indicated in Table 11.

Table 11 Nematodes of medical importance and their prevalence[1]

Subclass	Order (Suborder)	Superfamily	Genus and species	Probable prevalence in humans
Adenophorea	Enoplida	Trichuroidea	*Trichinella spiralis*	49 million
			Trichinella papuae	Thousands
			Trichinella zimbabwiensis	?
			Trichuris trichiura	500 million
			Capillaria hepatica	Rare
			Capillaria philippinensis	Thousands
Secernentea	Rhabditida	Rhabditoidea	*Strongyloides stercoralis*	70 million
	Strongylida	Ancylostomatoidea	*Strongyloides fulleborni*	Thousands
			Pelodera strongyloides	Rare
			Rhabditis spp.	Rare
			Ancylostoma duodenale }	700–900 million
			Necator americanus }	
			Ancylostoma caninum	Thousands
			Ancylostoma braziliense	Thousands
			Ancylostoma ceylanicum	Rare
			Ternidens deminutus	Thousands
			Oesophagostomum bifurcum	>250 000
			Syngamus laryngeus	Rare
		Trichostrongyloidea	*Trichostrongylus* spp.	10 million
		Metastrongyloidea	*Metastrongylus elongatus*	Rare
			Parastrongylus cantonensis	Thousands
			Parastrongylus costaricensis	Thousands
	Oxyurida	Oxyuroidea	*Enterobius vermicularis*	400 million
	Ascaridida	Ascaridoidea	*Ascaris lumbricoides*	800–1000 million
			Toxocara canis	Thousands
			Toxocara cati	Thousands
			Lagochilascaris minor	Rare
			Baylisascaris procyonis	Rare
			Anisakis spp.	Rare
			Pseudoterronova decipiens	Thousands
	Spirurida (Spirurina)	Spiruroidea	*Gongylonema pulchrum*	Rare
		Gnathostomatoidea	*Gnathostoma spinigerum*	Thousands
		Thelazoidea	*Thelazia callipaeda*	Rare
		Filarioidea	*Wuchereria bancrofti*	120 million[2]
			Brugia malayi }	6 million
			Brugia timori }	
			Loa loa	33 million
			Onchocerca volvulus	<17 million[3]
			Mansonella perstans	65 million
			Mansonella streptocerca	2 million
			Mansonella ozzardi	15 million
			Dirofilaria spp.	Rare
	Spirurida (Camallanina)	Dracunculoidea	*Dracunculus medinensis*	<3 million[4]

[1] The estimated prevalences of helminthic infections vary greatly. These figures and the figures in Table 12 are based on estimates by the WHO (1993).
[2] In 1998 it was estimated that 120 million people were affected with lymphatic filariasis of whom 40 million were seriously incapacitated. A global programme to tackle this disease has now been established.
[3] The Onchocerciasis Eradication Campaign that started in 1974 succeeded in interrupting transmission in all but one endemic African country, thus almost eliminating the numbers of new cases from about 17 million and preventing about 600,000 cases of blindness by 2005. Progress in Central America has been slower.
[4] As a result of the global Dracunculiasis Eradication Campaign that was established in 1986, the number of people exposed (120 million) and cases (3.5 million) fell drastically each year to 15,000 cases (all of them in Africa), by the end of 2004.

404–418 The eggs of helminths

The morphology of helminth eggs that are detected in urine, faeces, sputum, etc., is usually sufficient to establish a diagnosis. Here, the eggs of species described in Chapters 2, 3 and 4 are shown at a single magnification for comparison. (See **Table 11** for classification. The eggs of the last three species are very difficult to distinguish.) *Schistosoma haematobium* (**404**), *Schistosoma mansoni* (**405**), *Schistosoma japonicum* (**406**), *Fasciola hepatica* (**407**), *Ascaris lumbricoides* (**408**), *Ascaris* (infertile) (**409**), *Paragonimus westermani* (**410**), *Diphyllobothrium latum* (**411**), hookworm (**412**), *Trichuris trichiura* (**413**), *Enterobius vermicularis* (**414**), *Vampirolepis nana* (**415**), *Hymenolepis diminuta* (**416**), *Taenia* (**417**), *Opisthorchis sinensis, Opisthorchis felineus, Heterophyes heterophyes* (**418**). (× 380) (Note: *Vampirolepis nana* was formerly known as *Hymenolepis nana*.)

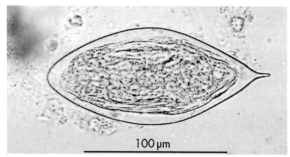

100 µm

404

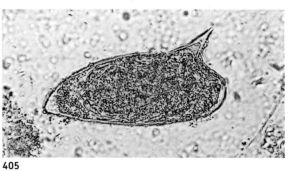

405

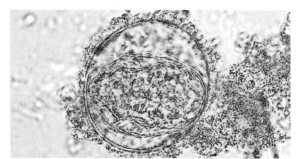

406

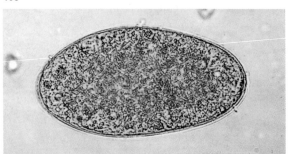

407

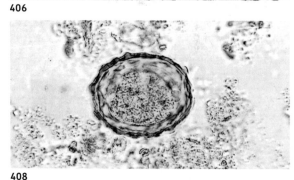

408

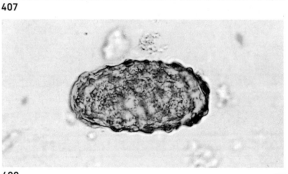

409

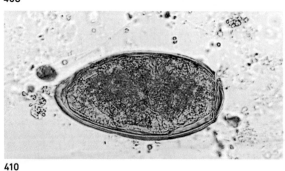

410

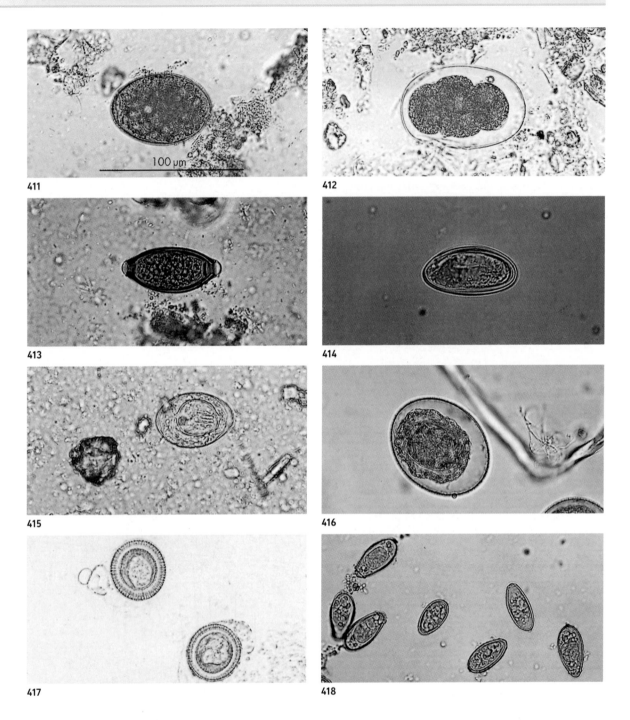

411

412

413

414

415

416

417

418

THE HOOKWORM INFECTIONS

Ancylostoma duodenale and *Necator americanus*

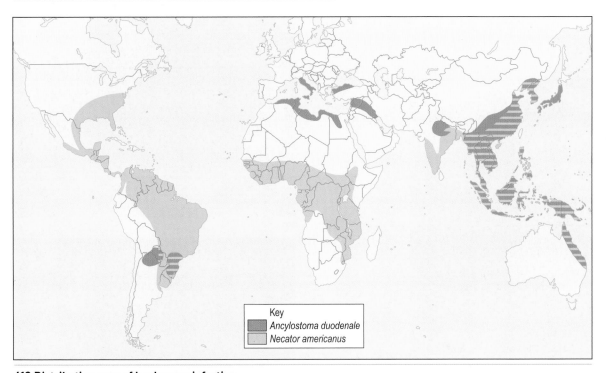

Key
Ancylostoma duodenale
Necator americanus

419 Distribution map of hookworm infection

The common hookworms of humans are *Ancylostoma duodenale and Necator americanus*. It is estimated that nearly a quarter of the world's population are infected. One species usually predominates in any one locality; the map shows the approximate areas in which one or other species dominates. Since the larvae can only develop in warm, moist soil, the distribution of the parasite is limited by climatic conditions.

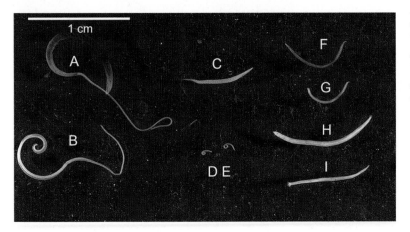

1 cm

420 Comparative size of nematodes

Trichuris trichiura ♀ ♂ **(A, B)**;
Enterobius vermicularis ♀ **(C)**;
Trichinella spiralis ♀ ♂ **(D, E)**;
Ancylostoma duodenale ♀ ♂ **(F, G)**;
Necator americanus ♀ ♂ **(H, I)**.

421–425 Identification of adult hookworms

Ancylostoma caninum (**421**) (× 280). *A. duodenale* (**422**) (× 630). *Ancylostoma ceylanicum* (**423**) (× 670), *N. americanus* (**424**) (× 470), *A. duodenale* (**425**) (× 470). The different species may be distinguished by the characteristic morphology of the head capsule (**421–424**) and male bursa (**425**), seen here in scanning electronmicrographs. The male bursae are distinguished by the numbers and pattern of the 'rays'.

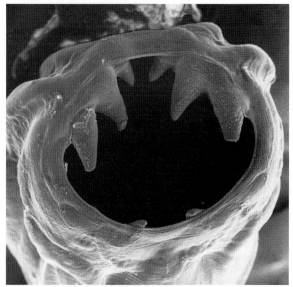

421

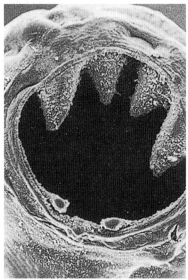

422

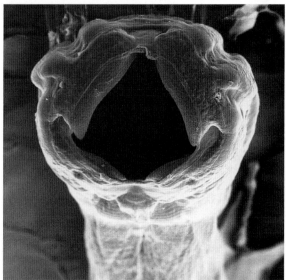

423

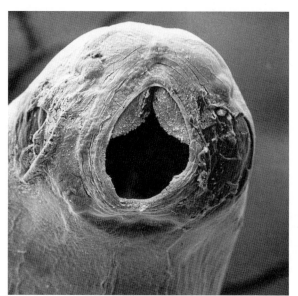

424

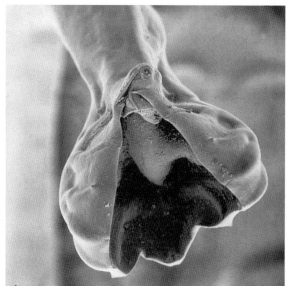

425

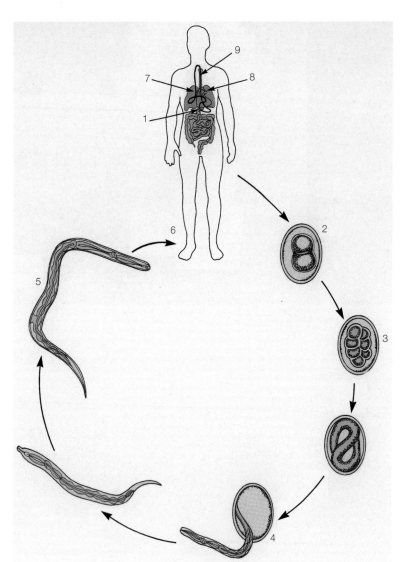

426 Life cycle of *Necator americanus* and *Ancylostoma duodenale*

Adults are attached to the walls of the jejunum (1) by the buccal capsule. Females lay large numbers of eggs, which are passed out with the faeces (2). The eggs mature through four-segment and eight-segment stages (3) to larvae, which hatch in the soil (4). There they feed on bacteria and undergo two moults to produce filariform, infective larvae (5). These penetrate the skin of a new host (6), usually on the feet. They migrate into venules, entering the right heart (7) and lungs (8). Here, they grow before penetrating from the capillaries into the alveoli. They enter the trachea (9), then the pharynx, are swallowed and pass into the small intestine (1), where they mature. *N. americanus* appears to enter the human body solely through the penetration of the skin by soil-dwelling, infective larvae. *A. duodenale*, on the other hand, is able to establish itself both percutaneously and via the ingestion of contaminated food and soil. It further differs from *N. americanus* in exhibiting the phenomenon of arrested development (i.e. the apparent ability to remain within the host at a larval stage for many months before finally reaching maturity). (See also **412** and **428–431**.)

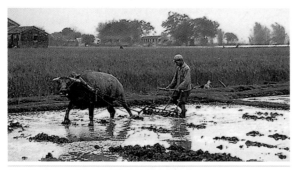

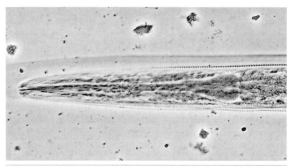

427 Ecology of geohelminth infection

In tropical and subtropical areas, wet soil (such as that found at the edges of rice fields, rubber plantations and the surroundings of villages in areas of high rainfall) supports the maturation of hookworm larvae from eggs deposited by indiscriminate defaecation; this limits their geographical distribution. In contrast, the well-protected eggs of nematodes with a direct cycle of transmission (*Ascaris lumbricoides*, *Trichuris trichiura*) can survive in drier conditions even at freezing temperatures. (See also **457**.)

428 Filariform larva of hookworm

Eggs (**412**) passed in the faeces hatch into rhabditiform larvae in damp soil; they feed and undergo two moults to produce an infective, sheathed filariform larva. (× *350*)

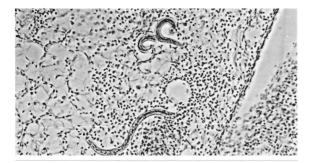

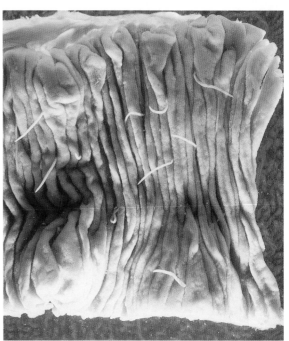

429 Larvae of hookworm in lung of dog

The infective larvae penetrate bare skin, usually of feet or legs, and, if they are in their correct host, enter the bloodstream to reach the lungs. The larvae then penetrate into the bronchioles, pass into the pharynx and are swallowed. They become attached to the small intestine and mature to adults. (× *100*)

430 Adult hookworms in situ

The worms are about 1 cm long and characteristically curved. They are attached by their buccal capsules to the villi of the small intestine. (*Natural size*)

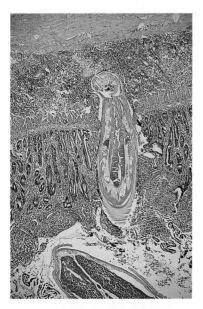

431 Section of adult *Ancylostoma duodenale* in situ

The hookworm feeds by sucking blood from the intestinal mucosa. It has been estimated that a single *A. duodenale* can withdraw as much as 0.2 ml a day while *N. americanus* withdraws 0.05 ml. (× *20*)

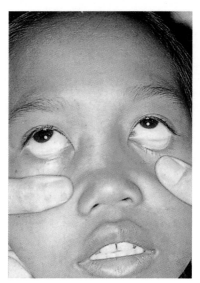

432 Hookworm anaemia

Severe anaemia is the classical feature of hookworm disease. This young Thai woman with a heavy load of *N. americanus* had a haemoglobin level of 22 g/l.

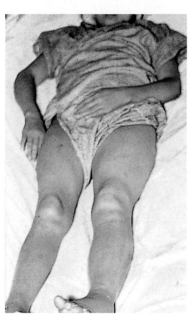

433 Clinical picture of gross hookworm disease

This results from a combination of a high hookworm load and low daily iron intake. The patients usually complain of lassitude and shortness of breath. Oedema and ascites as seen in this young patient also occur.

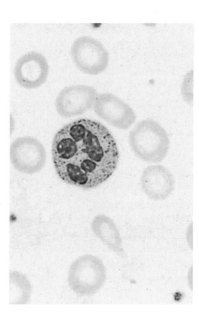

434 Blood film from a patient with hookworm anaemia

The typical anaemia resulting from severe hookworm infection is of the iron-deficiency type, with hypochromic, microcytic red cells, a low serum iron and low ferritin level. (× *1300*)

435 Cutaneous larva migrans ('creeping eruption') due to larvae of animal hookworms

Infective larvae of various species of animal hookworms (e.g. *Ancylostoma braziliense, Ancylostoma caninum, Ancylostoma ceylanicum*) frequently fail to penetrate the human dermis. They migrate through the epidermis leaving typical serpiginous tracks known also as 'creeping eruption'. Larvae of a free-living Rhabditoid nematode, *Pelodera strongyloides*, as well as *A. caninum*, can cause severe folliculitis rather than typical 'creeping eruption'. A severe eruption caused by ancylostome larvae is present on the toes of this patient who went for a beach holiday in the Bahamas. The patient was cured with a 3-day course of albendazole. (In a trial of mass treatment of over 500 residents of a poor community in north-east Brazil, a single or 2-day course of ivermectin reduced the prevalence rate of cutaneous 'creeping eruption' from 0.7% to zero over a 9-month observation period. In addition, the prevalence of hookworm was reduced from 28.5% to 7.7%, ascariasis from 17.1% to 7.2%, trichuriasis from 16.5% to 9.4% and strongyloidiasis from 11% to 0.7%. The prevalence of ectoparasitic arthropods was also significantly reduced.)

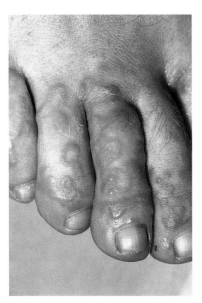

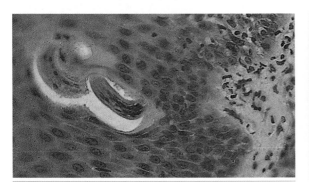

436 Larva of dog hookworm in the epidermis of a human foot

Portions of a larva are seen in longitudinal section. (*Haematoxylin and eosin (H&E) × 400*)

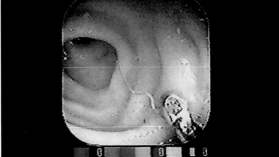

437 Adult *Ancylostoma caninum* in human ileum

In the humid north of Queensland, Australia, the larvae of this dog hookworm cause eosinophilic enteritis – a form of visceral larva migrans. The infection is probably acquired by the penetration of infective larvae from contaminated grass through the skin of the feet. Severe inflammatory lesions in the small intestine are associated with recurrent abdominal colic and sometimes diarrhoea, which is characterised by eosinophilia and is relieved by anthelminthic treatment. Resection of the severely inflamed segment of bowel shows oedema and eosinophilic inflammation of the wall. In the case seen here, the worm was situated in a nodule in the terminal ileum, from where it could be removed under visual control through a fibreoptic endoscope.

Strongyloidiasis

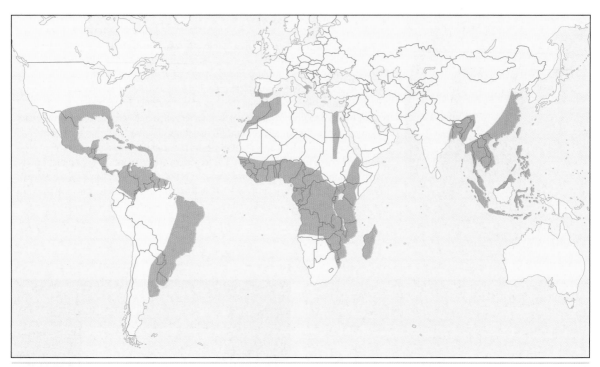

438 Distribution of strongyloidiasis
While mainly distributed in humid tropical and subtropical areas where its larvae can survive in the soil, *Strongyloides stercoralis* is also transmitted in some cooler areas (e.g. in warm and humid deep mines). It has also been reported to be spread on occasion from human to human by contamination with faeces containing infective rhabditiform larvae (e.g. in mental institutions and prisons). The map illustrates areas of high prevalence. There is an association between strongyloidiasis and human T-cell leukaemia virus (HTLV1) infection in the Caribbean and Japan.

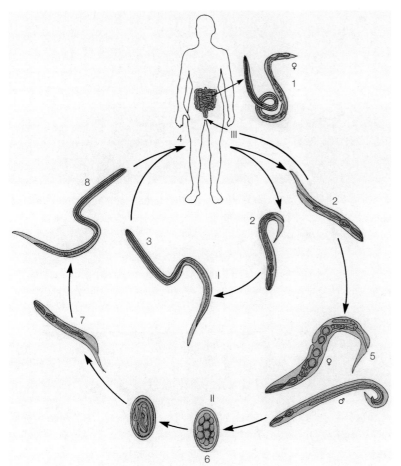

439 Life cycle of *Strongyloides stercoralis*

This tiny nematode has two generations: one free-living and the other parasitic. I. *The parasitic generation*. Males are rare and the females (1) are probably parthenogenetic, living in the mucosal glands of the small intestine. Eggs usually hatch in these glands into larvae, which are passed in the faeces (2). These rhabditiform larvae can develop into filariform larvae (3) in the ground, with the infective filariform larvae then penetrating the skin of a new host (4). The rest of the cycle in humans is as in hookworm infections. II. *Free-living generation*. Rhabditiform larvae (2) may develop into free-living males and females (5), which lay eggs (6) that hatch in the soil into rhabditiform (7), then infective filariform larvae (8). These too can penetrate the skin (4) and recommence a parasitic cycle in humans. III. *Autoinfection*. Rhabditiform larvae (2) can mature into filariform larvae in the intestine; these can directly penetrate the perianal skin, causing autoinfection. IV. *Hyperinfection*. Rhabditiform larvae may penetrate the intestinal mucosa, causing massive autoinfection, usually in people with diminished immune responsiveness and in those treated with steroids (cycle not illustrated here).

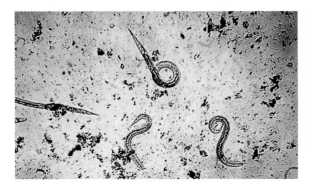

440 Rhabditiform larvae of *Strongyloides stercoralis* in *faeces*

The figure shows rhabditiform larvae, which are usually the only stage seen in faeces. Eggs, which are rarely seen, resemble those of hookworm but contain maturing larvae. Larvae of *S. stercoralis* can readily be distinguished (by their active, snake-like movements) from larvae of hookworms, which sometimes hatch in faecal specimens that have been left standing for some time. (× 60) (See also **452**.)

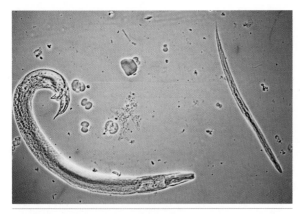

441 Adult male and free-living larva in soil
(× 65)

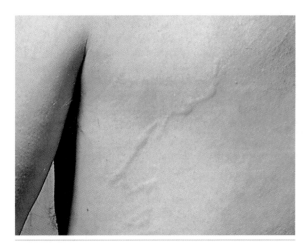

443 Migrating larvae of *Strongyloides stercoralis* in skin
Autoinfection can lead to severe 'creeping eruption' which usually occurs on the back. This may occur many years (30 or more) after initial infection. Deep migration of the larvae may be associated with an 'eosinophilic lung' type of syndrome.

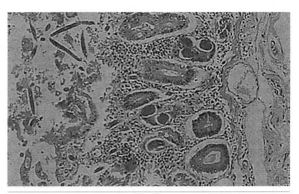

442 Sections of parasitic female and eggs embedded in jejunal mucosa
Free-living females (about 1 mm long) are smaller than the forms found in the intestine (up to 2.2 mm). Males are normally found only in the soil and are about 0.7 mm long. The parasitic females lying in the intestinal mucosa may reproduce parthenogenetically, with the eggs filtering through to the intestinal lumen or first hatching in the mucosa. (× *180*)

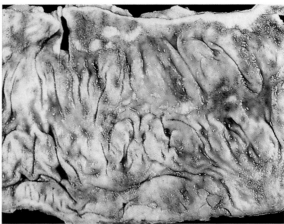

444 Post-mortem appearance of colon
The incidental administration of steroids and immunosuppressive agents may greatly enhance infection with *S. stercoralis*, which may even be fatal, as in this case. Note the multiple ulcerations and thickening of the wall of the colon. There is also evidence that concurrent infection with HTLV1 can be associated with an increased incidence of larvae in the faeces, possibly due to suppression of the normal IgE response to the helminths.

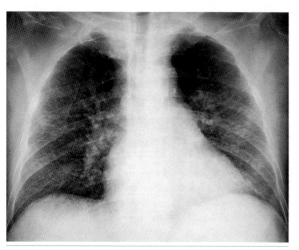

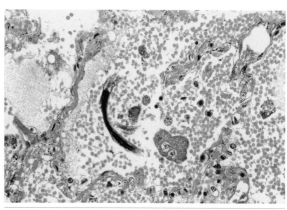

445 Haemorrhagic pneumonia in disseminated *Strongyloides stercoralis* infection

The chest radiograph shows bilateral, confluent, interstitial and alveolar infiltration.

446 Section of lung from a patient with disseminated *Strongyloides stercoralis*

At post-mortem the lungs of the patient whose chest X-ray is shown in **445** show haemorrhagic pneumonia with thickening of the alveolar walls, inflammatory infiltration with erythrocytes and eosinophils and sections of filariform larvae within an alveolus. In some cases eosinophils may be absent in this condition which is fatal in 50 to 75% of all cases, even with intensive anthelminthic therapy. (*H & E* x *100*).

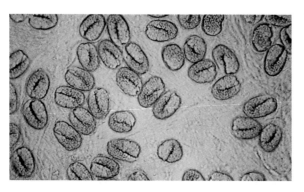

447 Eggs of *Strongyloides fülleborni* in faeces

S. fülleborni, a common intestinal nematode in African and Asian primates, is found in humans in a number of countries, including Zambia, where 10% of human *Strongyloides* infections may be caused by this species. Massive infections with a subspecies of this nematode, *S. fülleborni kellyi*, cause an often fatal illness in infants in the south and central parts of Papua New Guinea, a country from which monkeys are absent. This condition, known as 'swollen belly sickness', is characterised by respiratory distress, abdominal distension and generalised oedema. Very heavy egg loads, as seen here, occur in such cases. The custom of mothers carrying babies in a woven bag known as a 'billum', which is often lined with soggy material, encourages autoinfection and may account for the very heavy worm loads found in their infants. (x *300*)

Other phasmid nematodes of humans

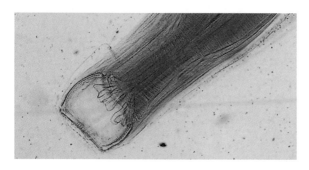

448 Head capsule of adult *Ternidens deminutus*

In some areas such as east Africa and Zimbabwe, infection commonly occurs with a hookworm-like parasite of monkeys, *Ternidens deminutus*, which also infects monkeys in Asia. The adult worm, which is about 1 cm long, is found at any level in the small and large intestine. Normally, infection is asymptomatic. (x *80*)

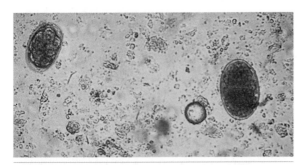

449 Eggs of *Ternidens deminutus* and hookworm compared
The eggs of *T. deminutus* (right) are usually mistaken for those of hookworm but the adults passed accidentally during hookworm therapy are distinctive (× *125*). (See also **412**).

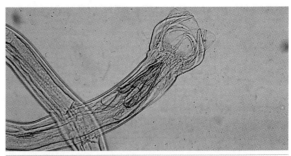

450 Adult male *Trichostrongylus*
Various species of *Trichostrongylus* inhabit the digestive tract of herbivores, burrowing into the mucosa (like hookworms) to obtain their nutrition. They have been encountered infrequently in humans but in many different countries, although in one Iranian town they were said to be present in 70% of the population. They are readily distinguished from human hookworms by their smaller size and more slender shape. The male bursa is different in form from that of *A. duodenale* (**425**). (× *100*)

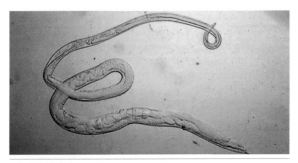

451 Adult female *Trichostrongylus*
The head of this tiny, very slender worm (about 0.5 cm long) lacks the distinct buccal cavity of the human hookworms (**421–424**). (× *50*)

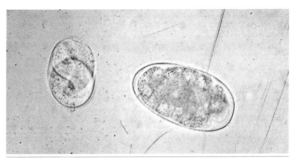

452 Eggs of *Trichostrongylus* and *Strongyloides stercoralis* in faeces
The hookworm-like egg of *Trichostrongylus* (right) is much larger (about 60 × 40 μm) than that of *S. stercoralis*, which contains an embryonic larva ready to hatch (× *250*).

Oesophagostomiasis

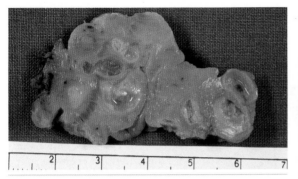

453 *Oesophagostomum bifurcum* **in the human colon**
Numerous human infections with this nematode occur in
localised areas of west and east Africa. A recent survey in
northern Togo and Ghana identified the larvae of *O. bifurcum* in
the faeces of up to 30% of the inhabitants of 65 villages. The
eggs, which resemble those of hookworms, mature in the soil
and produce infective third-stage larvae, which are
morphologically distinct in stool culture from those of the
common hookworms that frequently coexist. When swallowed,
the larvae develop into adults in the mucosa and submucosa of
the large intestine, where they produce small abscesses. After
maturation, the adults leave the abscesses to attach to the
colonic mucosa. The figure, which shows part of the wall of the
colon resected from a patient in northern Ghana, is
characteristic of the multinodular form of the infection, which
can give rise to intestinal obstruction necessitating surgery.
The numerous, pea-sized nodules each contain a juvenile
worm.

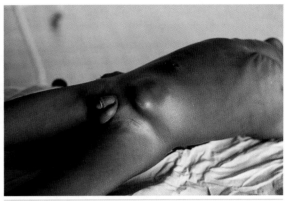

454 'Dapaong tumour' in a Togolese boy
At least 250 000 people are estimated to be infected with
O. bifurcum in the north of Togo and Ghana, with a prevalence
rate as high as 50% in some villages. In some individuals the
worms cause large abdominal masses in the epigastric or
periumbilical region, a condition known locally as 'Dapaong
tumour'. These abdominal masses may be large, inflamed and
painful, as in the child seen here, but are often smaller and less
prominent. They characteristically contain a single juvenile
worm about 10–12 mm long.

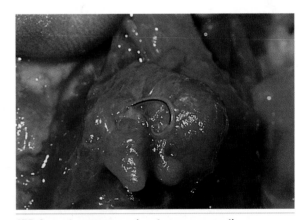

455 *Oesophagostomum* **in a human appendix**
The specimen seen here was found at operation for
appendicitis in a Ugandan patient. The species was probably
related to *Oesophagostomum stephanostomum* which is a
parasite of gorillas.

INFECTION WITH *ASCARIS* AND RELATED NEMATODES

Ascariasis

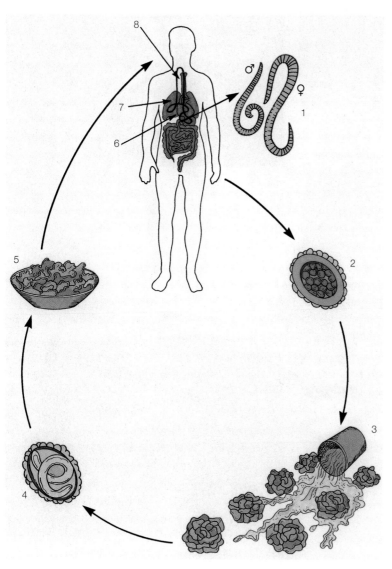

456 Life cycle of the roundworm: *Ascaris lumbricoides*

Adult worms (1) live in the small intestine where they lay large numbers of eggs (2) that are passed out with the faeces. In the soil, they can readily contaminate vegetables, for example, when night soil (3) is used as fertiliser. The larvae develop inside the eggs (4), which are swallowed when they are present in uncooked food (5). The eggs enter the jejunum (6) where the larvae hatch, penetrate the mucosa, and are carried through the hepatic circulation to the heart and lungs (7). There they grow, moulting twice before escaping from the capillaries into the alveoli. They again enter the stomach via the trachea and oesophagus (8), and thence pass to the small intestine where they grow to adulthood. (*See also* **408** *and* **409**.)

Infection with *Baylisascaris procyonis*

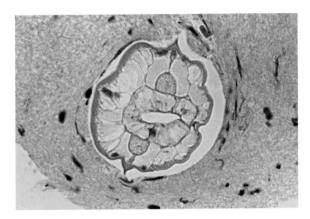

472 Cross section of a larva of *Baylisascaris procyonis* from a child with neural larva migrans

The parasite was discovered in a brain biopsy from a teenage boy with a history of pica living in California. The adult nematode is found in the small intestine of the majority of peridomestic raccoons in the western United States (80% or more in some areas) and the larva is an increasingly reported cause of visceral larva migrans. Infection is acquired when eggs on contaminated soil (raccoon 'latrines') are accidentally ingested. The larvae, measuring 1.5 to 2 mm in length, hatch in the stomach and migrate through the tissues but do not develop fully except in their natural host in which they produce typical, ascarid adults from 14 to 18 cm long. In accidental hosts such as humans, from 5 to 7% of larvae are believed to migrate to the eye and central nervous system where they can cause extensive lesions. (*H&E × 800*)

TRICHURIASIS

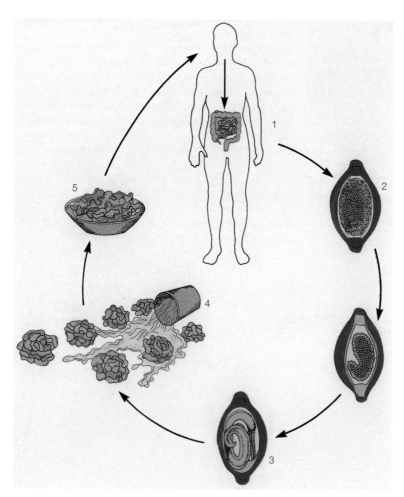

473 Life cycle of the whipworm Trichuris trichiura

Adults inhabit the caecum (1), and sometimes the colon and rectum where they are attached to the mucosa. Eggs passed with the faeces (2) mature in the soil to larvae (3), which remain in the eggs. Eggs can readily contaminate vegetables (e.g. when night soil is used as fertiliser (4) or when sanitary habits are otherwise primitive), and are then swallowed in uncooked food (5). The eggs hatch in the small intestine and the developing larvae pass directly to their attachment sites in the large intestine. Females commence egg-laying after about 3 months. (*See also* **413** *and* **420**.)

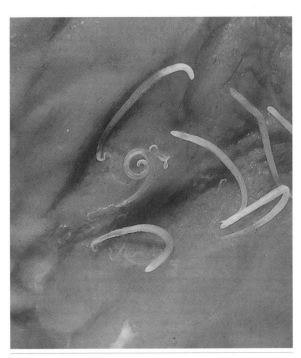

474 Adult morphology, females and males

Three to 10 days after the eggs are ingested, the young worms pass down to the caecum where the whip-like anterior portion becomes entwined in the mucosa. The adult worms are about 3–5 cm long, with the females being slightly larger than the males which are coiled. The adult worms (one male and several females) are seen in this figure of the caecal mucosa. (× 2) (AFIP No. 69–3583.)

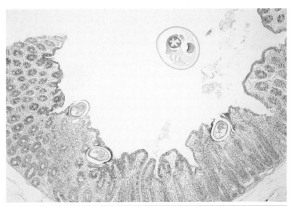

475 Cross-section of *Trichuris trichiura* associated with caecal tissue

The section shows a cross section of an adult worm free in the lumen and sections of the slender anterior end apparently inserted in the mucosa. (*H&E × 13*)

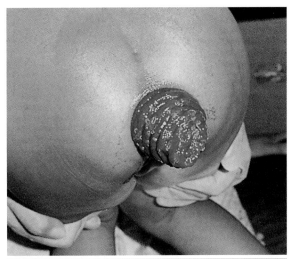

476 Rectal prolapse

Heavy infections may cause rectal prolapse following chronic bloody diarrhoea with abdominal pain in infants and children, especially if they are undernourished.

3. Mollusc-mediated helminthiases

With the exception of the angiostrongyliases (Ch. 4), which are nematode infections transmitted accidentally to humans in the course of their complex life cycles in rodents and other mammals, the important group of snail-transmitted helminthiases are all caused by trematodes (flukes), which undergo a complicated cycle involving various species of land or aquatic snail or, rarely, oysters.

A total of 600 million people are exposed to schistosomiasis and over 200 million are estimated to be infected, 120 000 showing symptoms. The three common species, *Schistosoma mansoni*, *Schistosoma haematobium* and *Schistosoma japonicum*, cause a heavy morbidity and contribute in certain areas to the high mortality rate found among adolescents and young adults. Infection with these parasites is a major cause of cancer in endemic countries. In the case of *S. haematobium* infection, for example, it has been estimated that its prevention would reduce the global rate of bladder carcinoma by 5000–10 000 cases annually. Since infection occurs by penetration of the skin by water-dwelling infective stages (cercariae), transmission tends to increase in parallel with the extension of land utilisation by irrigation. Hence, schistosomiasis is a positive obstacle to agricultural and economic development in many parts of the developing world. In 2002 a new Schistosomiasis Control Initiative was launched in order to coordinate and intensify global efforts to control this major public health problem.

Apart from schistosomiasis due to *S. haematobium* and *S. mansoni*, for which humans are the main reservoir of infection, *S. japonicum* has an important animal reservoir, while the other snail-mediated helminthiases are zoonoses. Like many zoonoses, they are relatively uncommon, with notable, highly localised exceptions. In spite of the availability of excellent molluscicides and antischistosomal drugs, up to now remarkably little overall success has met attempts to control the schistosomiases in many endemic countries, although significant progress has been made in reducing the morbidity and mortality they cause. In China a major project commenced in the mid-1950s and, supported by the World Bank from 1992, reduced the infection rates of *S. japonicum* by 55% in humans and 50% in livestock by 2002. The densities of infected snails in the region had decreased by 75%. However, in 2004 1 million Chinese were still believed to be infected and 65 million exposed to schistosomiasis. Natural floods, for example of the Yangtze River, as well as major dam construction projects favour the dissemination of the carrier snails and hence resurgence of the disease. Mass drug chemotherapy with praziquantel has made a major contribution to the reduction of all the schistosome species affecting humans, including *Schistosoma mekongi*. The localised African species, *Schistosoma intercalatum*, is, for reasons unknown, spontaneously decreasing in prevalence. Some progress has been made towards the development of antischistosomal vaccines but none is yet available for human use.

The public health importance of food-borne, intestinal liver-fluke and lung-fluke infections has, until very recently, been grossly underestimated; indeed, our knowledge of the epidemiology of some species is still limited. It is, however, now realised that at least 40 million people are infected with liver-dwelling and lung-dwelling trematodes. These flukes have a somewhat more complicated life cycle than the schistosomes, in that the cercariae develop a resting stage (the metacercaria), which, in turn, must be ingested for infection to occur. As the metacercariae are found usually on various water plants, on fish or on crustaceans, infection with these worms tends to be localised to areas in which particular local eating habits bring humans and the metacercaria together. Thus, clonorchiasis and opisthorchiasis are restricted to regions where raw fish is commonly ingested (notably in parts of south-east Asia and the former Soviet Union), fasciolopsiasis to regions where, for example, water caltrops and water chestnuts are eaten uncooked, and paragonimiasis to regions where the appropriate crustaceans form part of the human diet in one culinary delicacy or another. Most of these flukes are primarily parasites of animals other than humans (e.g. *Fasciola hepatica* is essentially a parasite of sheep that infects humans who eat watercress or other aquatic plants from contaminated, wet pastures). In certain villages in north-east Thailand,

Table 12 Digenetic trematodes of medical importance and their prevalence

Superorder	Order	Superfamily	Genus and species	Estimated cases*	No.
Anepitheliocystida	Strigeida	Schistosomatoidea	*Schistosoma mansoni*	57 million	1
			Schistosoma haematobium	78 million	2
			Schistosoma japonicum	69 million	3
			Schistosoma intercalatum	Thousands	4
			Schistosoma mattheei	Thousands	5
			Schistosoma mekongi	Thousands	6
	Gymnophalloidea	Gymnophallidae	*Gymnophalloides seoi*	>40 000	7
	Echinostomomida	Paramphistomatoidea	*Gastrodiscoides hominis*	Rare[†]	8
			Watsonius watsoni	Rare	9
		Echinostomatoidea	*Fasciola hepatica* ⎫	2.4 million	10
			Fasciola gigantica ⎭		11
			Fasciolopsis buski	0.2 million	12
			Echinostoma hortense ⎫	Thousands	13
			Echinostoma ilocanum[‡] ⎭		
Epitheliocystida	Plagiorchiida	Dichrocoelidea	*Dicrocoelium dendriticum*	Rare	14
		Plagiorchioidea	*Nanophyetus salmincola*	Rare	15
			Paragonimus westermani	21 million[§]	16
			Paragonimus africanus	Rare	17
			Paragonimus uterobilateralis	Thousands	18
			Paragonimus mexicanus ⎫	> 2 million	19
			Paragonimus ecuadoriensis ⎭		
	Opisthorchiida	Opisthorchioidea	*Opisthorchis felineus*	> 1 million	20
			Opisthorchis viverrini	10 million	21
			Clonorchis sinensis[¶]	35 million	22
			Heterophyes heterophyes	Thousands	23
			Metagonimus yokogawai	0.5 million	24

Note: The numbers in the right-hand column refer to **Table 13**, in which are indicated the molluscs that serve as intermediate hosts for these trematodes. Some species referred to as rare may occur in high prevalence in certain foci where local food habits make the intake of the infective stages more common. The list is by no means inclusive. At least 70 species of intestinal trematode have been recorded in humans.

* The estimated prevalences of helminthic infections vary greatly. These figures and the figures in **Table 11** are based on estimates by the World Health Organization (WHO 1993 The control of schistosomiasis. Technical Report Series No. 830. WHO, Geneva). Numerous other species rare in humans are listed in WHO 1995 Control of foodborne trematode infections. Technical Report Series No 849. WHO, Geneva. † Said to be common in Assam where a prevalence of over 40% was found in certain foci. ‡ Prevalence rates average 5% in northern Luzon (Philippines). § See other data in **Table 14**. The estimate of 21 million includes all *Paragonimus* species of humans. ¶ Now referred to by some authors as *Opisthorchis sinensis*.

for example, *Fasciolopsis buski* has been found to infect nearly 100% of the population and *Opisthorchis viverrini* 90%, even though they are zoonoses. An indication of the numbers of human infections with these trematodes is given in Table 12. With its wide geographical distribution, *O. sinensis* is estimated to infect 35 million people, 15 million of them in China.

The diagnosis of snail-mediated helminthiases rests mainly on the demonstration of the parasites (e.g. as eggs in urine or faeces), or on medical imaging techniques of adults within various tissues. Serological procedures and skin testing are of value in some types of infection.

SCHISTOSOMIASIS

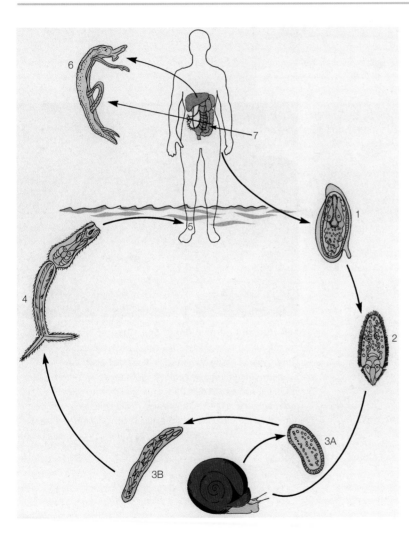

477 Life cycle of *Schistosoma mansoni*

The schistosomes provide a classic example of the life cycle of trematodes. The three common parasites of humans, *Schistosoma haematobium*, *Schistosoma japonicum* and *S. mansoni*, have a similar life cycle. Eggs (1) that are passed in urine (*S. haematobium*) or faeces (*S. japonicum* and *S. mansoni*) hatch in aggregations of water such as ponds, lake edges, streams and canals. From the eggs, miracidia (2) hatch into the water, where they penetrate into suitable snails. In the snails, they develop two generations of sporocysts (3A, 3B), the second of which produces fork-tailed cercariae (4). These cercariae penetrate the skin (5) when a new host comes into contact with contaminated water. Once through the skin, the cercariae shed their tails and become schistosomulae, which migrate through the tissues until they reach the portal venous system of the liver. Here, males and females (6) copulate before settling down in pairs in the venous system of the liver. From there *S. haematobium* usually migrates to the venous plexus of the bladder and other species (including the geographically localised *S. intercalatum* and *S. mekongi*) to the rectum (7), where eggs are laid. The eggs penetrate the bladder or rectum, from which they reach the exterior. Eggs laid by worms in the liver itself lead to local fibrotic changes and cirrhosis. (See also **404–406, 480–482, 484–492, 496, 506** and **535–538**.)

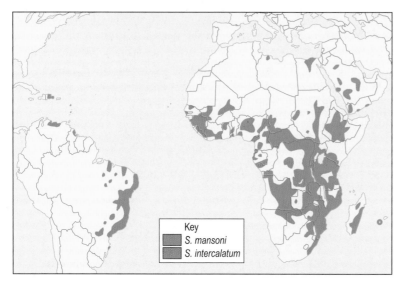

478 Distribution of *Schistosoma mansoni* and *Schistosoma intercalatum*

The distribution of schistosomiasis is regulated by both the presence of susceptible snail intermediate hosts and human sanitary habits. *S. mansoni* occurs in Africa, the Middle East, some Caribbean islands and in parts of South America. It was introduced from the Old World into the New World, where potentially susceptible species of *Biomphalaria* were already present. (Adapted from WHO Map No. 92720.)

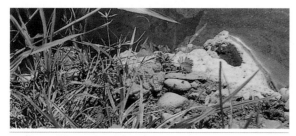

479 Ecology of intestinal schistosomiasis

Human faeces deposited at the edge of a pond in which snail hosts of *S. mansoni* were breeding. Eggs enter the water to hatch and perpetuate the cycle of transmission.

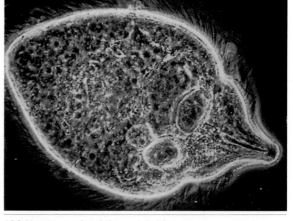

480 Hatched miracidium of *Schistosoma mansoni*

The three common species of schistosomes infecting humans have easily recognisable eggs, although those of *S. haematobium* may be confused with those of *S. intercalatum* (**535**). Miracidia can often be seen inside mature eggs. As many eggs deposited in the tissues in old infections may be nonviable, the detection of miracidia ('miracidia hatching test') in urine or stool specimens diluted in water can give a valuable indication of the activity of an infection. (× *600*)

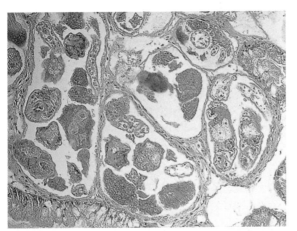

481 Section of 'mother' sporocyst in the hepatopancreas of a snail

The cycle in the snail is of variable duration, depending upon the species of parasite and host, and on the environmental conditions, but it is usually only 1 month. Cercaria develop in the second generation ('daughter') sporocysts. The figure shows several coils of the sporocyst in the hepatopancreas and sections of cercaria. (*Acetic carbol fuchsin × 130*)

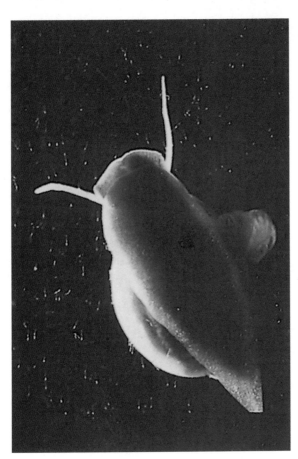

482 A snail 'shedding' living bifurcate cercaria of *Schistosoma mansoni*

Once snails start to 'shed' cercariae, they continue to do so during daylight hours for up to as many as 200 days. A heavily infected snail may shed 1500–2000 cercariae a day. (× 4.4)

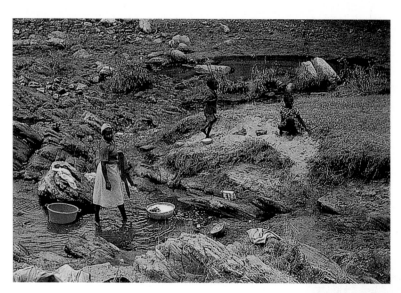

483 Site of human infection with *Schistosoma mansoni*

These women and their children became infected by cercariae while washing clothes in contaminated water. The provision of a piped water supply to the village drastically reduced the amount of transmission.

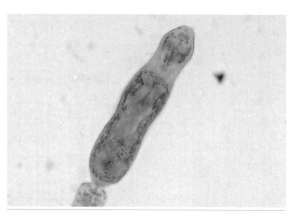

484 Head of cercaria

The apical and ventral suckers of the future schistosomule are clearly seen in this preparation. (*Mayer's haemalum × 310*)

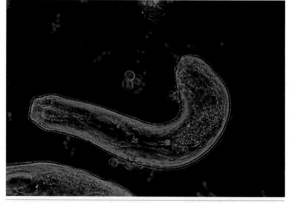

485 Schistosomule of *Schistosoma mansoni*

(*Phase-contrast × 350*)

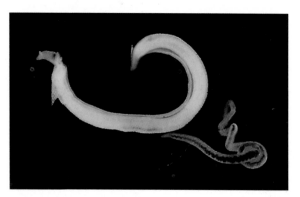

486 Living male and female *Schistosoma mansoni*

The slender female (right) is normally seen within the gynaecophoral groove of the male (left). (× *14*)

487–492 Morphology of adult schistosomes

Mature males and females live in copulating pairs. The common species are recognised by the characters shown in the figures. Testes of males: *S. haematobium* (**487**); *S. mansoni* (**488**); *S. japonicum* (**489**). Ovaries of females: *S. haematobium* (**490**); *S. mansoni* (**491**); *S. japonicum* (**492**). (× 25)

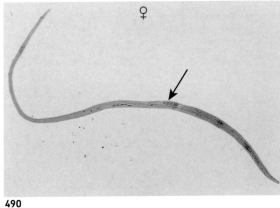

490

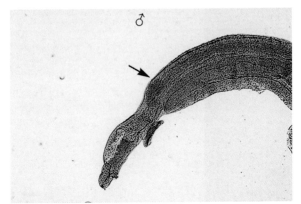

487

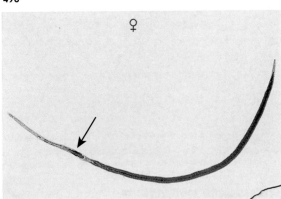

491

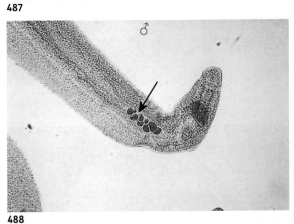

488

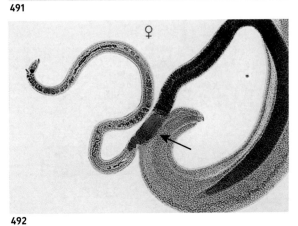

492

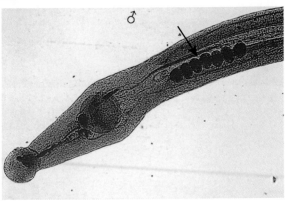

489

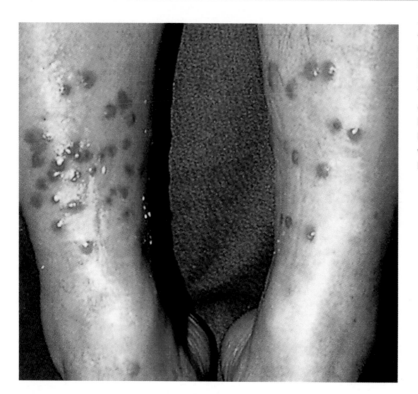

493 Dermatitis from avian cercariae in a Japanese patient
Penetration of the skin by cercariae may give rise to an itchy rash known as 'cercarial dermatitis'. This is occasionally seen in countries free of human schistosomiasis due to invasion by the cercariae of avian schistosomes which are otherwise nonpathogenic to humans.

Schistosoma mansoni

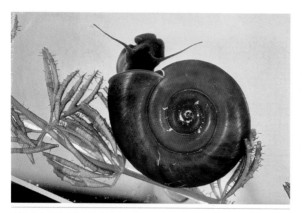

494 Intermediate host of *Schistosoma mansoni*
The snail intermediate hosts of *S. mansoni* are various species of *Biomphalaria*. (× 4) (See also **Table 13**.)

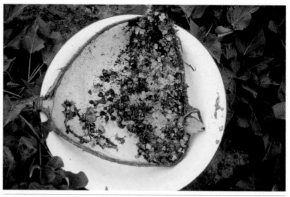

495 Sampling snail populations
A scoopful of *Biomphalaria sudanica*, a host for *S. mansoni* in Lake Victoria.

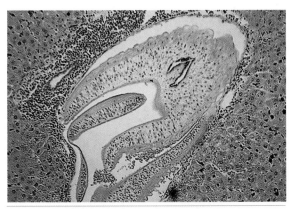

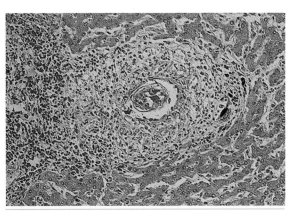

496 Adult *Schistosoma mansoni* in portal tract
Male and female schistosomes lodge *in copula* in the portal tract, mesenteric or vesical plexuses. The figure shows a cross-section of a male and female *S. mansoni* in a branch of the portal vein. (*H&E* × 44)

497 Granuloma surrounding egg of *Schistosoma mansoni* in liver
Eggs (**405**) may lodge ectopically in any tissues, where they cause characteristic granulomas. It has been suggested that toxic substances associated with the ova trigger the fibrotic process. In histological sections, the ova are seen in the portal and periportal regions. All types of reaction may be present from acute eosinophilic cellular infiltration (as seen here) to the dense collagenous deposition that leads to periportal fibrosis. (See also **509**.) (*H&E* × 90)

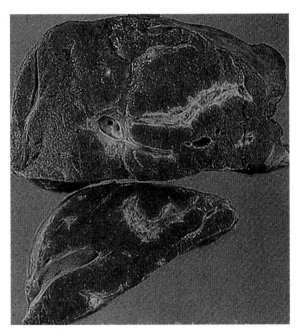

498 Periportal fibrosis of the liver
Periportal fibrosis ('pipestem fibrosis') is the classic pathological hepatic lesion. The white areas, which may be round, oval, or stellate, are due to the terminal fibrotic reaction originally caused by the presence of the ova in and around the portal venous radicles. (See also **531**.)

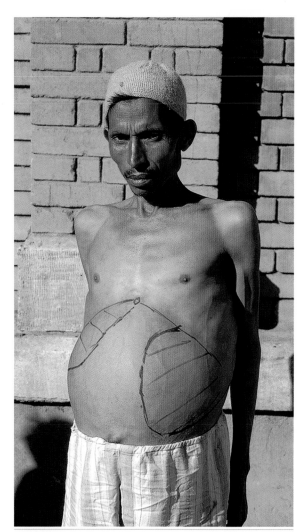

499 Egyptian splenomegaly
The combination of enlarged, irregularly fibrosed liver and greatly enlarged spleen is commonly called 'Egyptian hepatosplenomegaly'.

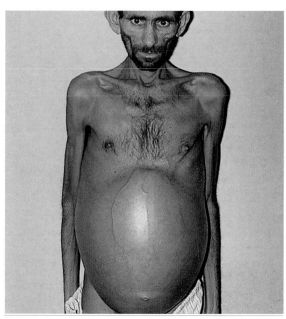

500 Ascites secondary to chronic portal hypertension in a Brazilian
The classic, clinical feature of chronic *S. mansoni* infection is portal hypertension. The opening up of a secondary, circulatory shunt leads to the development of varices in the oesophageal and gastric veins, ascites and gross splenomegaly.

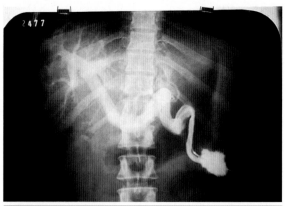

501 Angiogram showing portal hypertension caused by *Schistosoma mansoni*
This X-ray was taken before surgery in this Brazilian man.

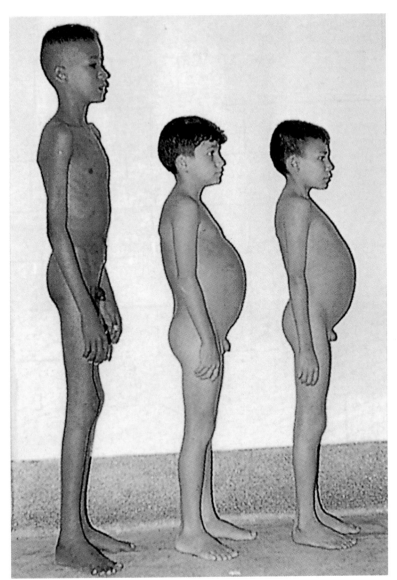

502 Growth retardation by chronic infection with *Schistosoma mansoni*
A combination of undernutrition and chronic infection with *S. mansoni*, especially around the time of puberty, can lead to significant retardation of growth. The boys seen here in the northeast of Brazil are (left to right) 14, 13 and 12 years old. The two on the right with hepatomegaly have schistosomiasis. Similar changes are seen in children infected with *S. japonicum*.

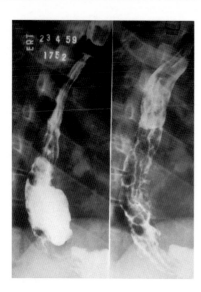

503 Radiograph of oesophageal varices

Oesophageal varices such as those shown in this Gastrografin swallow can rupture, leading to a fatal haematemesis.

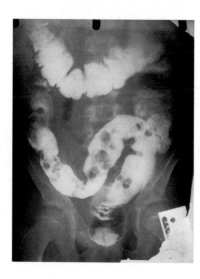

504 Barium enema of colonic polyposis

Diarrhoea is a common complaint in the early stages of *S. mansoni* infection. Extensive polyposis of the colon sometimes occurs. These lesions are reversible with antischistosomal drug therapy.

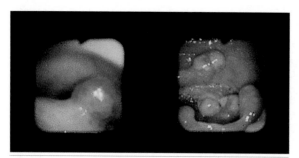

505 Sigmoidoscopic view of colonic polyps
Two views of polyps in the descending colon.

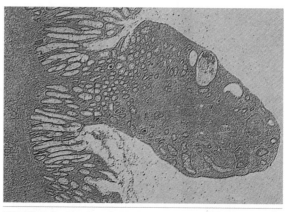

506 Biopsy showing *Schistosoma mansoni* eggs in a colonic polyp
Diagnosis is usually confirmed by demonstrating eggs of *S. mansoni* in the stool. The Kato–Katz technique is one of the simplest quantitative procedures to evaluate egg loads in faeces. However, intestinal biopsy through a proctoscope or sigmoidoscope is also an effective means of finding eggs and establishing a definitive diagnosis of *S. mansoni* infection. It may also be positive in patients with *S. haematobium* or *S. japonicum*. (See also note on the 'miracidia hatching test', **480**.) (*H&E × 25*)

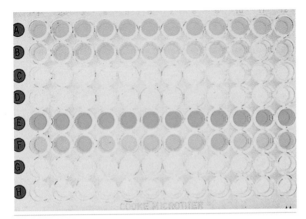

507 Enzyme-linked immunosorbent assay

This, one of the most sensitive tests currently available for the detection of antischistosomal IgG, IgM or IgE, is probably of most value for the screening of expatriates for recently acquired infection with any of the species of *Schistosoma*, and to distinguish acute from chronic infections. In this example of an IgG enzyme-linked immunosorbent assay (ELISA), alkaline phosphatase-*p*-nitrophenyl phosphate was used as indicator in rows A–D, and horseradish peroxidase in rows E–H, with different sera in each of the wells. A and E show a strong positive reaction, E and H a weak positive reaction, and C and G a negative reaction; D and H are the buffer controls. Circulating antigen detection with monoclonal antibodies is now shown to be more specific and sensitive both for diagnosis and for the confirmation of cure following intervention. Skin tests, which are relatively unreliable, have now been abandoned. However, a very sensitive and specific test, 'colloidal dye immunofiltration assay' (CDIFA), has been shown recently to offer a cheap and reliable method for screening for infection with *S. japonicum* in the field and reports of its potential value in other schistosome infections are awaited with interest.

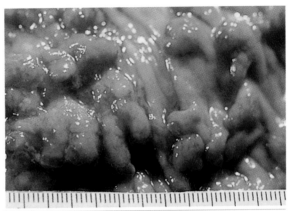

508 Polyposis of colon at post-mortem

Massive polyposis of the colon with fatal intestinal haemorrhage seen at post-mortem in an Egyptian farmer.

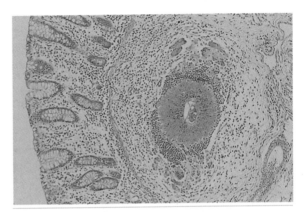

509 Hoeppli reaction

The fibrotic granuloma around this dead ovum in the colon is known as a Hoeppli reaction. (*H&E* × 70)

510 Ectopic infection – *Schistosoma mansoni* infection of lung

Typical eggs may appear in the sputum when the lungs are affected. Such ectopic lesions usually contain large numbers of ova in necrotic material surrounded by eosinophils, and multinucleated giant cells. They may also involve the central nervous system. (*H&E* × 100)

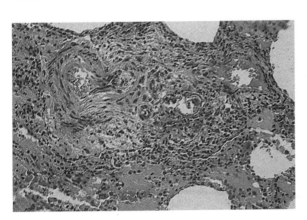

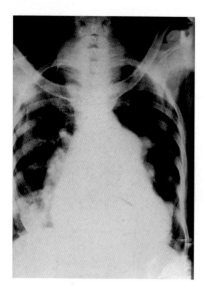

511 Radiograph of 'cor pulmonale' due to schistosomiasis
Eggs that reach the lungs by metastatic-blood spread lead to periarteritis. This is followed by fibrosis of the pulmonary arterioles with pulmonary hypertension and, finally, enlargement of the right heart (i.e. cor pulmonale).

Schistosoma haematobium

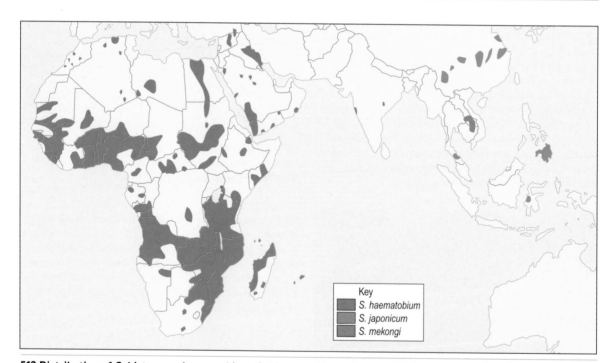

512 Distribution of *Schistosoma haematobium*, *Schistosoma japonicum* and *Schistosoma mekongi*
S. haematobium is found in Africa and the Middle East; *S. japonicum* is endemic in the Far East, south-east Asia and the Philippines; *S. mekongi* is limited to parts of Laos, Kampuchea and south Thailand, bordering the lower Mekong river basin. (Adapted from WHO Map No. 92721.)

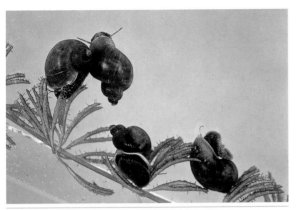

513 Intermediate hosts of *Schistosoma haematobium*
The intermediate hosts of *S. haematobium* are species of *Bulinus*. (× 3.5) (See also **Table 13**.)

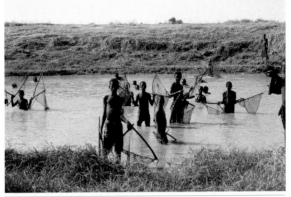

514 Ecology of *Schistosoma haematobium* infection
Increased land use through the development of irrigation projects (as in Egypt, the Sudan and Kenya), may result in an increasing incidence of *S. haematobium* transmission through *Bulinus* snails breeding in the irrigation canals, which are favourite swimming places for children. In this lake near their village in Niger children were infected while fishing. (Photo by Dr Albis Gabrielli; Schistosomiasis Control Initiative, courtesy of Professor Alan Fenwick.)

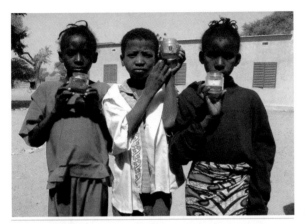

515 Children in a village in Niger with urine samples
Haematuria is often best seen at the end of urination and is a characteristic early clinical feature of infection with *S. haematobium*. (Photo by Dr Jurg Utzinger, Swiss Tropical Institute, courtesy of Professor Alan Fenwick.)

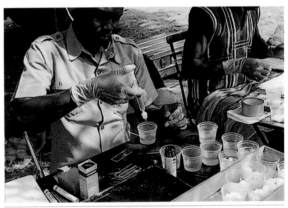

517 Village survey for urinary schistosomiasis
A simple and effective technique to detect eggs in urine is to pass samples through a nylon-mesh filter attached to a 10 ml syringe. The filter is removed and examined under the microscope using a × 10 objective, and the eggs collected on it are counted. A simple dipstick test for protein and blood is a useful supplementary method of assessing the prevalence of those passing eggs, and may even replace microscopy. This procedure, which saves labour, time and money, facilitates the delivery of treatment programmes in communities for which such intervention might otherwise be delayed (or not provided at all) and is valuable for assessing the effectiveness of such programmes.

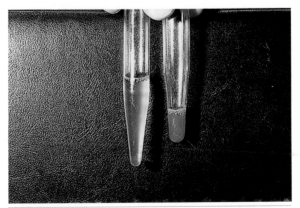

516 Haematuria in centrifuge specimen of urine
Typical, terminal spined eggs of *S. haematobium* (see **404**) may be found in the centrifuge deposit. (See also note on 'miracidial urination, haematuria hatching test', **480**.)

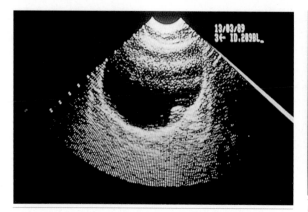

518 Ultrasonic probe of bladder in early infection
A large polyp can be seen in this ultrasonic probe of a bladder early in infection with *S. haematobium*. Unlike radiography, ultrasonography with portable equipment can readily be used in a simple peripheral medical centre or even under field conditions by specially trained personnel. It is an invaluable procedure for assessing morbidity in individuals or in community surveys (e.g. to evaluate the progress of control campaigns).

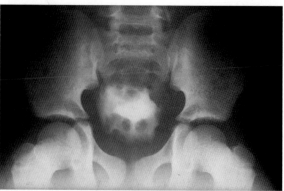

519 Bladder radiograph in early infection with *Schistosoma haematobium*
Active proliferating papillomatous or granulomatous lesions are responsible for the bladder-filling defects seen radiologically in the early stages of infection.

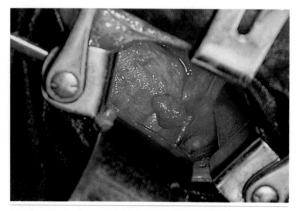

520 Nodules due to *Schistosoma haematobium*
The appearance of a nodular lesion in the vesical wall as seen at open operation is clearly shown here.

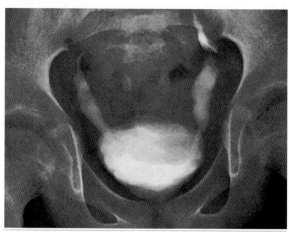

521 Intravenous urogram of dilated ureters
Gross tortuosity and dilatation of the ureters result from stenosis of the ureteric orifices, possibly due to calcification.

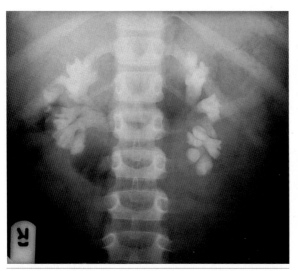

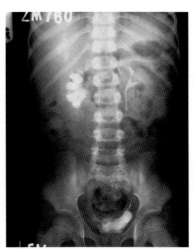

523 Persistent hydronephrosis in child
Hydronephrosis due to *S. haematobium* infection in children is often reversible with adequate antischistosomal drug treatment. In this 6-year-old child the lesion persisted despite therapy.

522 Renal radiograph showing bilateral hydronephrosis
Unilateral and bilateral hydronephrosis are not uncommon in haematobium infection.

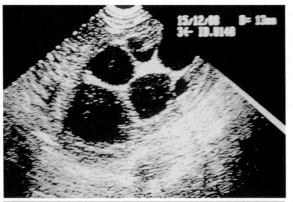

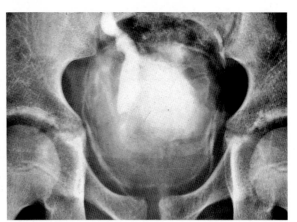

525 Radiograph of bladder with calcification
Widespread fibrosis and eventually calcification of the bladder wall result in this 'fetal head' appearance.

524 Ultrasound showing severe hydronephrosis
The noninvasive technique of ultrasonography has largely replaced urography in the investigation of severe urinary tract lesions due to *S. haematobium* in a hospital environment.

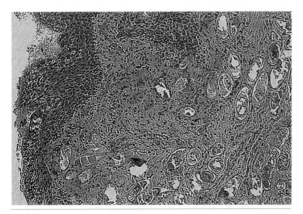

526 Eggs in section of bladder
Schistosome ova laid by female worms in the vesical plexus
are retained in the vesical tissues and later become calcified.
(*H&E × 50*)

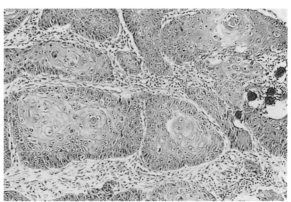

527 Squamous-cell carcinoma of the bladder
In areas where *S. haematobium* infection is intense, the
incidence of bladder cancer is high. Squamous-cell carcinoma
is the type most commonly found, and ova of *S. haematobium*
are often present in such tumours. Adenocarcinoma also
occurs. (*H&E × 90*)

Schistosoma japonicum and *Schistosoma mekongi*

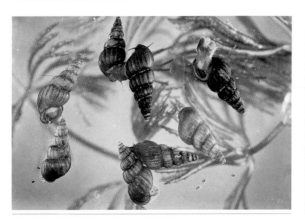

**528 *Oncomelania*: intermediate host of *Schistosoma
japonicum***
Various species of the amphibious genus *Oncomelania* serve
as intermediate hosts for *S. japonicum*. In the lower Mekong
river basin, a river-dwelling snail, *Tricula aperta*, is the
intermediate host for *S. mekongi* – a trematode closely related
to *S. japonicum*. (× 3) (See also **Table 13**.)

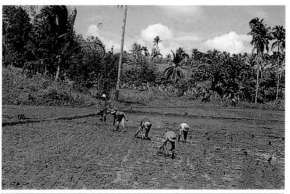

**529 Ecology of *Schistosoma japonicum* and
*Schistosoma mekongi***
These infections are zoonoses. *S. japonicum* is found in a wide
variety of vertebrate hosts, including domestic animals and
bovines. Human infection frequently occurs in farm workers
(e.g. when planting rice in contaminated paddy fields as seen
here) (see also **427**). In contrast, *S. mekongi* is associated more
with rivers; it is likely to increase as irrigation works in the
lower Mekong River basin are extended. In some Kampuchean
'floating villages', up to 47% of sampled villagers have been
found infected with this parasite.

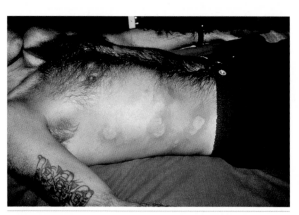

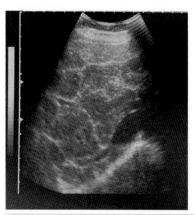

530 'Katayama fever'

The acute phase of moderate or heavy infection with schistosomes may present as a febrile reaction with hypereosinophilia that can last for a number of days or weeks. 'Katayama fever', which is the commonest in infection with *S. japonicum*, less common with *S. mansoni* and rarely seen with *S. haematobium*, appears with the onset of oviposition. It results from the formation and circulation of antigen–antibody immune complexes, which provoke a type of serum sickness, and may be complicated by glomerulonephritis. Massive giant urticaria occurred in this man soon after infection with *S. mansoni*.

531 Liver cirrhosis in a patient with *Schistosoma japonicum*

Severe hepatic fibrosis and massive splenomegaly occur in *S. japonicum* infection (in the same manner as in *S. mansoni* – see **499** and **500**), often with ascites. In this ultrasound scan, the presence of fibrosis around the portal tracts is seen as light-coloured lines in the liver, the so-called 'turtle shell' appearance. *S. mekongi* may also produce severe changes similar to these.

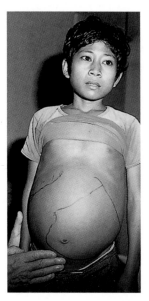

532 Philippino boy with gross splenomegaly

Advanced lesions due to *S. japonicum* may also be seen in children and adolescents.

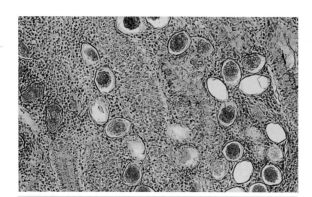

533 Eggs of *Schistosoma japonicum* in wall of colon

The adult worms do not invade the vesical plexus, but usually inhabit the mesenteric plexus. The diagnosis of *S. japonicum* can usually be made by finding typical eggs in the faeces. However, it is commoner for eggs of *S. japonicum* to be deposited in ectopic sites than those of other schistosome species. (*H&E × 150*)

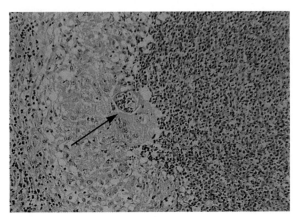

534 Ova of *Schistosoma japonicum* in spinal cord
Schistosomal lesions in the spinal cord or brain may contain large numbers of ova in necrotic material, often surrounded by eosinophils. Patients with cerebral schistosomiasis usually present with epileptiform attacks. This post-mortem specimen from a 24-year-old Japanese male shows marked cellular reaction, including a multinucleated giant cell round a dead ovum in the spinal cord. (*H&E × 200*)

Schistosomes found uncommonly in humans

535–538 Eggs of unusual schistosomes seen in humans
The eggs of *S. intercalatum* (**535**) are similar to those of *S. haematobium*, but are found only in the faeces. *S. mattheei* (**536**), which occurs in sheep and cattle, has been found in humans on rare occasions (× 290). *S. mekongi* (**537**) is easily mistaken for *S. japonicum*, which is shown here for comparison (**538**). (× 140) (*S. intercalatum* is decreasing in prevalence; the incidence of human infection with *S. mekongi* has been considerably reduced by mass chemotherapy but its main intermediate snail host, *Neotricula aperta* is difficult to control.)

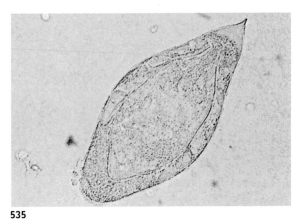

535

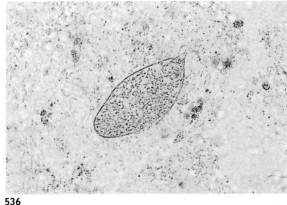

536

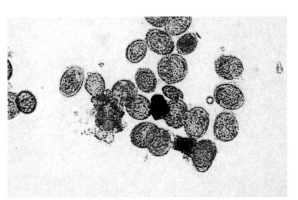

537

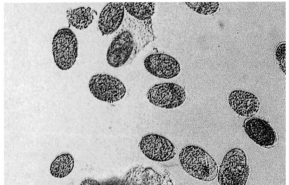

538

THE INTESTINAL FLUKES

See Tables 12 and 13.

Zoonotic intestinal infections have been recorded in humans with at least 70 species of trematode, most of which are acquired by eating raw or inadequately cooked fish that contains encysted metacercariae. In other species, the metacercariae are eaten with raw amphibians, aquatic arthropods, molluscs or plants.

Most infections are symptomless, and are revealed only during surveys or when the hosts are given drugs to expel the more important trematodes such as *Fasciolopsis buski*. Although many species

Table 13 Snails and other molluscs of medical importance (class Gastropoda)

Subclass	Order (Suborder)	Family	Genus and species	Helminths
Streptoneura	Prosobranchiata (fresh water)	Bithyniidae	*Bithynia* spp.	**19, 20, 21**, 22
			Parafossularis spp.	23
		Pamatiopsidae	*Oncomelania* spp.	**3**
			Tricula aperta	6
		Thiaridae	*Thiara granifera*	**16**, 24
		Pleuroceridae	*Semisulcospira libertina*	**16**, 24
		Pilidae	*Pila conica*	13
	(brackish and sea water)	Potamidiae	*Cerithidia cingulata*	23
			Pirenella conica	24
Euthyneura	Pulmonata (Basomatophora) (fresh water)	Planorbidae	*Biomphalaria* spp.	**1**
			Bulinus (Bulinus) spp.	**2**
			Bulinus (Physopsis) spp.	**2, 4, 5**
			Segmentina hemisphaerula	13
			Segmentina trochoideus	**12**
			Hippeutis cantori	**12**
			Hippeutis umbilicalis	14
			Gyraulus convexiusculus	13
			Gyraulus prashadi	13
			? *Indoplanorbis exustus*	8
		Ancylidae	*Ferrissia tenuis*	**2**
		Lymnaeidae	*Fossaria* spp.	**10**, 11
			Lymnaea spp.	**10**, 11
			Stagnicola bulimoides	**10**
			Pseudosuccinia columella	**10**, 11
	(Stylommatophora) (land snails)	Helicidae	*Helicella candidula*	14
		Enidae	*Zebrina detrita*	14
		Cionellidae	*Cionella lubrica*	14
			Achatina fulica ⎫	*
			Bradybaena similaris ⎬	
			Subulina octona ⎭	
	(Systellommatophora)	Veronicellidae	*Veronica leydigi*	
Pteriomorphia	Bivalvia	Ostreidae	*Crassostrea gigas*	7

The relation of the genera to the helminths that infect them is indicated by reference to the numbers in **Table 12**. The most important helminths are indicated in bold type.

* *Parastrongylus contonensis. Achatina fulica* may be kept in non-endemic areas as a 'pet'; care is needed to ensure that infected snails are not imported. The land planarian *Geoplana septemlineata* has also been found infected with this nematode. *Parastrongylus costaricensis* is acquired from the slug *Vaginulus plebeius*.

are minute, and hence frequently overlooked, their prevalence in endemic foci may be high. For example, *Echinostoma hortense* acquired from raw loach occurs in up to 22% of people in some villages of southern Korea, while *Echinochasmus lilliputanus* was found in a similar proportion of some villagers in parts of China. *Nanophyetus salmincola*, acquired by eating raw salmon or trout, is endemic in Khabarovsk territory (Russia), where up to 60% of local ethnic minorities may be infected in some villages.

The eggs of the minute intestinal trematodes are virtually indistinguishable by normal microscopy of stool specimens. **Table 13** includes only those species to which reference is most commonly made, and is by no means all-inclusive.

539–546 Snail intermediate hosts of trematode infections of humans

A number of the molluscs listed in **Table 13** are shown here: *Oncomelania nosophora* (× 7.7) (**539**); *Thiara granifera* (× 2.0) (**540**); *Biomphalaria glabrata* (× 4.1) (**541**); *Biomphalaria sudanica* (× 1.7) (**542**); *Bulinus (Bulinus) senegalensis* (× 4.8) (**543**); *Bulinus (Physopsis) globosus* (× 2.5) (**544**); *Segmentina* sp. (× 5) (**545**); *Lymnaea truncatula* (× 5) (**546**).

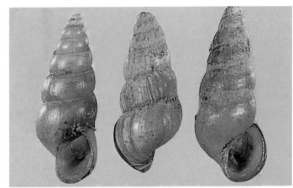

539

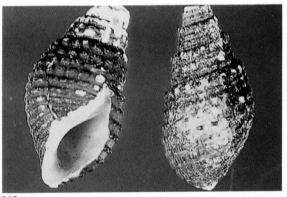

540

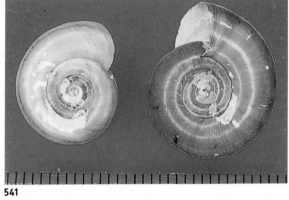

541

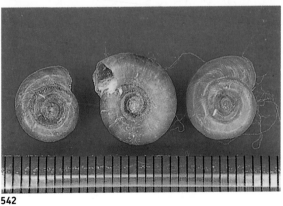

542

543

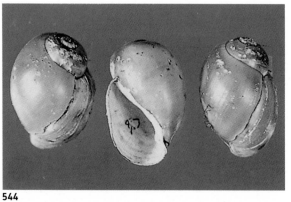

544

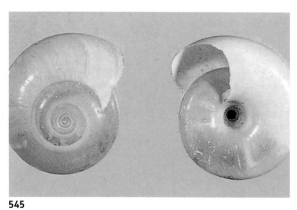

545

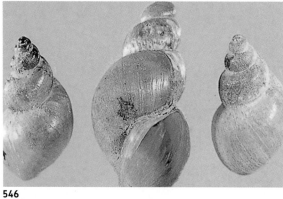

546

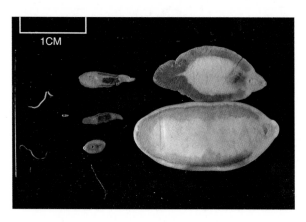

547 Comparative sizes of flukes
From left to right: first column – *S. mansoni* (♂) and (♀); second column – *H. heterophyes*; third column – *O. felineus*, *O. sinensis*, *P. westermani*; fourth column – *F. hepatica* and *F. buski*.

Fasciolopsiasis

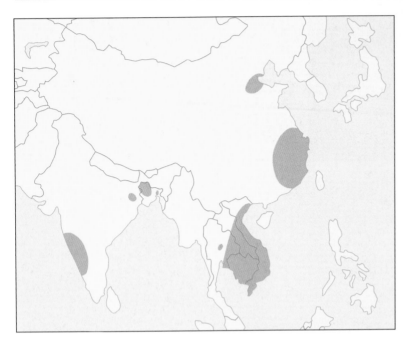

548 Distribution of *Fasciolopsis buski*

F. buski is limited to areas of the Far East and Kalimantan (Indonesia). In certain foci (e.g. in north-east Thailand), almost the entire population of some villages may be infected.

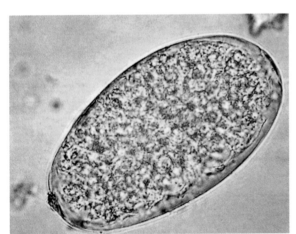

549 Egg of *Fasciolopsis buski*
Miracidia, hatching from eggs passed in the faeces after shedding their ciliated coats, invade snails of various genera, including *Segmentina* and *Hippeutis*. The reproductive cycle in the snail differs from that of the schistosomes. After development through the sporocysts and two generations of rediae (see **560**), cercaria emerge into the water. They then encyst on aquatic plants such as the water caltrop (**552**) and water chestnut (**571**). (× 240)

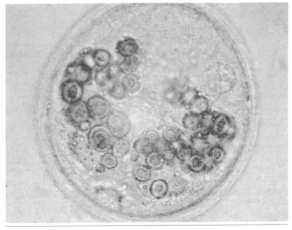

550 Metacercaria of *Fasciolopsis buski*
The metacercaria of *F. buski* with its cyst wall. (× 220)

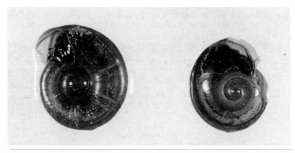

551 Segmentina hemisphaerula
This snail and a number of species of *Hippeutis* are the first intermediate hosts of *F. buski*. (× 2.7)

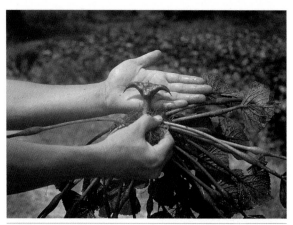

552 The water caltrop
'Plantations' of water caltrop are harvested in endemic areas. The characteristic fruits of this plant are commonly eaten raw, and the metacercariae are thus swallowed. Water chestnuts (**571**) also often serve as a source of infection to children who peel the raw plants with their teeth, thus ingesting the attached metacercariae.

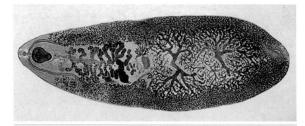

553 Adult *Fasciolopsis buski*
The adult *F. buski* is the largest parasitic trematode of humans and may reach 7.5 cm in length. Larvae mature in about three months when the adults attach to the mucosa of the duodenum and jejunum. They can produce local trauma or, in heavy infections, obstruction, together with toxic effects that may be due to absorption of their metabolic products and subsequent sensitisation of the host. The pig is the main animal reservoir of infection for humans. (*Natural size*)

Uncommon species

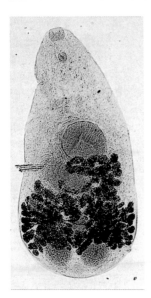

554 Adult *Heterophyes heterophyes*
This is a widely distributed (from Egypt to the Philippines), tiny trematode, one of the large family Heterophyidae, with a typical life cycle in brackish water snails (e.g. *Pirenella*) (see **Table 13**). Up to 1% of villagers in some foci in the northern Nile delta are infected, and rates as high as 24% have been recorded in foci in Khuzestan; elsewhere, it is usually rare. The cercariae encyst on fish such as the mullet, and infect humans when improperly cooked fish is eaten. The adult trematode shown here lives in the middle part of the small intestine. The eggs (see **418**) are very similar to those of *Clonorchis* and *Metagonimus*. (× 45)

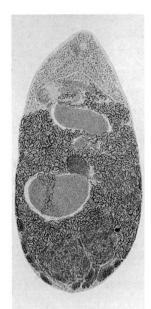

555 Adult *Metagonimus yokagawai*

This is the most common heterophyid fluke of the Far East but it is also found in the Mediterranean basin. The life cycle is similar to that of *Heterophyes*, and the eggs of the two genera can be differentiated only with difficulty. The adult worm shown here is also very small (1.4 × 0.6 mm) and lives in the upper and middle jejunum. Several genera of snails, including *Semisulcospira* (see **Table 13**), are the first intermediate hosts for the species. The prevalence rate in the Korean Republic averages 4.8%, with rates over 20% in several foci there and in the eastern provinces of the former Soviet Union. The cercariae encyst on various species of freshwater fish. (× 45)

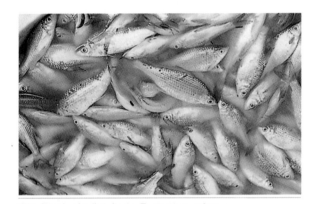

556 Cyprinoid fish in an Eastern market

The mullet and other fish living in fresh or brackish waters are common intermediate hosts for *H. heterophyes* and *M. yokagawai*. The metacercariae are attached under the scales or in the skin.

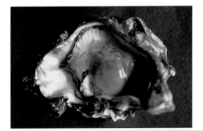

557 Pacific oyster, *Crassostrea gigas*

This widely distributed, large, edible oyster is the main intermediate host for the metacercariae of the minute, heterophyid trematode, *Gymnophalloides seoi*, which was discovered in 1993. Wading birds such as the Palaearctic oyster catcher, *Haematopus ostralegus*, are natural definitive hosts for this parasite which infects humans when he consumes uncooked oysters that bear metacercariae. (From Chai et al. Trends in Parasitology (2003) 19: 109–112. Fig. 2b.)

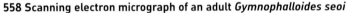

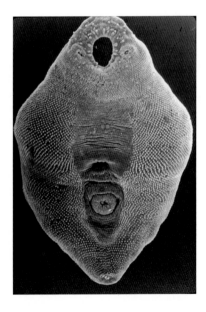

558 Scanning electron micrograph of an adult *Gymnophalloides seoi*

The adult trematode is only about 0.4–0.5 mm long and 0.2–0.3 mm wide. It is believed to live in the small intestine of humans, possibly infects the pancreatic duct and can infest a wide range of small mammals in the laboratory. The typical heterophyid eggs which are minute, about 20 µm long, are passed in the faeces. In some coastal villages of Korea this infection is highly endemic, up to half the villagers in some being infected. (× 150) (From Chai et al. Trends in Parasitology (2003) 19: 109–112. Fig. 1b.)

LIVER AND LUNG FLUKE INFECTIONS

Over 100 species of snails have been implicated as hosts of the four commonest liver flukes (see **Table 12**), while 150 species of freshwater fish, 60 species of crustacea and 20 species of plants are involved in the cycles of these and other trematode species which infect 40 million people.

Opisthorchiasis (excluding that caused by *O. sinensis*, of which there are 35 million cases), formerly believed to be most prevalent in south-east Asia, is now admitted to be extremely common in parts of the former Soviet Union, affecting about 1.2 million, with almost 100% infection rates in some foci, especially of western Siberia. Altogether, at least 10 million people have opisthorchiasis. As many as 10% of those infected may develop cholangiocarcinoma. A high proportion (up to 20%) of south-east Asian immigrants to Europe or North America have been found infected with *Opisthorchis* (or *Clonorchis*). Acute opisthorchiasis has also been identified in immigrants to the USA from Siberia who consumed illegally imported carp from that country where *O. felineus* is common. Moreover, it is now estimated also that the lungs of about 21 million individuals are infected with various species of *Paragonimus*, which is frequently mistaken (and thus wrongly treated) for pulmonary tuberculosis. In part of north-eastern India, for example, 60% of patients receiving such therapy were found to have pulmonary flukes, while in Ecuador, where at least 2 million are infected, 13% in one clinic had paragonimiasis, not tuberculosis.

Opisthorchis sinensis

(Previously called *Clonorchis sinensis*. The infection is still commonly referred to as clonorchiasis.)

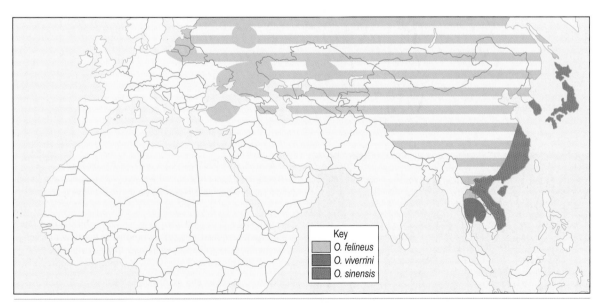

Key
O. felineus
O. viverrini
O. sinensis

559 Distribution map of *Opisthorchis* species of humans
Parasitic food-borne trematodes of this genus are very widely distributed in the Old World. *O. sinensis* is also known as the Chinese or oriental liver fluke; it is found in humans and also in other fish-eating mammals in the areas shown. *Opisthorchis felineus* is now known to have a much wider distribution, whereas that of *Opisthorchis viverrini* is localised in parts of Thailand and neighbouring countries. Of the estimated 35 million people infected with this species globally, 15 million live in China.

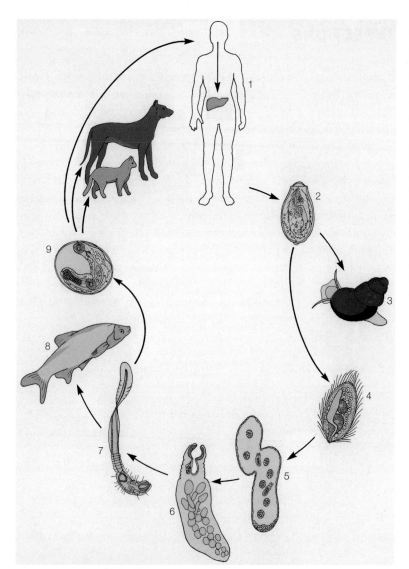

560 Life cycle of *Opisthorchis sinensis*

The adult flukes living in the biliary tree of the liver (1) produce operculated eggs (2) which are passed in the faeces. When ingested by the snail host (3), miracidia (4) hatch from the eggs to produce sporocysts (5) in which develop a single generation of daughter cells (rediae) (6). Within these develop lophocercous (i.e. single-tailed) cercariae (7), which leave the snails to enter various freshwater fish (8), in which they encyst to form metacercariae (9). When the fish is eaten by a carnivore, the young trematodes emerge and eventually pass up the common bile duct, finally reaching the smaller branches of the biliary tree, where they mature. (See also **418**.)

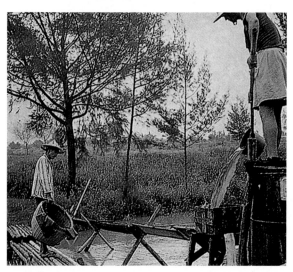

561 Ecology of *Opisthorchis sinensis* infection

Latrines used to be built over the edges of fishponds into which faecal material containing helminth eggs would drop. This provided an ideal way of infecting cultivated fish and perpetuating the cycle of transmission. While this practice has been greatly reduced, it is still common practice to pour fresh night soil into fishponds, as seen here. The control of this infection must include health education aimed at improved disposal of night soil and aquiculture practices.

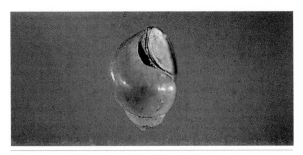

562 Intermediate host of *Opisthorchis*
Bithynia funiculata is one of the species of this genus in which *O. sinensis* will develop. Other molluscan genera (see **Table 13**) can serve as intermediate hosts. (× 3.2)

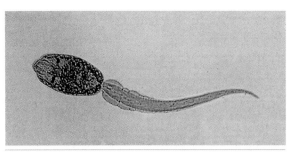

563 Cercaria of *Opisthorchis sinensis*
The lophocercous cercariae escape from the snail to encyst under the scales of various species of freshwater cyprinoid fish. (× 62)

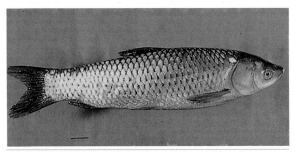

564 *Ctenopharyngodon idellus*
This fish is a common host for metacercariae of *O. sinensis*.

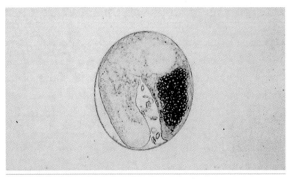

565 Metacercaria in fish
Humans are infested by eating raw or incompletely cooked fish, a common delicacy among many Chinese. Metacercariae are thus ingested and excyst in the duodenum. (× 160)

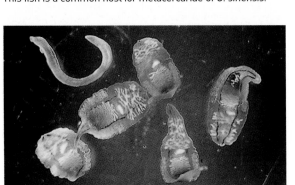

566 Living adult *Opisthorchis sinensis*
The young worms migrate up the common bile duct to the liver. At maturity they may reach 2 cm in length. (× 2.5)

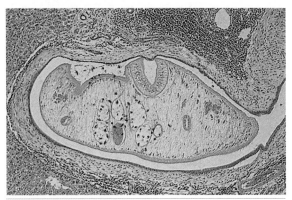

567 Section of *Opisthorchis sinensis* in bile duct
Direct mechanical damage and possibly toxic effects of the adult worms lead to fibrotic changes in the bile ducts. (× 25)

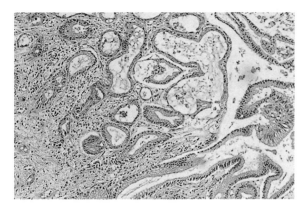

568 Cholangiocarcinoma of the liver

Severe chronic infection with *O. sinensis* may lead to marked pericholangitic fibrosis and finally multifocal cholangiocarcinoma of the liver. In this case, metastases were widely distributed throughout the body. (*H&E × 80*)

Opisthorchis felineus and Opisthorchis viverrini

The distribution is shown in **559**. *O. felineus* is common in domestic cats, dogs, and some other animals in eastern and south-eastern Europe, as well as many parts of the former Soviet Union. In the Far East, it is largely replaced by *O. viverrini*, which occurs mainly in north-east Thailand, where it infects up to 90% of the population in some villages. Cats, as well as humans, serve as reservoirs of infection. The life cycles are similar to that of *O. sinensis*, with snails of the genus *Bithynia* serving as intermediate hosts (see also **562**).

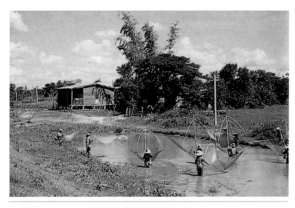

569 Ecology of Opisthorchis viverrini

Humans are infected by ingesting the metacercaria in cyprinoid fish. The figure shows a typical village fishpond in north-east Thailand. Both the snail and fish populations of the ponds increase during the rainy season.

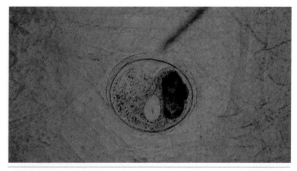

570 Metacercaria in fish

Most infection is from uncooked fish. In north-east Thailand, the fish sauce *koipla* is the most important source. (× 230)

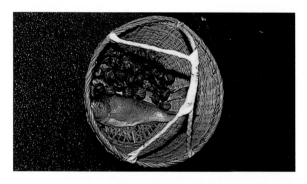

571 *Cyprinus carpio*: host for metacercariae of *Opisthorchis felineus*

These freshwater fish are often infected in the Far East and are a common source of infection in north-east Thailand. This Shanghai shopper's basket also contains water chestnuts, on which metacercariae of *F. buski* may encyst (see **550**).

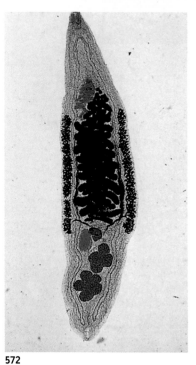

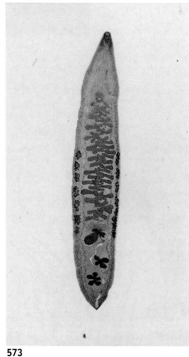

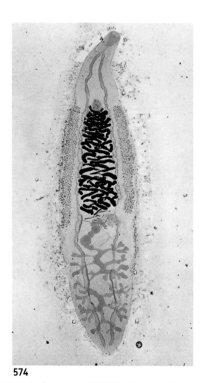

572   573   574

572–574 Adult flukes of *Opisthorchis felineus*, *Opisthorchis viverrini* and *Opisthorchis sinensis*

The adults of *O. felineus* (**572**, left) and *O. viverrini* (**573**, centre), which are similar to those of *O. sinensis* (**574**, right), live in the bile ducts and produce similar pathological changes. They can be distinguished by such structural details as the numbers, positions and shapes of the testes in the posterior parts of the worm (the lower thirds in these figures). (× 7.7)

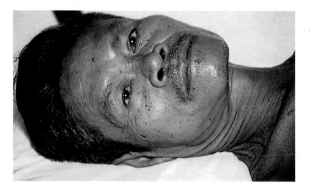

575 Jaundice in a patient with opisthorchiasis

This adult Thai was heavily infected with *O. viverrini*.

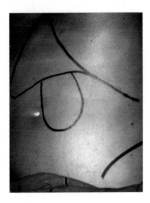

576 Gross enlargement of the gall bladder in opisthorchiasis
This figure shows the grossly enlarged gall bladder of the patient seen in **575**.

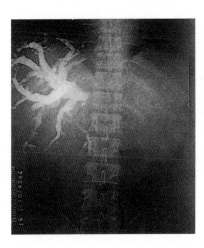

577 Cholangiogram of patient with opisthorchiasis
This X-ray shows dilatation of the main bile ducts and disorganisation of the biliary tree.

Dicrocoelium dendriticum

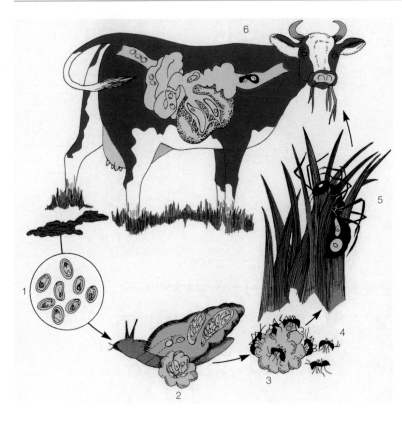

578 Life cycle of *Dicrocoelium dendriticum*
The only trematode of medical importance in which the life cycle involves insects is a cosmopolitan parasite normally found in the biliary tract of sheep. It has evolved a bizarre method to ensure its transmission. (1) Eggs passed by infected sheep are eaten by various species of land snail, in the intestine of which miracidia hatch. (2) The miracidia form several generations of sporocysts and finally tailed cercariae, which accumulate near the snails' surface. (3) This leads to their ejection by the molluscs in small balls of slime, each of which may contain several hundred cercariae. (4) The slime balls are eaten by ants, the second intermediate hosts, in the body cavities of which most of the parasites encyst as metacercariae. However, a few encyst in the suboesophageal ganglion. (5) Their presence causes the ants to behave in a remarkable fashion, climbing to the tips of vegetation where they remain overnight, ready to be ingested by grazing animals in the cooler hours. The next day when the temperature increases, they descend to the shelter of the cooler microclimate provided near the soil. (6) Once taken up by the herbivore (or, accidentally, by humans), the parasites excyst in the duodenum, from where they migrate to their definitive sites in the smaller bile ducts.

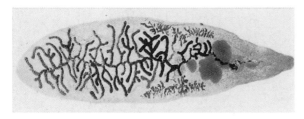

579 Adult *Dicrocoelium dendriticum*
Maturation of the flukes takes between 6 and 7 weeks and individual animals may harbour as many as 50 000 adult flukes. The adult, which grows up to 1.5 cm long, lives in the biliary tract, especially the small bile ducts. The eggs are similar to those of the *Opisthorchis* group (see **418).** Infection in humans, understandably, is rare. In west Africa, zoonotic infection with *Dicrocoelium hospes* has been reported, with species of *Dorylus* and *Crematogaster* serving as secondary hosts. (× 4.5)

Fasciola hepatica and *Fasciola gigantica*

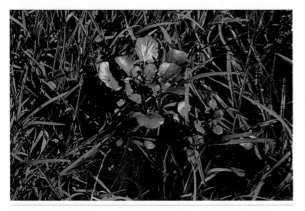

580 Watercress: a source of infection of fascioliasis
Infection with *F. hepatica* is cosmopolitan in herbivores that graze in wet pasturage where the intermediate hosts – snails of the genus *Lymnaea* – are found. About 2 million people are believed to be infected with *Fasciola* acquired from metacercaria-infected aquatic plants. In temperate climates, humans are most often infected by eating wild watercress on which metacercariae have encysted. It grows commonly in swampy pasture by small streams. *F. gigantica*, the common liver fluke of cattle in the Middle East, much of Africa and Asia, occasionally infects humans.

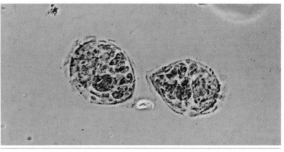

581 Miracidia of *Fasciola hepatica*
Motile miracidia hatch from eggs passed in faeces and infect snails of the genus *Lymnaea*. (× 225)

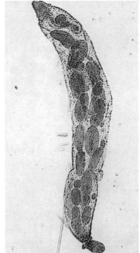

583 Redia from intermediate host
These develop in the hepatopancreas, with the formation of cercariae. (× 30)

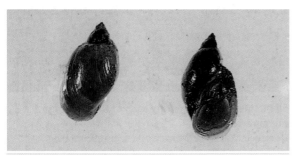

582 *Lymnaea swinhoei*
This snail is a host for *F. hepatica* in parts of China. In Europe, the usual intermediate host is *L. truncatula* (see **546**). (× 7)

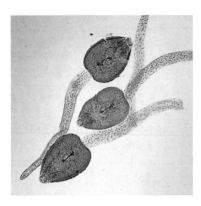

584 Cercaria of *Fasciola hepatica*
The cercariae, which have unforked tails, encyst on aquatic vegetation to form metacercariae. (× 85)

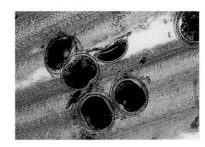

585 Metacercariae on grass
These are found on grass or other moist herbage such as watercress (**580**). When the metacercariae are ingested, the cycle recommences. (× 75)

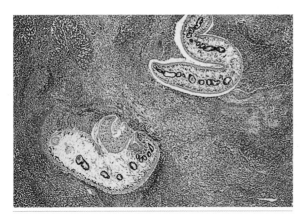

586 Migrating flukes in liver
After being swallowed, the metacercariae pass through the intestinal wall and penetrate the liver capsule to enter the liver parenchyma. The figure shows a sheep liver with migrating, immature flukes. (*H&E × 20*)

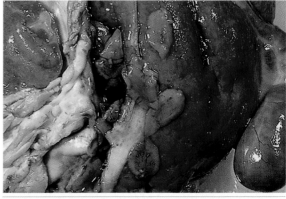

587 Adult flukes in bile ducts of a sheep liver
The adult flukes penetrate into the bile ducts, where they cause damage to the biliary tract. Eggs (see **407**) are passed with the bile into the faeces. (*Natural size*)

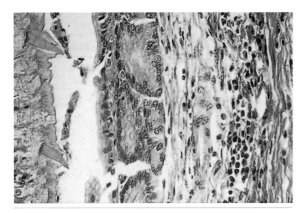

588 Adult *Fasciola hepatica* in section of liver
The surface spines of the adult fluke produce mechanical damage to the biliary epithelium. (*H&E × 350*)

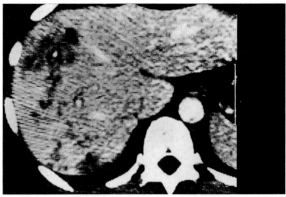

589 Computed tomography scan of *F. hepatica* in human liver
Using contrast, cystic filling defects suggestive of this trematode infection can be visualised. They usually disappear after therapy.

Paragonimiasis

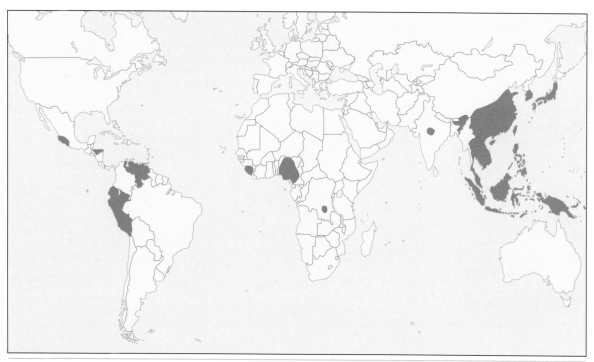

590 Distribution of lung flukes

Paragonimiasis, affecting over 20 million people worldwide, is caused by numerous species of lung fluke (see **Table 14**). *Paragonimus westermani* is the commonest parasite responsible for human infection in the Far East, where it has a wide range of mammalian reservoirs. Human infections with *Paragonimus heterotremus* are well known in Thailand and with *Paragonimus pulmonalis* in the Far East. *Paragonimus africanus* and *Paragonimus uterobilateralis* have a focal distribution in humans in west Africa. *Paragonimus mexicanus* and other species commonly produce human infection in parts of Central and South America. The so-called 'lung flukes' have the further distinction of becoming localised at times in the brain, where they may give rise to major neurological symptoms.

Table 14 Species of *Paragonimus* recorded in humans

Species	Geographical area	Natural final hosts*
Asia and Pacific		
Paragonimus westermani westermani	China, Thailand, Malaysia, Sri Lanka	Dog, wild canids, cat, wild felids, civets, mongooses, macaques
P. westermani japonicus	Japan	Mainly raccoon dog, fox
P. westermani filipinus	Philippines, Taiwan	Dog, cat, rat
P. westermani ichunensis	Northern China, former Soviet Union	Dog, cat, tiger, raccoon dog, wolf
Paragonimus pulmonalis	China, Taiwan, Korea, Japan	Dog, cat, tiger, wild boar
Paragonimus miyazakii	Japan	Dog, cat, weasel, sable, wild boar, raccoon dog, badger
Paragonimus heterotremus (= *P. tuanshanensis*)	China, Laos, Thailand	Dog, cat, leopard, rat, bandicoot
Paragonimus skrjabini (= *P. szechuanensis*)	China	Cat, dog, ? weasel, masked palm civet
Paragonimus hueitungensis	China	
Paragonimus ohirai	Japan	Rodents, insectivores, dog, raccoon dog, badger, pig, wild boar, weasel
Paragonimus iloktsuenensis	Taiwan, Japan	Dog, weasel, rodents, insectivores
Paragonimus sadoensis	Japan	Weasel, cat
Africa		
Paragonimus africanus	Cameroon, Zaire, Nigeria, Ghana	Dog, civet, mongoose, drill, potto
Paragonimus uterobilateralis	Cameroon, Nigeria, Guinea, Ivory Coast, Liberia	Dog, civet, mongoose, rat, shrew
North and South America		
Paragonimus mexicanus	Mexico, Guatemala, Costa Rica, Panama, Peru, Ecuador	Opossum, wild felids, canids, coati, raccoon, skunk
Paragonimus caliensis	Panama, Colombia, Peru	Opossum
Paragonimus peruvianus	Peru	Opossum, cat
Paragonimus ecuadoriensis	Ecuador	Coati

* In addition to humans. Other species occur only in domestic or wild animals.

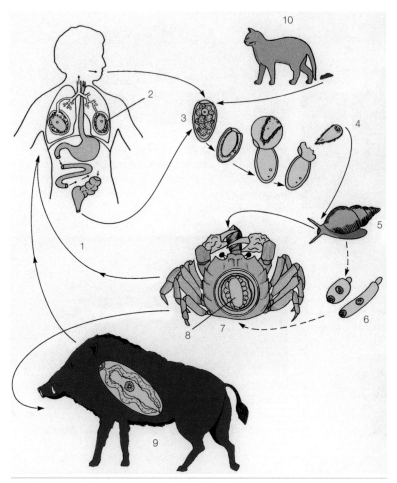

591 Life cycle of *Paragonimus pulmonalis*

This may be taken as a typical example of the genus. (1) Humans, a definitive host, are infected when they eat the flesh of crustacea containing living metacercaria. The metacercariae hatch in the duodenum and the young flukes penetrate the gut wall, the mesentery and the diaphragm to the pleural cavity. Within 2–3 weeks, the worms, which are hermaphroditic, penetrate beneath the lung capsule, where they meet and cross-fertilise. Adult trematodes (2) become partly encapsulated in the parenchymal tissue, where they lay eggs (3) that pass into the alveoli and are coughed up or swallowed. Eggs that reach water hatch into miracidia (4), which penetrate snails of an appropriate species. These are the first intermediate hosts. In the snails (5), they form sporocysts from which develop two generations of daughter cells (rediae), which give rise in about 3 months to very short-tailed (microcercous) cercariae (6); after emerging into the water the cercariae seek their crustacean (secondary intermediate) host (7) into which they penetrate to encyst in the gills or muscles as metacercariae (8). *P. pulmonalis* can also be acquired by eating uncooked flesh of the wild boar (9), which serves as a paratenic host of this species (i.e. a supernumerary intermediate host). Domestic cats (10) and dogs can also serve as definitive hosts for numerous species of *Paragonimus* in the Far East and in west Africa. Like *P. westermani*, *P. heterotremus* may invade the brain and subcutaneous tissues but often only causes a type of larva migrans in humans.

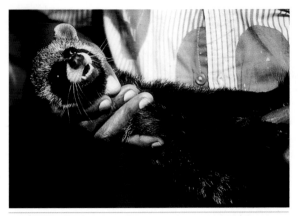

592 African civet cat, *Viverra civetta* (Viverridae)
This carnivore is a primary reservoir host for both *P. africanus* and *P. uterobilateralis* in west Africa. The west African long-nosed mongoose, *Crossarchus obscurus*, is also an important host for *P. uterobilateralis* in Liberia as well as being infected by *P. africanus* in countries further east. The palm civet, *Paradoxurus hermaphroditus* (Viverridae) is one of the feral reservoir hosts of *Paragonimus* in Thailand and other Far East countries.

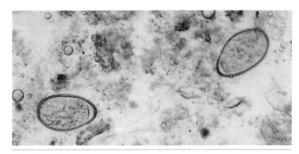

594 Eggs in human sputum
Eggs are passed in the sputum or swallowed to be passed later in the faeces. The miracidia hatching from the eggs penetrate snails of various genera, including *Semisulcospira* and *Thiara* (see **Table 13**). After the usual cycle of development in the snail, microcercous cercariae emerge and encyst inside freshwater crayfish and crabs. Various crab-eating carnivores thus become the natural reservoirs of *Paragonimus* species. (See also **410**.) (× *150*)

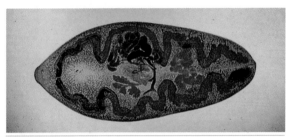

593 Adult *Paragonimus westermani*
The adult fluke normally lives in the lungs. It is rather lemon-shaped and about 1 cm long when alive (see **600**). Preserved specimens, as seen here, become flattened and distorted during preparation (× *5.2*).

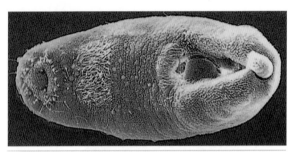

595 Microcercous cercaria of *Paragonimus pulmonalis*
Ventral view of the cercaria of this species, which is widely distributed in Korea, China (including Taiwan) and Japan, where the infection is acquired from crabs or crayfish. (*Scanning electron microscopy × 510*)

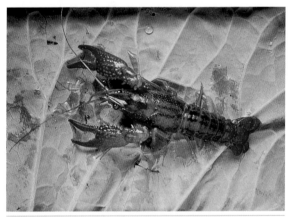

596 *Procambarus clarkii*, an intermediate host of *Paragonimus pulmonalis*
This crayfish, which is a popular item of food in parts of Japan, is an intermediate host for the metacercarial stage of this trematode.

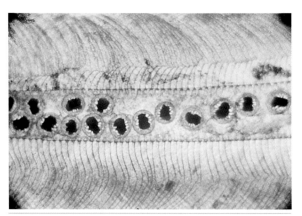

597 Metacercaria of *Paragonimus pulmonalis* along a gill bar of the crab *Eriocheir japonicus*
Compare with the smaller metacercaria of *O. sinensis* (**565**). (× 7)

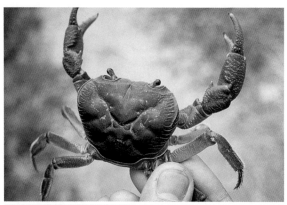

598 *Ranguna smithiana*: a host of lung fluke
Crabs are commonly eaten raw or in the form of an uncooked paste, with which the metacercariae are ingested. This species is a host of *P. westermani* and *P. heterotremus* in Thailand.

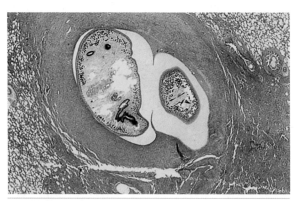

599 Section of lung
The figure shows a section of lung containing encapsulated, adult *P. westermani*. (*H&E* × 20)

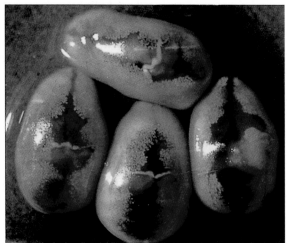

600 Living adult *Paragonimus westermani*
Compare the appearance with that of the prepared specimen in **593**, which is the condition figured in most textbooks. (× 4.3)

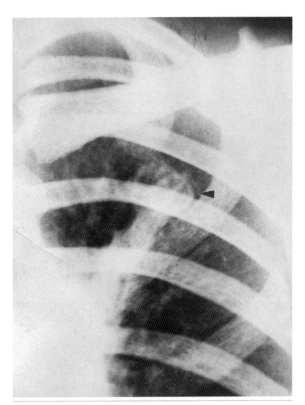

601 Chest radiograph
Human infection is manifested by cough, haemoptysis, and other signs and symptoms, which are commonly confused with those of tuberculosis. Typical shadows caused by the encysted adult trematodes may be seen on this X-ray of a 7-year-old Japanese girl who was infected with *P. pulmonalis* after eating the flesh of the crab *Eriocheir japonicus*. Note the ring shadow in the left lobe. There were also nodes in the hilar area. Numerous eggs were present in her brown-coloured sputum.

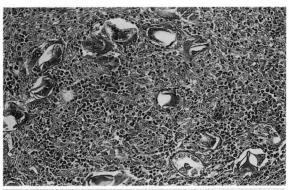

602 Eggs in mesenteric lymph node
In this section, several disintegrating eggs of *P. westermani* are seen in a granuloma containing numerous eosinophils in a mesenteric node. (*H&E × 120*)

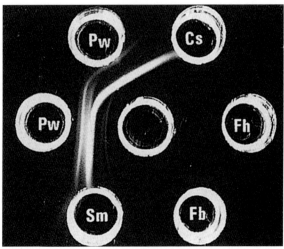

603 Gel diffusion test for paragonimiasis
The reaction of antigen derived from adult worms with serum antibodies can be a useful diagnostic aid. More sensitive tests now include a dot-ELISA, based on a specific monoclonal antibody, which detects *Paragonimus* antigens in the serum.

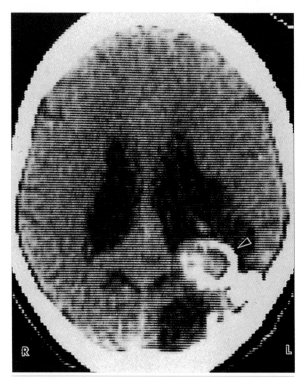

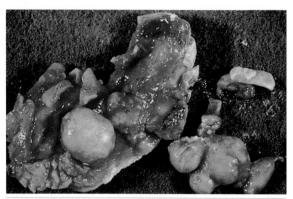

605 *Paragonimus* cyst extracted from brain
A cyst of *P. westermani* found at autopsy in the brain of a
21-year-old Japanese girl. Unlike the patient in **604**, such
individuals usually present with epilepsy occurring for the first
time in adult life.

604 Cyst of *Paragonimus* in the brain
This patient, a 59-year-old woman who lived in China as a
teenager, presented with a history of epileptic convulsions once
or twice a year for over 40 years. They followed an initial
pulmonary infection that was probably acquired when she was
about 16 years of age. A computed tomography scan revealed a
large, calcified mass caused by encystation of an adult fluke,
probably *P. westermani*, in the left occipital region. The
peripheral brain tissue was shrunken and the left lateral
ventricle dilated.

4. Infections acquired through the gastrointestinal tract

Many of the important pathogens that gain entry through the gastrointestinal tract are cosmopolitan in their distribution. They include viruses, bacteria, protozoa, helminths and endoparasitic arthropods. The first three of these can be directly infectious for humans when they are passed in the faeces but, in the case of helminths, the eggs may become infectious only after maturation in the soil (e.g. *Ascaris lumbricoides*) or after passing through an intermediate host (e.g. *Taenia saginata*). (Helminthiases acquired from the soil are included in Chapter 2, and those requiring a snail intermediate host in Chapter 3. A number of the latter are also acquired via the oral route.) Some of the pathogens pass from the intestinal tract to cause systemic infection and may localise in other organs (e.g. poliomyelitis, acute viral hepatitis (see **Table 15**), trichinosis). Localised infection of the gastrointestinal tract itself with pathogenic viruses or bacteria (see **Table 16**) accounts for a high proportion of deaths in infants and young children in developing countries where the standards of hygiene and nutrition are often already at very low levels. Rotavirus-related diarrhoea is estimated to have killed over 600 000 children under 5 years of age between 2000 and 2004.

The most important pattern of transmission is the passage of infective material from human faeces into the mouth of a new host, which is known as 'faeco-oral' transmission. This occurs mostly through inapparent faecal contamination of food, water and hands – the three main points of contact with the mouth. Some of the pathogens that infect through the mouth are not excreted in the faeces (e.g. Guinea worm infection is acquired by drinking contaminated water, but the larvae escape through the skin). On the other hand, while the ova of *Necator americanus* are passed in the faeces, the route of human infection is by direct penetration of the skin by the larvae after a period of incubation of the egg in the soil.

A number of the infections that are acquired through the gastrointestinal tract, such as cholera and typhoid, characteristically occur in epidemic form. The spread of cholera, for example, is facilitated by the potentiating combination of a symptomless carrier state with widescale local and international travel. It was feared that the pandemic of the E1 Tor biotype would soon be replaced by the more virulent O:139 serovar, which appeared in south-east Asia in the early 1990s, although so far this has not been realised. Typhoid continues to appear in epidemic form where poor sanitary conditions and inadequate fresh water supplies coexist. In the Democratic Republic of Congo, for example, between September 2004 and January 2005, 42 564 cases with 214 deaths were officially reported and these entailed nearly 700 cases with severe intestinal perforation. Globally it has been estimated that about 16 million cases and 600 000 deaths due to typhoid occur yearly, 70% of the deaths being in Asia. Even the protozoal pathogen *Cryptosporidium hominis* (formerly known as *Cryptosporidium parvum*) may cause severe, waterborne epidemics, as occurred in the USA in 1993 and more recently elsewhere. Other infections may be more localised, affecting persons from the same household or institution (e.g. amoebiasis or enterobiasis); hospitals housing the mentally subnormal are particularly vulnerable to such conditions.

The importance of some of the rare, protozoal infections such as the microsporidia is only being appreciated now that they are appearing as concomitant infections in people with depressed immune responsiveness (e.g. in acquired immuno-deficiency syndrome, AIDS).

VIRAL INFECTIONS

Poliomyelitis

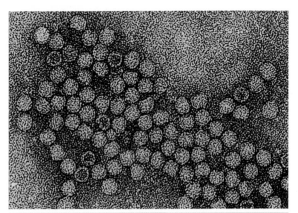

606 Ultrastructure of poliomyelitis virus
Spherical particles measuring 25 nm in diameter are apparent in this electron micrograph; both 'full' and 'empty' particles are shown. Once considered to be mainly a disease of the industrialised world, poliomyelitis, thanks to effective vaccination, is now mainly a problem in the developing countries throughout which it was, until very recently, widespread. (× 126 000)

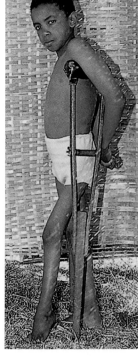

607 Ethiopian boy with paralysis of left leg
Today, young indigenous children in the developing countries are predominantly affected, along with nonimmunised expatriates of all ages. Since humans are the only reservoir of the polio virus from which so-called 'wild virus' originates, vaccination of all susceptible people should, in principle, result in the eradication of human infection and its resultant acute flaccid paralysis. A global campaign to eliminate the disease in developing countries made spectacular progress in its first decade. In India alone, for example, 200 000 cases were reported in 1989. By 1993, only 8000 new cases were reported globally to the WHO, and 141 countries were apparently free of the disease.

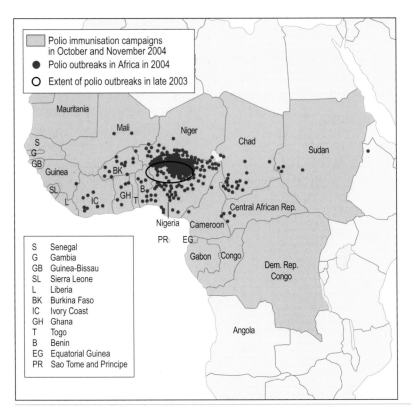

Legend:
- Polio immunisation campaigns in October and November 2004
- Polio outbreaks in Africa in 2004
- Extent of polio outbreaks in late 2003

S   Senegal
G   Gambia
GB   Guinea-Bissau
SL   Sierra Leone
L   Liberia
BK   Burkina Faso
IC   Ivory Coast
GH   Ghana
T   Togo
B   Benin
EG   Equatorial Guinea
PR   Sao Tome and Principe

608 Residual and new foci of poliomyelitis in Africa

The figure summarises the locations of polio outbreaks in Africa up to early 2005 and the area in which intensive immunisation campaigns were reinstalled late in 2004. A global campaign that was commenced in 1988 to eradicate poliomyelitis by mass vaccination with three oral doses succeeded in reducing the number of endemic countries from more than 125 to six by 2003. However, during that year 10 countries reported the importation of wild polio virus, nine of them in Africa, where there were over 8000 cases. After the vaccination programme was intensified to cover 415 million infants under 5 years of age in 55 countries, there was a further dramatic fall to 1600 in the global number of cases of acute flaccid paralysis that were due to the polio virus (AFP) as confirmed by the detection of virus in stool samples. During 2004 the numbers of cases again fell dramatically, except in Nigeria, in the north of which the local religious authorities had refused to permit the extension of the vaccination programme. From Nigeria the virus rapidly spread back to some neighbouring countries, especially along the highways of the Sahel, to Sudan and Egypt, south to Botswana and, via pilgrims on the Haj, as far east as Saudi Arabia, especially via the Sudan. By mid-2004 polio had returned to 22 countries, of which 10 had been polio-free the previous year. Civil unrest in a country such as Sudan poses a major threat to the global progress of the eradication campaign, to which US$2 billion has already been committed, and from that country there is a great risk of further spread to such countries as Chad and Ethiopia. Of the three types of wild polio virus (WPV), type 1 has returned to the Yemen but type 2 has not been reported anywhere in the world since 1999 and type 3, although not identified in humans for several years, may still be circulating cryptically in some areas. In early 2005 cases of AFP caused by WPV type 1 were identified in Indonesia after an infection-free interval of 10 years, the virus probably having been imported by pilgrims returning from the Haj or by expatriate workers from Saudi Arabia. (Adapted from Anonymous 2005 Polio spread in Africa. Crunch time for polio. *New Scientist*, 8 Jan, p 26.)

Acute viral hepatitis

Acute viral hepatitis and its sequelae are a major problem, particularly in the tropics and subtropics, although the viruses are cosmopolitan. The viruses so far identified are reviewed in **Table 15**.

Hepatitis A (HAV) and hepatitis E (HEV), formerly called HNANB(E), are transmitted by the faeco-oral route. HBV (hepatitis B virus), HCV, HDV and HFV are transmitted by parenteral infection; they are dealt with in Chapter 10 (see 1190–1196). Yellow fever is highlighted in Chapter 1 (**13–22**). Hepatitis may also be associated with cytomegalovirus, Epstein–Barr virus and filoviruses (see **Table 26**). HAV is commonly acquired from contaminated food, with shellfish being a notorious source of infection. It can occur in epidemic fashion and may affect more than 90% of the adult population in some developing countries. It does not usually have serious consequences.

Table 15 Hepatitis viruses[1]

Name	Type or genus	RNA/DNA	Transmission mode	Course of infection	Notes
HBV	Orthhepadnavirus (similar to retroviruses)	DNA	Via blood and blood products, usually by inoculation; perinatal infection from mother	Incubation 1–3 months, then immune-mediated acute hepatitis	High proportion become chronic carriers; chronic active infection leads to cirrhosis, hepatocellular carcinoma (i.e. oncogenic)
HCV = HNANB(P)	Hepacivirus Togavirus	RNA	As HBV plus other modes (90–95% of transfusion induced HNANB)	Incubation 2 months; hepatitis less severe than HBV infection	May give chronic carrier state with same sequelae as HBV
HDV (delta)	Deltavirus 'Defective virus'	RNA	Transfusion, heterosexual transmission	Incubation 2–12 weeks; requires HBs antigen; ('piggy-back virus'); superinfection may give fulminating hepatitis	Commonest in Africa and South America – probable cause of Labrea fever
HAV	Hepatovirus Heparnivirus ('enterovirus 72')	RNA	Faeco–oral route; water, shellfish, etc.	Incubation 2–4 weeks often mild infection with or without jaundice	Can give epidemic spread, >90% of adults infected in developing countries
HEV = HNANB(E)	Hepivirus[1] Calicivirus	RNA	Faeco–oral route; mainly water; may be zoonotic	Incubation 6–8 weeks; mild except in pregnancy	Mortality up to 20% in pregnancy
HFV	Not known	?	Accounts for 5–10% of HNANB(P) infections	Little known	Little known
Yellow fever	Togavirus	RNA	Vector-borne	Incubation period 3–6 days; usually severe hepatitis, high mortality rate	See **18–21**

[1] Hepatitis may also be associated with infection by cytomegalovirus, Epstein–Barr virus and filoviruses (see **Table 25**).
[2] The precise systematic status of Hepivirus remains to be defined.

HEV may be the commonest agent of acute viral hepatitis in developing countries and can result in serious disease in pregnant women. In addition to its spread through contaminated water supplies, HEV has been reported as a zoonotic infection from inadequately cooked wild boar or domesticated pigs in Japan and elsewhere.

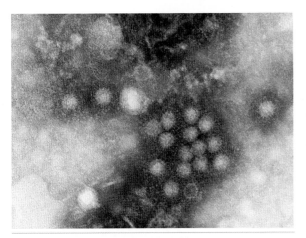

609 Ultrastructure of hepatitis A virus
The electron micrograph of this enterovirus shows the particles (27 nm in diameter) that were found in faecal extracts from an adult volunteer during the acute phase of HAV infection after inoculation with serum. The particles are heavily coated with antibody present in convalescent serum. The incubation period is between 2 and 4 weeks and the infection, which may be with or without jaundice, is frequently mild. HEV is a calicivirus with a longer incubation period. Although usually producing a mild illness, the infection can be particularly dangerous during pregnancy, when it may cause a high mortality. ($\times$ 220 000)

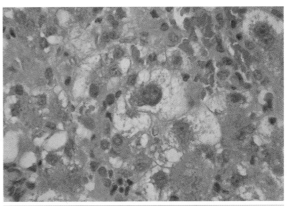

610 Section of liver in acute viral hepatitis
The changes seen here are found in both HAV and HBV infection. Marked swelling of the hepatocytes (which have indistinct or lysed membranes) and loss of cytoplasmic contents cause this 'ballooning degeneration'. ($\times$ 1200) (AFIP No. 71–1396) (see also **1194**.)

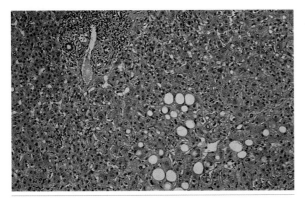

611 Acute spotty hepatitis
This liver in mild viral hepatitis (which was caused by HEV or HCV) shows macrovesicular fat in the centrilobular area and diffuse microvesicular fat with infiltration of inflammatory cells in the portal triad. (*Haematoxylin and eosin (H&E)* $\times$ 100) (See also **1194**.)

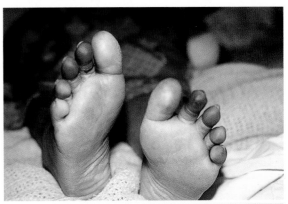

612 Peripheral vasculitis in a patient with hepatitis C
Hepatitis C is produced by a positive single-stranded RNA virus of the Flaviviridae family. It is a common viral infection of the liver and can occasionally present with systemic features of a vasculitis, as demonstrated here, with severe involvement of the terminal digits of the foot due to an immune-related, essential, mixed cryoglobulinaemia.

Acute viral gastroenteritis

Acute viral gastroenteritis is a major cause of morbidity and mortality, especially in infants and young children in the developing countries, where it is the leading cause of death in those under 4 years of age. It has been estimated that over 500 million children are infected and about 2.4 million under 5 years of age die yearly from infectious gastroenteritis. Self-limiting but highly infectious outbreaks of Norovirus are not infrequent on passenger ships, causing major disruption but relatively few major pathological effects.

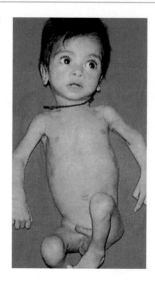

613 Infant with viral gastroenteritis
Among the viruses that have been identified as responsible for acute gastroenteritis in children are a variety of rotaviruses, adenoviruses, astroviruses and caliciviruses including Norwalk and Norwalk-like virus (see **Table 16**). Infection results in severe dehydration which calls for energetic oral replacement therapy, with glucose and electrolytes or parenteral rehydration in the most severe cases. Malnourished infants are at particular risk. Note here the flaccidity and other signs of dehydration in this infant.

Table 16 Major viral and bacterial pathogens causing acute diarrhoea*

Pathogen	Pathogenesis	Notes
Viruses		
Rotaviruses (Rotaviridae)	Destroy tips of microvilli; new cells absorb less water, salts and sugars	Global. Cause 140 million cases and 1 million deaths yearly. Major cause in developing countries
Adenoviruses (Adenoviridae)	Less severe but more prolonged than above. Types 40, 41 main pathogens	Second most important agents developing countries
Astroviruses (Astroviridae)	Mild gastroenteritis, may occur in outbreaks	Mainly children <7 years
Caliciviruses (Caliciviridae)	Mild gastroenteritis, may occur in outbreaks	Older children
Norwalk and Norwalk-like viruses (Caliciviridae)	Mild gastroenteritis, may occur in outbreaks	Older children and adults; common in closed environments e.g. cruise ships
Bacteria		
Salmonella species (except *S. typhi, S. paratyphi*)	Invade lamina propria of ileocaecal region; prostaglandins released, trigger cyclic AMP; active fluid secretion	Were commonest in Western world; mainly zoonotic
Escherichia coli		
– enterotoxigenic	Pili bind bacteria to mucosal cells, secrete exotoxins; these increase cyclic GMP, causing fluid secretion	Major cause in children in developing countries and of 'turista'
– enteropathogenic	Adhere to enterocytes, destroy microvilli	Babies and infants in developing countries
Helicobacter pylori	Stomach is normal site, invades mucosa	High prevalence in adults in developing world; associated with gastric adenocarcinoma
Vibrio cholera	Biotypes of serovar 0:1 vary in virulence factors and toxin production; toxin activates cyclic AMP, blocks absorption of salt, increases fluid secretion	E1 Tor replaced classic biotype but virulent serovar 0:129 now spreading
Shigella species	Enteropathogenic, causing ulcers in distal ileum and colon	Major cause in young people in developing countries
Campylobacter species	Cause acute gastroenteritis, colitis	A common cause of travellers' diarrhoea; mainly *C. jejuni*

*Excluding typhoid and paratyphoid, which cause systemic infection. See also Protozoal Infections, Table 17.

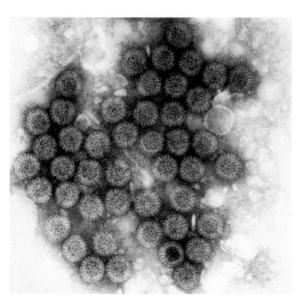

614 Rotavirus causing viral gastroenteritis

Rotaviruses, of which at least seven groups and two subgroups can infect humans, are responsible for about 20% of all diarrhoeal infections in developing countries. This electron micrograph shows particles approximately 75 nm in diameter that were found in faeces. They have a characteristic, wheel-like appearance. (*Electron microscopy (EM) × 125 000*)

BACTERIAL INFECTIONS

Salmonellosis – typhoid (enteric) fevers

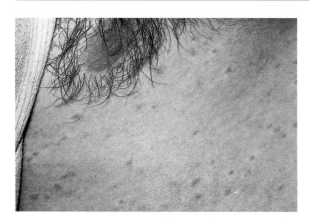

615 Rose spots

Species of *Salmonella* cause only a small proportion of the diarrhoeal infections (about 2.5%) in developing countries. The most important member of this genus is *Salmonella typhi*, the cause of typhoid (enteric fever). The classic rose spots of typhoid (1–3 mm in diameter) may appear irregularly, usually on the abdominal wall, the lower thorax and the back of the trunk.

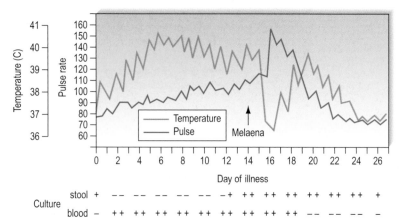

616 Temperature chart

The fever, which often rises in a stepwise fashion, is high and accompanied by confusion and severe prostration ('typhoid state'). There is often a dissociation between pulse and temperature (Faget's sign), and an accompanying leukopenia. The tongue is frequently coated (in contrast to kala-azar, when it is usually clean – see **262**).

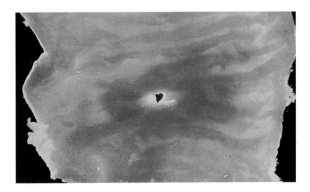

617 Ulceration of Peyer's patches
Intestinal haemorrhage and perforation are the two most serious complications of typhoid fever. They are due to ulceration of Peyer's patches.

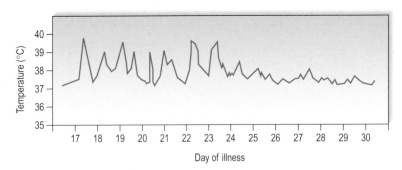

618 Temperature chart in salmonellosis associated with *Schistosoma mansoni* infection
An association exists between fever occurring in chronic *Salmonella typhi* infection and concomitant *S. mansoni*. In such cases, clearance of the helminth infection is needed before the *Salmonella* organisms can be eliminated.

'Nonspecific' acute infectious diarrhoea

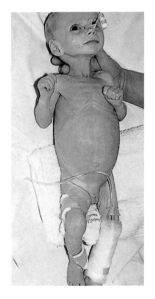

619 Dehydration due to gastroenteritis
Severe dehydration due to diarrhoea and vomiting is the salient diagnostic feature of acute infectious diarrhoea of bacterial origin. As in the treatment of viral gastroenteritis, oral rehydration with a solution containing salts and glucose and intravenous fluid replacement have revolutionised the treatment of 'nonspecific' diarrhoeal diseases of bacterial origin.

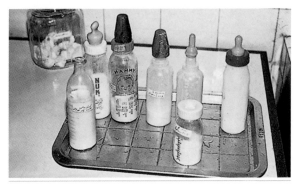

620 Sources of infantile infectious diarrhoea
Gastroenteritis due to a variety of bacteria, as well as to viruses (see **613** and **614**), is one of the major causes of childhood mortality in the tropics. The substitution of the milk bottle for breast feeding is increasing, rather than decreasing, the problem. Mismanagement of artificial feeding is a serious cause, due to contamination of feeds with pathogenic organisms.

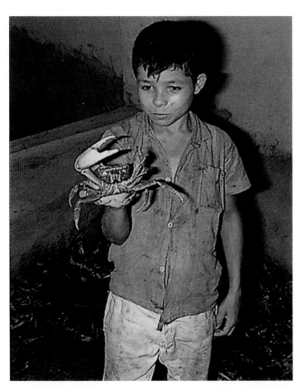

633 Seafood as a source of cholera infection

Raw or improperly cooked seafood (e.g. shellfish and crabs) has been incriminated as a source of infection with El Tor cholera. Infections arose in the USA in 1991 in individuals who ate crabs such as these that were imported by travellers from Ecuador. Endemic cholera is also known to exist in some coastal areas of North America, China and a few other countries where the vibrios have been identified in brackish coastal waters. *Cyclops* water fleas have been shown to harbour the organisms, which produce a chitinase that may permit them to attach to the hosts. The water fleas are consumed by larger arthropods such as crabs and crayfish. These, and various molluscs such as oysters, may form part of the natural cycle of some strains of *V. cholerae*, which could account in part for the transcontinental spread of the vibrios, probably in ships' ballast tanks. Other species of vibrio that may be acquired by eating raw, contaminated seafood are *Vibrio vulnificus* and especially *Vibrio parahaemolyticus*. The first of these has caused occasional deaths off the Gulf coast of the USA. In 2005 the latter organism infected 6300 people in Chile and even affected some oyster farms in Alaska. The wild population of *V. cholerae* is probably kept in check by different bacteriophages, especially in fresh water. However, their dilution by, for example, monsoon or spring rain flooding may be a trigger for the increase of the bacteria and the resurgence of human infections. The massive inundation of exposed coastal regions by a tsunami may also produce conditions favourable to the multiplication of *V. cholerae*.

Helicobacter pylori

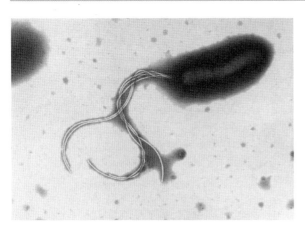

634 *Helicobacter pylori*

This microaerophilic, Gram-negative bacterium with a complex terminal flagellum occurs on the mucosa of the stomach and duodenum of up to 80% of adults living in developing countries, where the incidence increases with decreasing socioeconomic status and poor nutrition. The prevalence is much lower in the Western world. *H. pylori* is associated with peptic ulceration and is the probable cause of the high rate of gastric adenocarcinoma in developing countries. (× 11 000)

Shigellosis

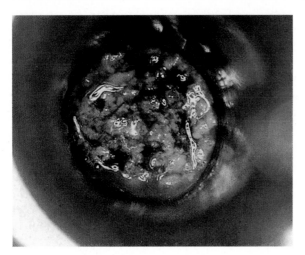

635 Shigellosis affecting the sigmoid colon

Like *V. cholerae*, the bacteria causing shigellosis produce an enterotoxin. Transmission is mainly faeco-oral and is associated with poor hygienic conditions. Not surprisingly, shigellosis is most prevalent in the poorer developing countries. Four species are responsible for most human infection, *Shigella dysenteriae*, *Shigella flexneri*, *Shigella sonnei* and *Shigella boydii*. They affect initially the distal small intestine, causing painful cramps, fever and bloody diarrhoea. Once in the colon they multiply in the lamina propria and destroy the overlying mucosa. The figure shows a sigmoidoscopic view of colonic mucosa from a fatal case of *S. dysenteriae* infection.

Enteritis necroticans ('pigbel')

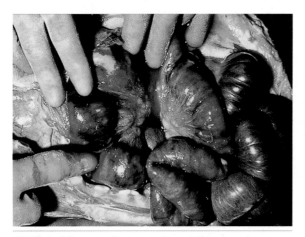

636 Enteritis necrotica seen at operation

'Pigbel' is a segmental disease of the intestine (usually the ileum), most commonly seen in the highlands of Papua New Guinea; it is caused by infection with a widely distributed soil organism, *Clostridium welchii* type C. A carrier state clearly exists as the organisms can be found in the faeces of 70% of highland villagers, although human-to-human transmission does not seem to occur. The infection is acquired by eating improperly cooked, infected pig meat, usually at ceremonial feasts, in an area where the diet (consisting mainly of baked sweet potatoes) is usually very low in protein. Vaccination with *C. welchii* type C β toxoid gives protection lasting a few years.

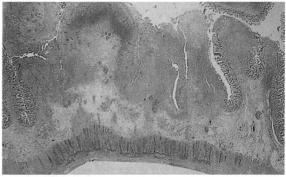

637 Necrosis of small intestine in 'Pigbel'

The main lesion is patchy necrosis of the small intestine, starting in the mucosa and extending through to the serosal wall, as seen here. Resection of the infected segment is indicated. (*H&E* × *150*).

Brucellosis

Goats, sheep, cows, pigs and camels are the common animal reservoirs of infection with *Brucella abortus*, *Brucella melitensis* and *Brucella suis*. Infection is commonly acquired by drinking unpasteurised milk or milk products. Brucellosis is an important cause of morbidity in the Middle East, especially for many desert-dwelling pastoralists.

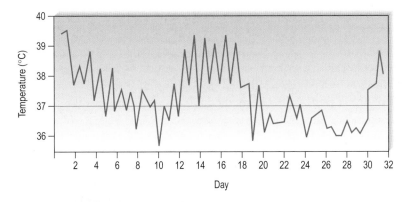

638 Temperature chart

Common initial symptoms of brucellosis are fever, which may be intermittent or undulant (as illustrated here). Moderate leukopenia with a relative lymphocytosis and hepatosplenomegaly are frequently encountered. In some areas, the fever is atypical. A persistent raised IgM is suggestive of brucellosis but a high *Brucella* agglutination titre or positive blood culture will confirm the diagnosis.

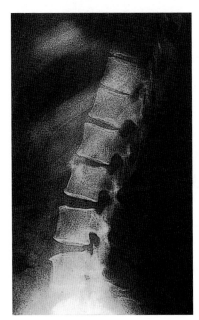

639 Radiograph of *Brucella* spondylitis

The earliest symptom of this condition is pain localised to the affected region of the spine (commonly the lumbar spine). Radiologically, one sees narrowing of the disc spaces, erosion of the vertebral margins, collapse of the vertebrae and, characteristically, the development of proliferative changes with unison of osteophytes. While such arthritic changes are common manifestations of chronic brucellosis, the infection may also present protean neurological signs, sometimes suggestive of disseminated sclerosis. Acute meningoencephalitis with fatigue, demyelinating neuropathy and spastic paraplegia are usually forms of presentation of neurobrucellosis.

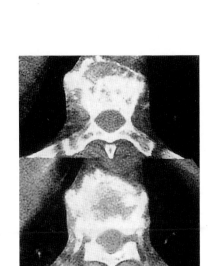

640 Computed tomography scan of *Brucella* spondylitis

This figure illustrates typical degenerative changes in the bones associated with spondylitis in a Kuwaiti patient with chronic brucellosis.

Melioidosis

This disease, which occurs mainly in south-east Asia and northern Australia, is due to infection with *Burkholderia* (formerly *Pseudomonas*) *pseudomallei* (Whitmore's bacillus). Diabetes mellitus and chronic renal disease are common predisposing factors. The route of infection is uncertain but it may be water-borne or air-borne, or may be acquired by contamination of wounds with soil. Inapparent infections are probably widespread as surveys, for example in Thailand, have shown that 30–50% of those examined are seropositive but asymptomatic. The disease may present as acute septicaemia followed by multiple organ abscess formation, or may be subacute from the start. Septicaemic melioidosis carries a 40% mortality rate. Chronic infections in children may present as a parotid abscess. Pulmonary infection may follow either direct aspiration of the bacteria, as happened in Thailand following the 2004 tsunami, or via soil-contaminated wounds. The diagnosis is indicated by a positive haemagglutination test or IgG-based enzyme-linked immunosorbent assay (ELISA), and is confirmed by culturing the organism from different body fluids on a selective medium such as Ashdown's.

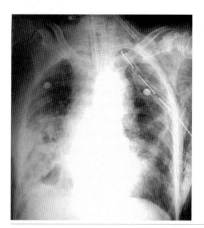

641 Bilateral pneumonia due to melioidosis
This is the chest X-ray of a 71-year-old Thai woman with no known underlying disease, showing extensive bilateral lung involvement in melioidosis. She was acidotic and hyperglycaemic on admission. Her sputum grew *B. pseudomallei* that was sensitive to ceftazidime but despite treatment she died 8 days later. (Courtesy of Dr Wirongrong Chierakul.)

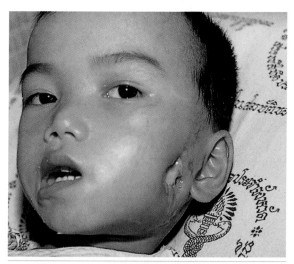

642 Parotid abscess caused by *Pseudomonas pseudomallei*
The parotid gland is a common site for localised melioidosis in children, with other common sites being the skin and soft tissues, liver, spleen and lymph nodes. This Thai boy shows a suppurating left parotid abscess. (© D A Warrell.)

Leptospirosis (Weil's disease) See Table 4.

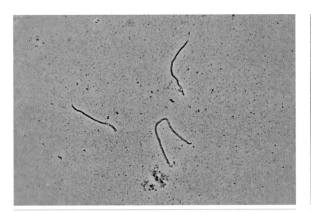

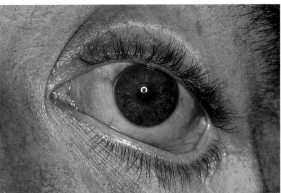

643 *Leptospira interrogans*
Leptospirosis is a zoonotic infection with one of a variety of organisms of the *Leptospira interrogans* species complex. The spirochaetes are readily seen in silver-stained preparations, especially with a phase-contrast microscope. The disease is usually acquired from either contact with infected animals or, more commonly, from water contaminated with animal urine. The commonest source of human infection is from rats or mice (serotype *Leptospira icterohaemorrhagiae*), and occasionally from dogs (serotype *Leptospira canicola*). The disease is global in distribution but commoner in tropical areas. (× *1050*)

644 Subconjunctival haemorrhages in leptospirosis
The infection can follow one of three courses. Asymptomatic or atypical infection occurs in probably 90% of cases and, in some tropical areas, leptospirosis may account for up to 15% of all patients with undiagnosed pyrexia. While this form can be mild, the infection may develop into a generalised septic form within 1–2 weeks. This is characterised by fever, myalgia and often subconjunctival haemorrhages. The photograph shown here was of a patient in the second week following the onset of symptoms. The most dangerous form (Weil's disease) may be very severe and can involve several organs, with jaundice, renal failure, haemorrhage and vascular collapse.

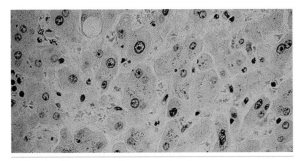

645 Hepatic changes in leptospirosis
In severe cases – even where hepatic dysfunction and jaundice are present – hepatocellular necrosis is unusual but large amounts of bilirubin can be seen in the hepatocytes. After specific chemotherapy, the liver function usually returns to normal. (*H&E* × *300*)

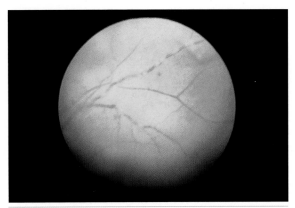

646 Uveitis in leptospirosis
During the recovery phase of leptospirosis, iridocyclitis or uveitis (as seen here) may be associated with the immunological response, often several weeks or months following the initial infection. This photograph of the fundus was taken 3 months after the patient developed acute systemic leptospirosis.

PROTOZOAL INFECTIONS See Table 17.

Table 17 Protozoa (phyla Ciliophora and Sarcomastigophora, subphylum Sarcodina) of medical importance

Phylum	Subphylum, etc.	Order	Genus and species
Apicomplexa (see **Table 5**)			
Ciliophora	Rhabdophora	Vestibuliferida	*Balantidium coli*
Sarcomastigophora	Mastigophora (see **Tables 7, 8, 9** and **18**) Sarcodina Superclass Rhizopodea	Amoebida	*Entamoeba coli* *Entamoeba histolytica** *Entamoeba dispar** *Entamoeba gingivalis* *Endolimax nana* *Iodamoeba bütschlii* *Acanthamoeba culbertsoni*[†] *Acanthamoeba polyphaga*[†] *Acanthamoeba castellani*[†] *Acanthamoeba hatchetti*[†] *Blastocystis hominis*[‡]
		Schizopyrenida	*Naegleria fowleri*[†]
		Leptomyxida	*Balamuthia mandrillaris*[†]

* *E. histolytica* causing human amoebiasis, is clearly distinguishable by isoenzyme and genomic characters from *E. dispar*, which is non-pathogenic in humans. † Pathogenic 'free-living' species. The other amoebae are obligatory parasites. ‡ This anaerobic, gut-dwelling protozoan has recently been ascribed to the order Amoebida.

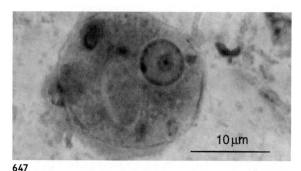

647

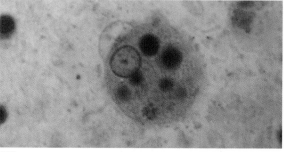

648

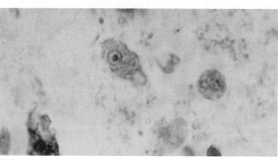

649

647–651 Trophozoites of intestinal protozoa
Entamoeba coli (**647**), *Entamoeba histolytica* or *Entamoeba dispar* (**648**), *Entamoeba nana* (**649**), *Iodamoeba bütschlii* (**650**), *Dientamoeba fragilis* (**651**). *E. histolytica* cannot be distinguished morphologically from *E. dispar*. (**647** and **648** trichrome stain; **649–651** haematoxylin). (× 1500) [*D. fragilis* is now classified in the order Trichomonadida. It has been shown to have significant clinical importance as a cause of acute and chronic abdominal pain but its life history remains unknown (*see* Stark *et al*; 2006 in Bibliography).]

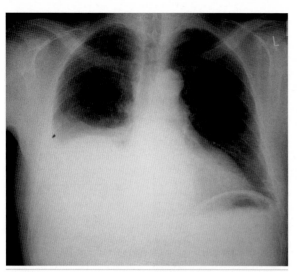

668 Chest radiograph in a patient with amoebiasis
One of the characteristic findings in a patient with amoebic liver abscess is a raised right hemidiaphragm, often with adjoining pulmonary collapse.

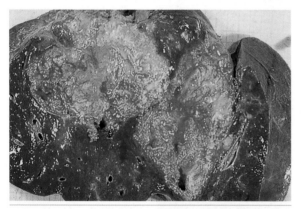

670 Macroscopic appearance of liver abscess at autopsy
The shaggy, irregular periphery consists of stroma and layers of compressed liver parenchyma.

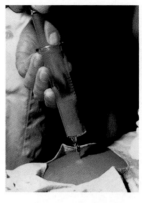

669 Aspiration of liver abscess
Aspiration of large abscesses is sometimes needed as an adjunct to specific chemotherapy for successful treatment, especially when the abscess is very large or close to the surface of the liver, with the risk of rupture. The pus is said to be 'chocolate-coloured'; some have likened it to 'anchovy sauce'.

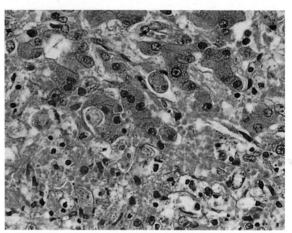

671 Section of amoebic liver abscess
Trophozoites, some containing ingested red blood cells, are seen in the tissues at the edge of the abscess and may be found in the pus if it is examined immediately after aspiration. (*H&E × 150*)

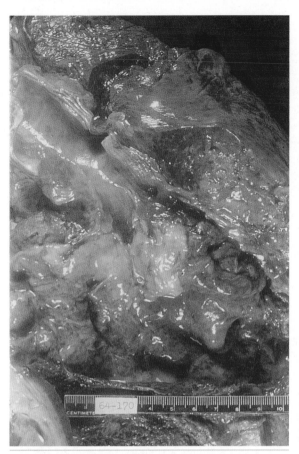

672 Amoebic abscess of lung

Extraintestinal infections occur commonly in the liver, but any site of the body may be affected. The lung and the pericardium are sometimes affected by rupture of a hepatic abscess through the diaphragm. Typical amoebic pus may be coughed up in the sputum.

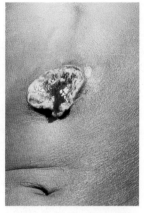

673 Amoebiasis of the skin

Amoebic infection of the skin may arise by direct spread from a primary abscess. This patient was erroneously operated on for a perforated duodenal ulcer and no antiamoebic drugs were given. Sloughing of the skin occurred and amoebae were recovered from the skin lesion.

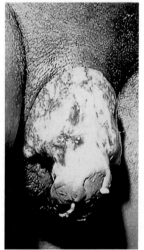

674 Amoebic balanitis

Amoebic infection of the genital organs can result from sexual intercourse. Although cysts are exceptionally common in homosexual males, the majority are attributable to nonpathogenic *E. dispar*.

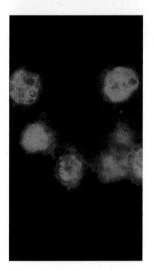

675 Fluorescent antibody staining of *Entamoeba histolytica*

The fluorescent antibody test (FAT), which is the most sensitive immunodiagnostic test available for invasive forms of amoebiasis, has proved a valuable adjunct to direct microscopical diagnosis. Fluorescence of cultured *E. histolytica* exposed to serum from a patient with hepatic involvement is seen in this figure. (× 780)

Giardiasis

Table 18 Protozoa (class Zoomastigophorea) of medical importance

Phylum/subphylum	Class	Order	Genus and species
Sarcomastigophora Sarcodina (see **Table 17**) Mastigophora	Zoomastigophorea (no vector)	Retortamonadida Diplomonadida Trichomonadida	*Chilomastix mesnili* *Giardia lamblia* *Trichomonas vaginalis* *Trichomonas hominis* *Dientamoeba fragilis**
	(invertebrate vector)	Kinetoplastida	*Leishmania* spp. (see **Tables 8** and **9**) *Trypanosoma* spp. (see **Table 7**)

* This parasite is now considered to be a flagellate and not an amoeba.

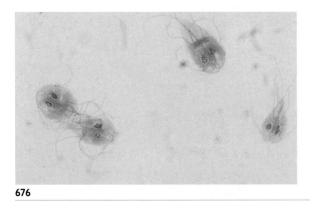

676

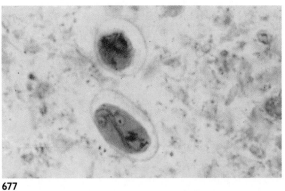

677

676 & 677 *Giardia lamblia* trophozoites and cysts

Giardiasis is probably the commonest globally distributed, water-borne protozoal infection. It has been estimated, for example, that 2 million new infections may be acquired in the USA each year from contaminated water. The flagellated trophozoites (**676**, left) attach by their suckers to the surface of the duodenal or jejunal mucosa. The ovoid cysts in faeces (**677**, right) have a very distinctive structure. They are able to survive standard chlorination procedures and filtration is required to ensure their exclusion from the drinking water supply. (**676** *Giemsa* × *1000*; **677** *trichrome* × *1230*)

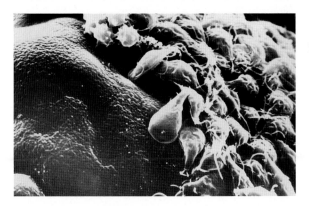

678 Scanning electron micrograph of *Giardia lamblia* in jejunal biopsy

The trophozoites are attached to the surface of the jejunal epithelium by sucker-like organelles that leave pit marks when they detach. Their ability to produce at least 12 variable surface proteins assists the trophozoites to evade host antibodies. Infection may therefore become chronic. (× *1000*)

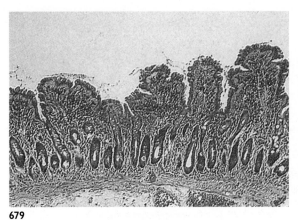

679

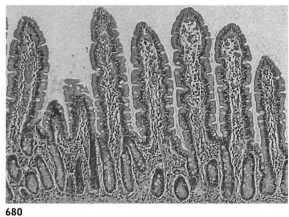

680

679 & 680 Jejunal epithelium

Severe infection with *G. lamblia* can result in partial villous atrophy of the duodenum or jejunum, with resulting flattening of the villi (**679**, left), compared with the normal pattern (**680**, right). Although the organism is commensal in many individuals, it is considered particularly pathogenic in children in the New World, and is a common cause of diarrhoea and a malabsorption syndrome characterised by steatorrhoea in travellers. Although in severe infections the trophozoites or cysts can usually be found in the faeces, they may be very sparse in chronic infections. The trophozoites can sometimes be obtained via a duodenal aspirate but serological methods have also been developed. An ELISA to detect IgM in serum provides evidence of current infection. A polyclonal antigen-capture ELISA can be used to demonstrate submicroscopic infections in faeces and an IgA-based ELISA will detect specific antibodies in saliva. (*H&E × 40*)

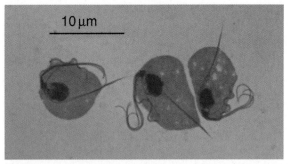

681

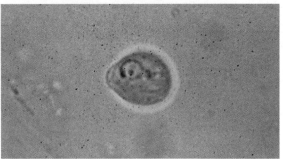

682

681–683 Other parasitic flagellates

Trichomonas vaginalis trophozoite as seen in culture (**681**) (see also **925**); *Cheilomastix mesnili* trophozoite (**682**) and cyst (**683**). *C. mesnili* is nonpathogenic. (Trophozoites *Giemsa*, cyst *eosin × 1800*)

683

Coccidial Infections See **Table 5**.

Most of the coccidial infections in humans are zoonoses. In immunocompetent individuals, they usually produce mild, self-limiting infection. However, toxoplasmosis in pregnancy poses a serious danger for the fetus, while most, if not all, of the parasites are able to cause serious pathological changes in immunocompromised people – notably those with human immunodeficiency virus (HIV) infection, of whom, for example, as many as 10% may pass oocysts of *Cryptosporidium hominis* (formerly known as *C. parvum*) (see **690–692**).

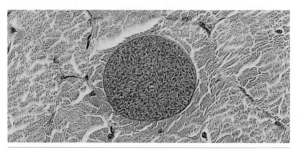

684 Section of sarcocyst in human muscle
In the muscles of the intermediate host, *Sarcocystis* forms fusiform cysts containing large numbers of bradyzoites. Although it is rarely diagnosed in life, this condition may be common in humans, who harbour the sarcocysts of a number of different species, none of which has so far been identified. 'Sarcocystis lindemanni' is no longer considered to be a valid species but is thought to represent accidental zoonotic infection with a variety of species of this genus. (*H&E × 375*)

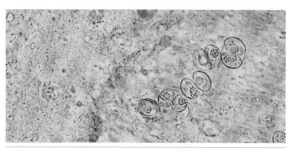

685 *Sarcocystis hominis*-like oocysts in intestinal epithelium
This coccidian parasite is common in humans and is acquired from the consumption of raw or inadequately cooked beef in which the sarcocyst stage occurs. In this case, humans are the definitive host. Sporulated oocysts or single sporocysts are passed in the faeces. *Sarcocystis suihominis* is acquired from pork. (*Phase contrast × 400*)

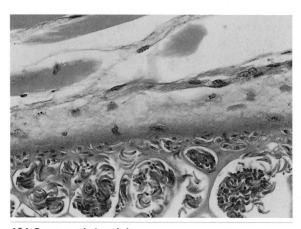

686 *Sarcocystis hominis*
The individual bradyzoites are seen within a large, fusiform sarcocyst in bovine muscle. (*H&E × 400*)

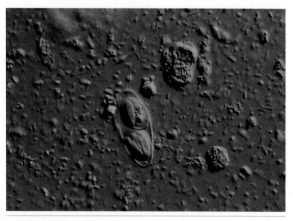

687 *Isospora belli* oocysts
Unsporulated oocysts of this species are passed in the faeces but they sporulate on storage to form eight sporozoites (of which five can be seen in this figure). The infection may be associated with diarrhoea, due to development of the parasite in the intestinal epithelium, or may be symptomless. Coccidian oocysts stain dark red with a modified Ziehl–Neelsen stain. (*Nomarksi optics × 450*)

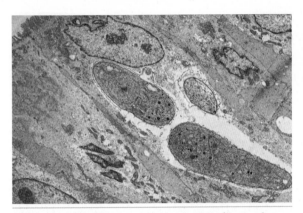

688 *Isospora belli* in a mucosal cell of the ileum of a patient with AIDS

The intracellular position of an immature oocyst containing sections of three sporozoites is clearly seen in this electron microscope image. In such immunocompromised individuals extraintestinal tissue cysts may also be located in lymphatic tissues such as those in liver, spleen and lymph nodes. (× 6300)

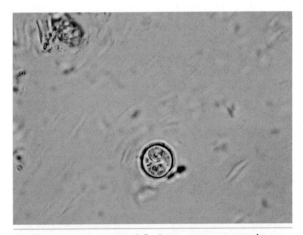

689 Sporulated oocyst of *Cyclospora cayetanensis*

This eimeriid parasite, which was first described in Peru in children with mild diarrhoea, has now been identified in countries as disparate as Mexico and the USA, the UK, Haiti, Nepal and Australia. Schizogony occurs within epithelial cells of the small intestine. When allowed to sporulate, for example in dichromate solution at 25–30°C for 1–2 weeks, *C. cayetanensis* produces two sporocysts, each with two sporozoites. Mixed infections with *Cryptosporidium* are common, and the two infections were formerly confused, especially since both may be associated with mild but chronic diarrhoea. Both are probably acquired from oocyst-contaminated water. A zoonotic reservoir of *C. cayetanensis* has not yet been identified. (*Saline* × 900)

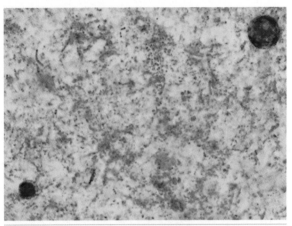

690 Oocysts of *Cryptosporidium hominis* and *Cyclospora cayetanensis* compared

C. hominis is enzootic in young calves. It is usually passed to humans in water containing oocysts, which survive normal chlorination and filtration. It causes outbreaks of self-limiting, mild diarrhoea in infants and small children (e.g. in day-care centres) but can also affect older people. Surveys have demonstrated a high level of seropositivity in normal, asymptomatic adults, over 50% in one outbreak. Rates as high as 75% have been recorded in young adolescents in rural China and 90% of infants in a Brazilian 'favela' were seropositive by the age of 1 year. In 1993 over 400 000 people suffered from diarrhoea when lake water near Milwaukee became contaminated following heavy rains. The use of the Ziehl–Neelsen stain on faecal smears or concentrates (made by sugar flotation) is a valuable technique both to detect the oocysts and particularly to reveal the existence of mixed infections. Both parasites stain red with Ziehl–Neelsen stain. However, *C. cayetanensis* typically takes up variable amounts of the stain and the oocysts are larger (8–10 µm, compared with 4–6 µm). The irregular staining helps to distinguish *C. cayetanensis* from the same-sized oocysts of *Toxoplasma gondii*, which are, of course, not found in human faeces (*Ziehl–Neelsen* × 850)

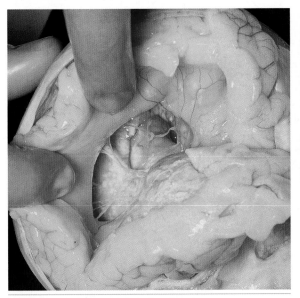

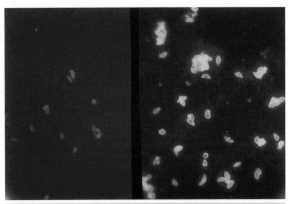

703 Post-mortem appearance of brain
Irregular areas of calcification in the lateral ventricles are seen in this brain of a 7-week-old child with toxoplasmosis. Mental disorders and blindness are common in children who survive. (See also **698** and **699**.)

704 Serological tests for toxoplasmosis
(Negative control, left; positive, right.) The Sabin Feldman dye test was formerly widely employed. Methylene blue stains *T. gondii* tachyzoites obtained from mouse peritoneal exudate but, in the presence of antibody-containing serum, the uptake of dye is inhibited by 50% or more. High titres occur in acute infections but a low positive titre remains indefinitely (see comment in **694**). Other useful serological tests are the complement fixation test (CFT), direct agglutination test and toxoplasmin skin test. The most direct test is the indirect fluorescent antibody test (IFAT) shown here, in which antigen consists of cultured tachyzoites.

Microsporidiosis

The medical importance of microsporidial infections in humans has only recently been highlighted by the frequent recognition of these parasites in material from patients with HIV infection and AIDS (see **Table 19**).

Table 19 Microsporidiosis in humans

Genus and species	Sites	Geographical distribution	Notes
Pleistophora spp.	Striated muscle	USA	Two cases, immunocompromised ♂ ♂, one HIV⁺, one HIV⁻
Encephalitozoon cuniculi	Brain, kidney, liver,	? Global	Very rare, four cases HIV⁻ or HIV⁺
Encephalitozoon hellem	Systemic spread to nose, eye, lung, kidney, etc.	? Global	May be transmitted via sputum, urine, nasal aerosol; known only from HIV⁺ patients
Enterocytozoon bieneusi	Small and large intestine, gall bladder, bile duct, lung, nasal epithelium	Global	Found in 6–30% of all AIDS patients with chronic diarrhoea; one case HIV⁻

continued

Table 19 Microsporidiosis in humans—*cont'd*

Nosema corneum	Eye		Single case, HIV⁻
Nosema ocularum	Eye		Single case, HIV⁻
Nosema connori	Striated and smooth muscle, generalised	USA	Single, immunodeficient (athymic) infant
Septata intestinalis	Small and large intestine, kidney, liver, gall bladder, bronchial epithelium, systemic spread	Global	Found in about 2% of all AIDS patients with chronic diarrhoea
'*Microsporidium africanum*'	Eye	Botswana	Single case, adult ♀
'*Microsporidium ceylonensis*'	Eye	Sri Lanka	Single case, 11-year-old ♂

The classification of some species is still disputed. Infections with other species in immunocompromised individuals have been reported recently.

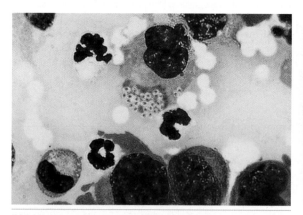

705 Microsporidia in a plasmacytoma cell
A clump of spores, probably of a species of *Encephalitozoon*, is seen in the cytoplasm of a macrophage in this bone marrow smear from a patient with a plasmacytoma. This is a rare case of microsporidiosis being detected in an immunocompromised but HIV-negative patient. (*Giemsa × 1800*)

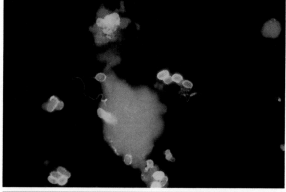

706 *Encephalitozoon hellem* in cell culture
This parasite produces a disseminated infection in immunocompromised patients. *E. hellem* causes severe keratoconjunctivitis and has also been found in the urine in patients with signs of urinary tract disease. Spores have been identified, moreover, in sputum, nasal swabs and faeces. Some of the spores seen here in tissue culture and stained with a specific antibody have extruded their polar filaments. (*IFAT × 2000*) (See also **900**.)

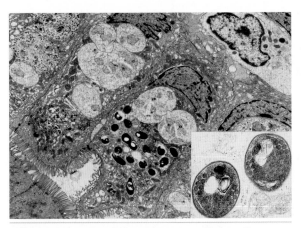

707 Mature spores of *Enterocytozoon bieneusi* in human jejunal enterocyte

Previously considered to be nonpathogenic in humans, infections are now being detected (particularly by biopsy) in individuals with chronic enteritis, cholangitis and cholecystitis who are immunocompromised, especially by AIDS (see also **901**). Their possible pathogenic role has, however, not yet been determined. Microsporidia are also suspected as a cause of ill-defined neurological manifestations. Note that the coils of the spiral filament of the spores seen in this biopsy lie in two rows in cross-section. The parasite develops in direct contact with the host cell cytoplasm. (Main section × *2800*; inset × *14 000*)

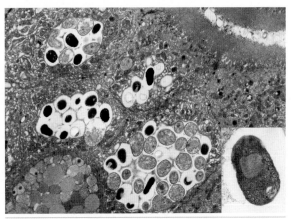

708 Mature spores of *Septata intestinalis*

This microsporidian is associated with nephritis and can also produce a similar clinical picture to that seen with *E. bieneusi*. Like that parasite, *S. intestinalis* develops in small-intestinal enterocytes but within a type of parasitophorous vacuole. The cross-section of a spore shows the coils of spiral filament lying in a single row. (Main section × *2800*; inset × *14 000*)

Balantidiasis

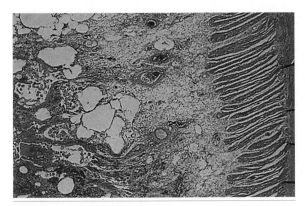

709 Balantidial ileitis

Balantidium coli is a common commensal of the large intestine of wild and domestic pigs but is pathogenic to humans and other primates, in which it causes severe diarrhoea. Active, flagellated trophozoites and cysts are readily found in fresh faecal specimens. Numerous trophozoites are seen invading the submucosa in this section of human ileum. (*H&E* × *10*)

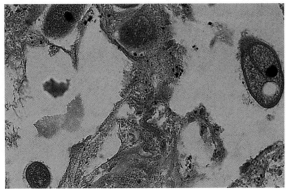

710 Trophozoites of *Balantidium coli*

Extensive ulceration of the ileum, colon and rectum may occur in severe cases. The characteristic morphology of *B. coli* trophozoites with their macronuclei and micronuclei is seen in this section. (*H&E* × *160*)

HELMINTHIASES – NEMATODES

See **Table 11** for classification and **404–418** for eggs.

Trichinosis

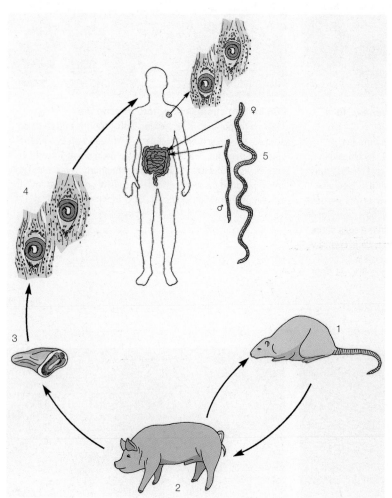

711 Life cycle of *Trichinella spiralis*
This nematode is a zoonotic infection that circulates between rats (1) and various carnivores. Trichinosis in humans commonly results from eating raw or inadequately cooked pork or pork products such as sausages. Domestic pigs (2) and wild boar usually acquire the infection by eating infected rats (1). Cycles of infection also exist in wild Canidae and other carnivores that eat rodents. Infection is acquired by eating muscle (3) containing the encysted larvae (4). These excyst in the small intestine and develop into minute adults (5) in the mucosa. About 5 days after infection, the females, now mature, deposit larvae, which migrate through the tissues to reach skeletal muscles, in which they again encyst. Larviposition may continue for a week or more. Finally, the larvae become calcified. Three other species (or subspecies) that can infect humans have been described in this genus: *Trichinella nelsoni* in parts of Africa and southern Europe, *Trichinella nativa* in the Arctic region and *Trichinella pseudospiralis*, which is now known to be widely distributed. In 1999 *T. pseudospiralis* was responsible for a number of human infections acquired from wild boar in the south of France.

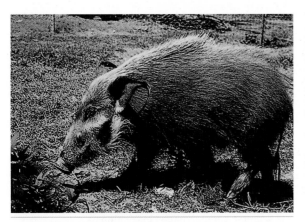

712 Wild reservoir of trichinosis
A common reservoir of infection is the wild pig, such as the African bush pig seen here. The flesh of other carnivores, such as the bear, has also served to initiate isolated outbreaks of human infection, following hunting parties for example. Recent epidemiological surveys have shown that human trichinosis is increasing in all continents. In Chile, for example, calcified *T. spiralis* larvae were found in 2% of all autopsies in 1992.

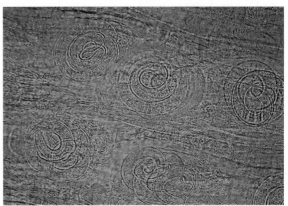

713 *Trichinella spiralis* larvae in crush preparation
The larvae are easily seen in pieces of muscle by crushing the tissue between two glass plates and inspecting it through a 'trichinoscope' (a simple magnifying system). (× *175*)

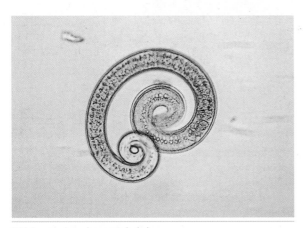

714 Larva free in gastric juice
The larvae can be freed for detailed examination by digesting a piece of contaminated muscle in artificial gastric juice. (× *175*)

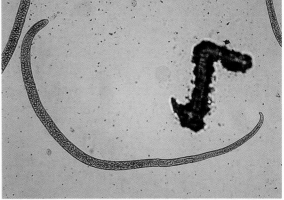

715 Parasitic female *Trichinella spiralis*
The adult female worm is about 2–3 mm long and 90 µm in diameter; the male 1.2 mm by 60 µm. (× *45*)

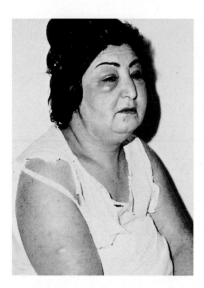

716 Patient with acute trichinosis

The four cardinal features of the disease are fever, orbital oedema, myalgia and eosinophilia.

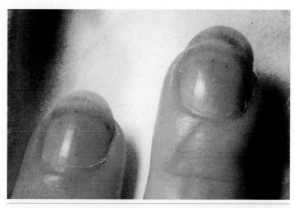

717 Splinter haemorrhages in trichinosis

Nailbed haemorrhages are a frequent sign in acute trichinosis.

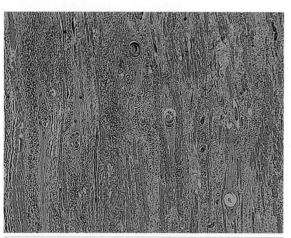

718 Larvae in muscle from a fatal human case

Many infections remain asymptomatic but heavy infections may lead to fatal myocarditis or encephalitis. Encysted larvae are found in the muscles at biopsy (or post-mortem). Calcification of the encysted larvae occurs after about 18 months in less severe infections and may be detected on X-ray, but the encysted larvae remain alive for years. (*H&E × 16*)

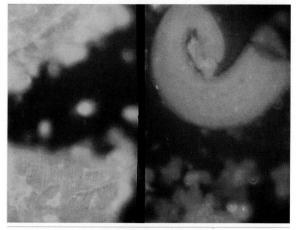

719 Fluorescent antibody test

Although immunity is largely cell-mediated, circulating antibodies to *T. spiralis* appear from 2–4 weeks after infection. Refined diagnostic antigens for their detection are currently being developed. For the present, a simple IFAT employing fragments of larvae as antigen is a useful diagnostic tool. Bentonite and latex tests with extracted larval antigens have also proved valuable in the acute stage, during which high antibody titres develop. An ELISA is also available. (Right, negative control.)

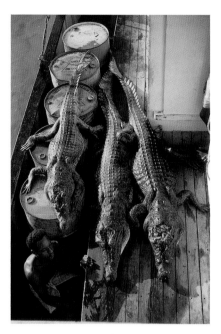

720 *Crocodylus porosus*, the estuarine crocodile

A number of species of aquatic reptiles harbour species of *Trichinella*. Antibodies to a newly described parasite of the saltwater crocodile *C. porosus*, *Trichinella papuae*, have been identified in nearly one-third of villagers, two-thirds of them males, in an area in the south-west corner of Papua New Guinea. The source for humans is the wild pig. In the same area, larvae of this nematode have been found in nearly 9% of wild pigs, which are widely hunted and often consumed inadequately or uncooked. Domestic pigs in that area have also been found infected. Another parasitic nematode of this genus, *Trichinella zimbabwensis*, has been recorded in 40% of farmed Nile crocodiles (*Crocodylus niloticus*). This African parasite has also been found in a number of wild mammals, which it readily infects. Since crocodile farming is increasing it is likely that these parasites will be identified in future years in humans with clinical evidence of trichinosis unless precautions are taken such as the screening of reptiles for larvae in tissues or the freezing of the meat. By 1998 national breeding programmes established in 30 countries were already generating an income equivalent to US$60 million.

Capillariasis

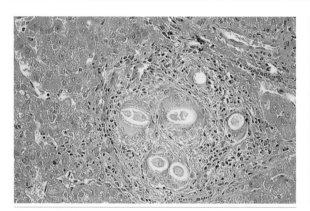

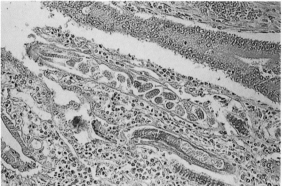

721 *Capillaria hepatica* in liver section

Human infection with this rodent nematode is very rare. In the rat, the worms have a direct life cycle resembling that of *Trichuris*. The adults live in the portal tracts. Eggs, also resembling those of *Trichuris* (see **413**), are infective only after undergoing maturation in the soil. Adult worms in the liver cause hepatic enlargement and severe parenchymal damage. Note the giant-cell reaction around the eggs. (*H&E × 150*)

722 *Capillaria philippinensis* invading small intestine

This species, the adults of which live in the upper small intestine, has occurred in epidemic form. A chronic malabsorption syndrome, which is sometimes fatal, develops in heavy infections. The parasites are acquired by eating raw, infected fish, which are the intermediate hosts. Monkeys appear to be the normal definitive host. Individual cases have been reported from a wide geographical area: from the Philippines as far west as Iran, the United Arab Emirates and Egypt. (*H&E × 150*)

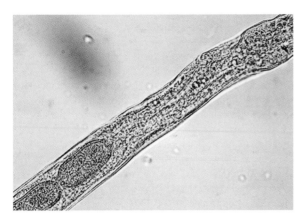

723 Female *Capillaria philippinensis* from human faeces
The figure shows the vulval region of the female in which two typical eggs can be seen. (× *300*)

Parastrongyliasis and eosinophilic meningitis

(The species *Angiostrongylus cantonensis* and *Angiostrongylus costaricensis* have been reclassified in the genus *Parastrongylus* – see **Table 11**. The term 'angiostrongyliasis' should, therefore, now be replaced by 'parastrongyliasis'.)

Species of *Parastrongylus* that infect humans could be classified as being 'mollusc-transmitted' but are grouped in this section for convenience. The main cause of eosinophilic meningitis is infection with larvae of the rat nematode *Parastrongylus cantonensis*. Originally common throughout southeast Asia, this parasite has spread geographically in recent years with the dissemination of one of its best intermediate hosts, the giant African land snail (*Achatina fulica*), which is a popular item of food in some countries. Rats or humans are infected by eating infected molluscs or food contaminated by the snails' bodies.

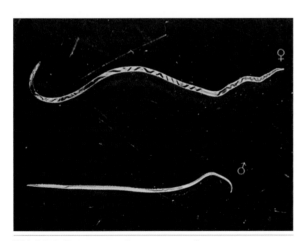

724 Adult *Parastrongylus cantonensis*
The adult worm, about 1–2 cm long, is a common parasite of rodents in the Far East and the Pacific. It lives in the pulmonary arteries and arterioles. (× *3.5*)

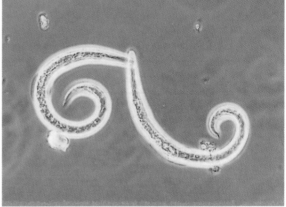

725 First-stage larvae of *Parastrongylus cantonensis* in rat faeces
The eggs, passed in the bloodstream, break through the pulmonary tract, are swallowed by the rodent and are passed in the faeces, in which they may hatch to first-stage larvae. (× *160*)

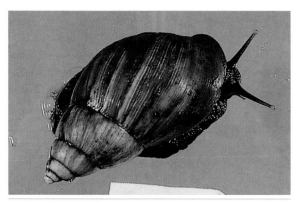

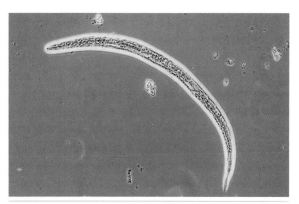

726 *Lissachatina fulica*, an intermediate host of *Parastrongylus cantonensis*
The first-stage larvae in rat faeces are eaten by snails of various genera (including *Lissachatina, Cipangopaludina* and *Bradybaena*) as well as by some slugs and land planarians in which the larvae develop to the third stage. *L. fulica* is sometimes kept in vivaria as a 'pet' or for educational purposes in schools. It is important to ensure that such molluscs are locally bred and not imported from countries where *P. cantonensis* is enzootic. (*Half life-size*)

727 Third-stage larvae in *Lissachatina fulica*
New rats become infested when they eat snails containing third-stage larvae. (× *100*)

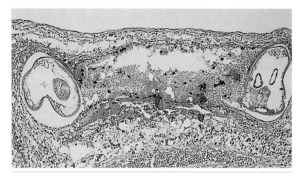

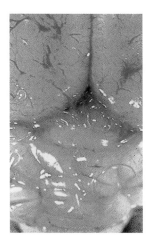

728 Larvae of *Parastrongylus cantonensis* in rat brain
The thread-like larvae can be seen in the subarachnoid space covering the base of this rat brain. Here, they mature to young adults, which migrate to the pulmonary arteries via the cerebral veins.

729 Section of *Parastrongylus cantonensis* larvae in meninges of human brain
Humans may be infested by eating freshwater prawns but how these come to contain larvae is uncertain. Infection may also be acquired by eating molluscs that contain larvae, or food contaminated with crushed molluscs. The larvae migrate to the brain, where they cause eosinophilic meningitis or meningoencephalitis. The diagnosis is aided by the serological examination of paired specimens, using a specific antigen from adult worms. (× *60*)

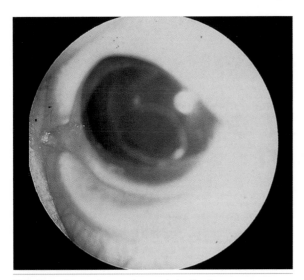

730 *Parastrongylus cantonensis* in the human eye
The adult nematode is seen floating in the anterior chamber of the eye of a 15-month-old Taiwanese child suffering from eosinophilic meningoencephalitis.

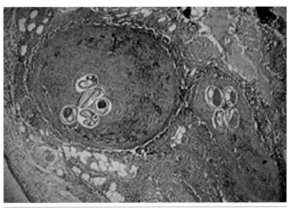

731 *Parastrongylus costaricensis* in a mesenteric vessel
This enzootic of cotton rats, black rats and other species of rodent as well as, on occasion, larger animals, is widely distributed in the New World and has also been found in Africa. Slugs are the intermediate hosts. Humans are occasionally infected by eating fruit or vegetables contaminated by infective larvae that have been shed by slugs with their mucus. In parts of Central America up to 85% of the slug *Vaginulus plebeius* have been found to be infected. In Costa Rica the prevalence of human infection has been estimated as 18 cases per 100 000 inhabitants. The larvae develop into adults in the mesenteric blood vessels (in contrast to *P. cantonensis*) and give rise to eosinophilic granuloma masses, a condition also known as Morera's disease. The symptoms, which include abdominal pain, vomiting and diarrhoea, and anorexia, are often mistaken for those of appendicitis, while abdominal masses may arouse suspicion of a malignancy. The presence of a high eosinophil count is a guide to the diagnosis. This figure shows cross-sections of adult worms in a mesenteric vessel occluded by a thrombus and surrounded by inflammatory exudate and eosinophils. (*H&E* × 25)

Enterobiasis

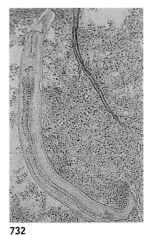

732

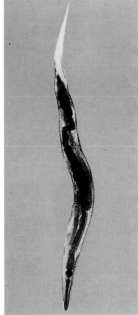

733

732 & 733 Adult Enterobius vermicularis

These 'pinworms' are small, white and thread-like. The males (**732**, left) have coiled tails and measure 2.5 mm in length. The females (**733**, right), which are about 10 mm long, emerge to the perianal region, where they lay some 10 000–15 000 eggs and then die. In the process, they cause severe pruritus. The embryonated eggs, which are directly infectious on ingestion, hatch in the duodenum; the larvae pass to the caecum where they mature. (♂ × 20; ♀ × 11)

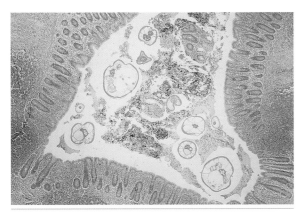

734 Adult pinworms in appendix

The worms are occasionally found in the appendix but their role as a cause of acute appendicitis is uncertain. Sections of several adult worms are seen here (*H&E* × 13)

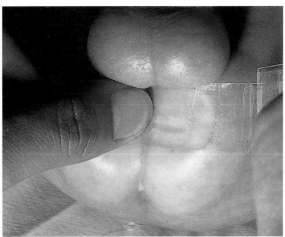

735

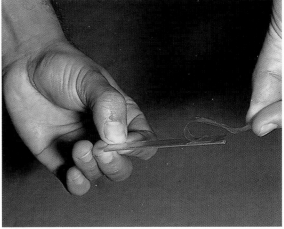

736

735 & 736 Scotch-tape swab to demonstrate perianal eggs

The eggs (see **414**) are found on the perianal skin. They adhere to the Scotch tape, which can then be placed on a slide and examined directly under a microscope. Because of severe pruritus ani, children frequently reinfect themselves from eggs under their fingernails. Bedding is also a source of infection, which tends to persist in households and institutions such as orphanages.

Anisakiasis

This term is used for human infection with the larvae of *Anisakis simplex* or *Pseudoterranova decipiens*. These are common nematode parasites the adults of which live in the stomach of marine mammals. There the worms produce eggs that are discharged with the faeces. The first-stage larvae progress to the second stage in the egg and these hatch when the eggs are eaten by krill. In these invertebrates they mature to the third stage, which encyst in the viscera or muscles of sea fish or squid that eat the krill.

A. simplex infects numerous species such as salmon, pollack, herring (hence the term 'herring worm' in Holland) or mackerel. *P. decipiens* mainly parasitises cod and halibut. Infection is acquired by consuming uncooked and even pickled fish – a custom that is very popular in countries such as Japan but that is no longer prevalent in Europe. In humans the larvae may moult to the fourth stage but they do not mature into adults.

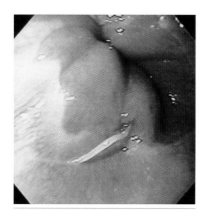

737 Third-stage larva of *Anisakis simplex*

This figure shows the larva as visualised through an endoscope in the stomach of a 39-year-old Japanese woman. The consumption of raw fish is very popular in some countries of the Far East, especially Japan. Various symptoms may develop following infection with *Anisakis*, depending upon the location of the larvae as they move further down the intestine. The most common site to be invaded is the gastric mucosa. This causes severe gastric pain within about 6 hours after the larvae are ingested. If the condition is diagnosed early, surgical removal is called for. The consumption of pickled herring in Holland used to be associated with anisakiasis ('green herring disease') but the compulsory freezing of all herring prior to consumption has now all but eliminated the condition there.

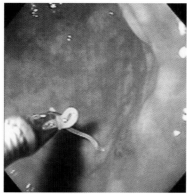

738 Removal of fourth-stage larva of *Anisakis simplex*

The third-stage larvae may moult to the fourth stage in the human host. The figure shows the removal with biopsy forceps through an endoscope of a fourth-stage larva from the gastric mucosa of an 80-year-old Japanese woman.

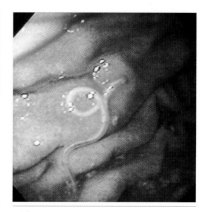

739 Larval *Pseudoterranova decipiens*

The whitish-coloured third-stage larvae, about 2 cm long, are less invasive than those of *A. simplex* but may invade the gastric mucosa, causing acute epigastric pain within a few hours of their being ingested. Frequently they are vomited before invasion occurs. This third-stage larva in the stomach of a 59-year-old Japanese woman has burrowed into the mucosa.

Gnathostomiasis

740 Life cycle of *Gnathostoma spinigerum*

Several species of the spirurid genus *Gnathostoma* are responsible for zoonotic infections in humans. The larvae of *G. spinigerum* are acquired mainly from various freshwater fish, especially in Thailand and Japan. Those of *Gnathostoma hispidum* are acquired from inadequately cooked pork. In the definitive hosts, which are usually carnivores such as cats (1), tigers, leopards and dogs, the adult nematodes live in nodules in the stomach wall. Eggs (2) passed in the faeces develop and sheathed first-stage larvae hatch when they reach water; when these larvae (3) are ingested by species of *Cyclops* (4) they moult to produce second-stage larvae in these first intermediate hosts. When the *Cyclops* are swallowed by fish (5) or frogs (6), the larvae pierce their gastric wall and develop into the third-stage larvae, which become encysted. If eaten by the definitive hosts, the third-stage larvae penetrate into their stomach walls and there mature to adults. If infected fish or frogs are eaten by other vertebrates, which act as paratenic hosts (see **587**), such as

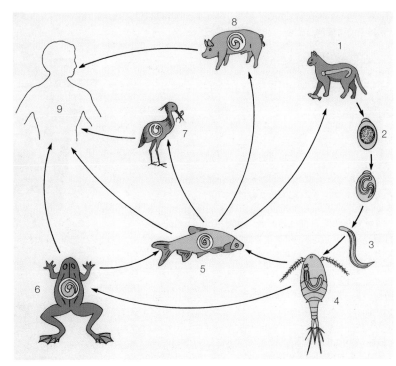

herons (7), pigs (8) or humans (9), they do not mature but migrate through the subcutaneous tissues, where they are manifested as 'larva migrans'. In a lakeside village the consumption of a popular raw fish dish infected with *Gnathostoma doloresi* caused a minor outbreak of acute gnathostomiasis, the first recorded on the American continent. A serological survey of 309 local villagers exposed a positivity rate of 35%.

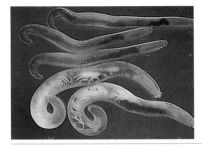

741 Living adult *Gnathostoma spinigerum*

The male worms have a red tail and the larger females a more curled one. (× 1.3)

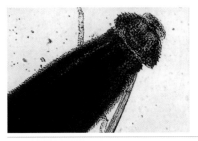

742 Head of adult *Gnathostoma spinigerum*

The adult usually lives in the stomach of dogs, cats and wild felines. It is found throughout south-east Asia. There are two intermediate hosts. Humans acquire infection by eating fermented fish (a delicacy in Thailand) or any other form of raw fish. The parasite cannot mature in humans but migrates, causing cutaneous and visceral larva migrans. (× 30)

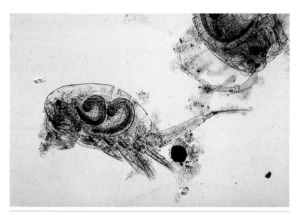

743 Early third-stage larvae of *Gnathostoma nipponicum* in a *Eucyclops serrulatus*
Several species of *Gnathostoma* have been incriminated in human infection in different continents. They include this species, for which a definitive host is the Japanese weasel. Larvae hatching from eggs that are passed with faeces into fresh water infect *Cyclops* water fleas and, later, fish that eat the *Cyclops*. The early third-stage larvae develop in the body cavity of the copepod within 7–10 days. They remain in this stage until the crustacean is ingested by a vertebrate host such as a freshwater fish, frog or possibly a small rodent. The larvae then penetrate from the intestine to take up a position in the new (second intermediate) host's muscles, where the late third-stage larvae form cysts about 1 mm in diameter. (× 75)

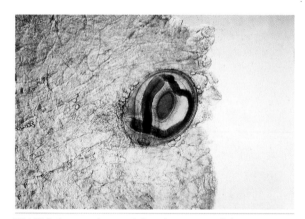

744 Third-stage larva of *Gnathostoma spinigerum* encysted in fish muscle
Spiced raw fish known as *somfak* and fermented fish such as that sold in Thai markets are a potential source of several helminths, including *G. spinigerum*. Infection may also be acquired from paratenic hosts that devour small fish that harbour the third stage larvae, for example, crabs, larger fish, amphibia, reptiles, rodents or chickens. Successive passages to paratenic hosts may occur, including, of course, to humans who also serve (with rare exceptions when the adult stage develops in the stomach) as a paratenic host if they consume, uncooked, any other animal harbouring third-stage larvae.

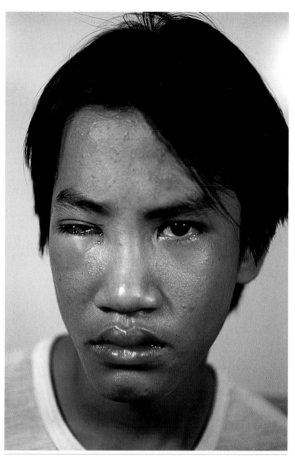

745 Periorbital larva migrans
One of the characteristic clinical features is a migrating subcutaneous swelling associated with boring pain and eosinophilia. Third-stage *Gnathostoma* larvae may be recovered surgically from swellings in suitable locations. Cerebral lesions with focal signs are not uncommon in Thailand.

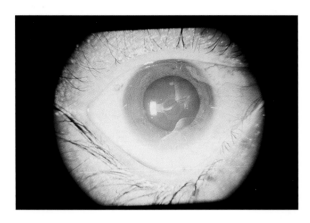

746 Late third-stage larva of *Gnathostoma spinigerum* in the eye

The figure shows a migrating third-stage larva of *G. spinigerum* in the anterior chamber of the eye of a Thai patient.

Dracunculiasis (dracontiasis, Guinea worm infection)

The 'Medina worm', so called because of its former frequency in that Arabian city, used to be widely distributed across Africa, the Middle East and south Asia. Small zoonotic foci also existed in parts of South America; in North America it is enzootic in various carnivores. Since the introduction of improved water supplies and the start of a global eradication campaign in 1986, its distribution and the numbers of cases in formerly afflicted regions have decreased rapidly. A major impact on transmission was made when a simple water filter was introduced to sieve out copepods from contaminated water (see **751**). In the 1980s, when 120 million people were at risk, the annual global incidence fell from about 3.5 to 2 million, and Guinea worm disease has now been eradicated from Pakistan, India, Yemen, Senegal, Cameroon, Chad, Kenya and Uganda. The numbers have also decreased spectacularly in some of the previously most highly infected parts of Africa, where, by the end of 2004, only 15 187 cases were reported in the remaining 11 endemic countries. In five of these fewer than 100 cases were notified and, in another four, fewer than 500 cases. Only Sudan and Ghana still reported about 7000 cases each. On a global basis a total of a mere 15 000 cases was recorded, a massive fall below the 1986 level and total eradication appears to be within reach. However, an infection was discovered in a domestic dog in Pakistan several years after human dracunculiasis had been declared to have been eradicated there. As this animal may have acquired the infection via an unidentified human carrier, vigilance must be maintained in such 'clean' areas in order to detect other possible residual infections in the human community.

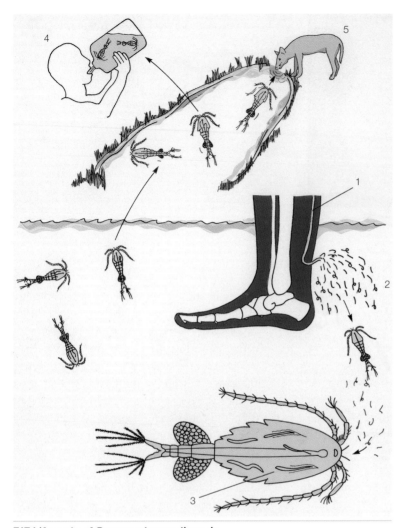

747 Life cycle of *Dracunculus medinensis*
(1) The mature female worm in the subcutaneous tissues of the human host causes
the formation of a blister, which bursts when the skin is immersed in fresh water and
through which the female's uterus releases large numbers of active, rhabditiform
larvae (2). Larvae that are swallowed by copepods present in the water penetrate the
gut wall and enter the new host's body cavity, where they grow and undergo two
moults (3). When infected water fleas are swallowed by humans in untreated drinking
water (4), the larvae are released to penetrate the wall of the duodenum. They
migrate through the body and, after undergoing two further moults, males and
females mate in the subcutaneous tissues, the males subsequently dying. Fertilised
females migrate along the muscle planes and finally reach the subcutaneous tissues,
commonly those of the lower limbs but sometimes the upper limbs or other parts of
the body. They are ready to oviposit about 1 year after reaching the human host. Other
animals that can be infected include dogs (5), horses, cows and some species of
monkey.

Dipylidium caninum (dog tapeworm)

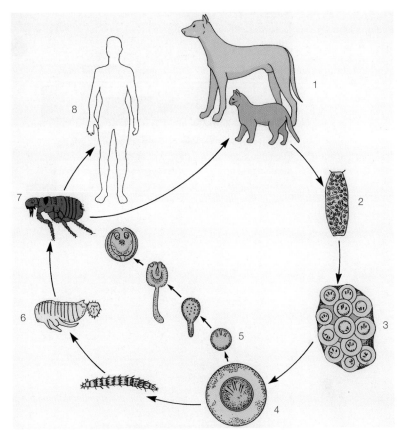

761 Life cycle of *Dipylidium caninum*
(1) The adult cestode (length 10–70 cm) in the small intestine of dogs, cats or wild canids produces proglottids, which may be passed in the faeces intact (2) or may degenerate, releasing clusters of encapsulated eggs (3). Oncospheres (4) hatching from eggs ingested by flea larvae remain undeveloped until the larvae pupate, whereupon they develop into cysticercoids (5). The cysticercoids undergo a complicated metamorphosis in the body cavities of the pupal (6) and adult fleas (7) and (8, 1) pass into the small intestine of the definitive host when it accidentally ingests the fleas, there everting the hooked rostellum to attach to the gut wall, where it will mature into an adult.

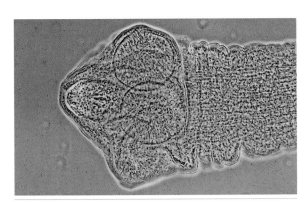

762 Scolex of *Dipylidium caninum*
This cestode, the adult of which reaches a length of 10–70 cm, is the common tapeworm of domestic and wild canines and felines. (× *15*)

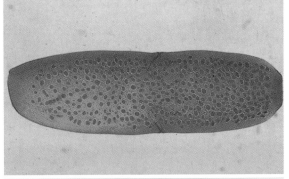

763 Mature segment of *Dipylidium caninum*
The cestode sheds whitish, mature segments, which are passed in the faeces or escape from the anus. The segments are visibly but slowly motile. (× *9*)

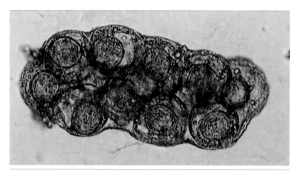

764 Egg capsule

In addition to mature segments, encapsulated clusters of eggs in which larval hooks may be seen are passed as the mature segments disintegrate. (× *240*)

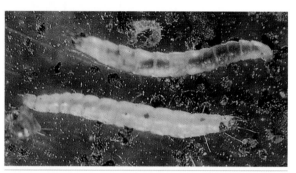

765 First instar larvae of *Ctenocephalides felis*

The eggs are ingested by larval cat, dog, or human fleas. They develop first procercoid, then cysticercoid larvae in the haemocoel of the insects, in which they remain when the fleas grow to the adult stage. These are cat flea larvae. (× *12*)

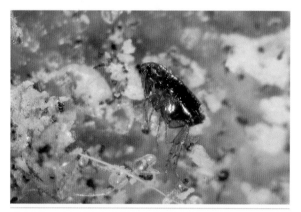

766 Male cat flea: *Ctenocephalides felis*

Humans becomes infected by inadvertently swallowing infected fleas from dogs or cats. (× *14*).

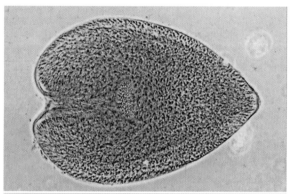

767 Immature cysticercoid from dog flea
(× *100*)

Vampirolepis nana (dwarf tapeworm)

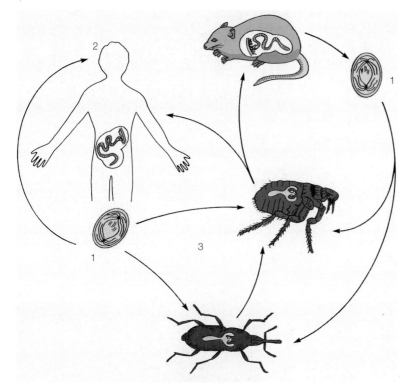

768 Life cycle of *Vampirolepis nana*

(1) Eggs released from mature proglottids in the upper ileum are passed in the faeces. (2) If ingested by another person, they hatch to yield hexacanth oncospheres, which burrow into the villi of the small intestine. There they mature into tailless cysticercoids (oncocysts), which migrate towards the ileum, where the scolices become attached to commence the formation of proglottids. (3) Eggs that are ingested by such insects as fleas, beetles or cockroaches hatch to form tailed cysticercoids, which remain unmodified as long as they are within the insect's body cavity. (4) If infected insects are accidentally ingested, the cysticercoids pass down the intestine to establish themselves in the ileum of the new vertebrate host. In this way rodents, as well as humans, may be infected, although the commoner parasite of rodents is *Vampirolepis nana* var. *fraterna*.

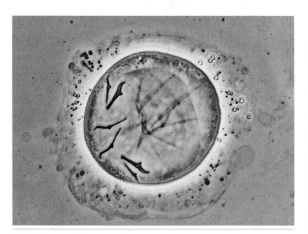

769 Hexacanth oncosphere

This cosmopolitan tapeworm reaches only 2.5–4 cm in length. Human infection is usually acquired directly by ingesting eggs. After ingestion by a mammal or by certain insects, the eggs (see **415**) hatch into the hexacanth oncospheres. (*Phase contrast × 1150*)

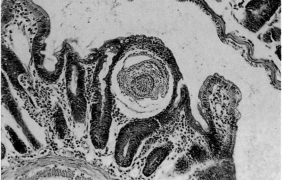

770 Cercocyst in intestinal villi

In the mammal, the oncospheres penetrate into the villi of the small intestine. There they mature into tailless cysticercoids (cercocysts), which leave the villi, move further down the gut and become attached to other villi, where they mature to adult tapeworms. (× *140*).

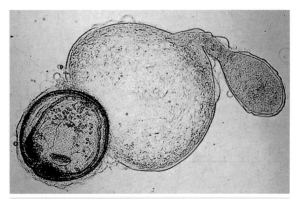

771 Cysticercoid in insect
If the egg is eaten by an insect, the oncosphere
metamorphoses to form a tailed cysticercoid in the insect's
body cavity. Further development takes place if the insect is
ingested by humans. (× 90)

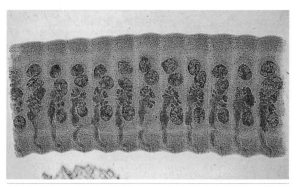

772 Mature proglottids
Humans are the only important source of human infection,
since rodents are parasitised normally by a strain that does not
develop in humans. (× 25)

Hymenolepis diminuta (rat tapeworm)

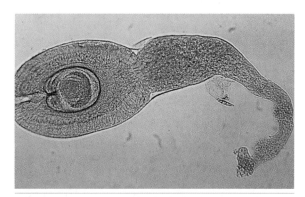

**773 Cysticercoid of *Hymenolepis diminuta* in an
arthropod**
The adults of this, the common cestode of rodents, are 20–60 cm
long. Their eggs (see **416**) resemble those of *Vampirolepis
nana* but lack the polar filaments. An intermediate insect host is
essential in this life cycle and a wide variety of coprophagic
arthropods serve as intermediate hosts. Occasionally humans
are infected by accidentally swallowing infected arthropods
(e.g. rat fleas, or larvae of grain moths and beetles). (× 90)

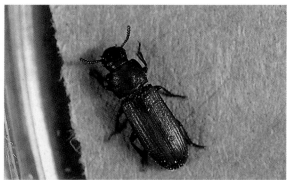

774 *Tribolium confusum*
These grain pests are typical intermediate hosts of *H. diminuta*.
(× 6.5)

Taenia solium (pork tapeworm)

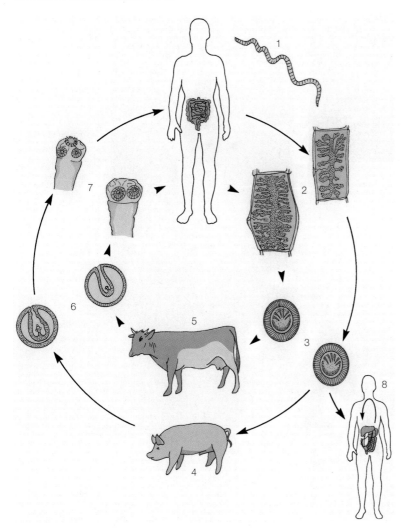

775 Life cycle of *Taenia solium*, *Taenia asiatica* and *Taenia saginata*
The adults (1) of both species live in the small intestine of humans, the definitive host. The gravid segments (2) are very active and escape through the anus, releasing large numbers of eggs (3) in the perianal region or on the ground, where they can survive for long periods. Faecal egg loads are, therefore, relatively light. When ingested by pigs (4) (*T. solium, T. asiatica*) or cattle (5) (*T. saginata*), the eggs hatch, each releasing an oncosphere, which migrates through the intestinal wall and blood vessels to reach striated muscle within which it encysts, forming cysticerci (6). When inadequately cooked meat containing the cysts is eaten by humans, the oncospheres excyst (7), settle in the small intestine and develop there into adult cestodes (1) over the next 3 months or so. The segments of *T. solium* are somewhat less active than those of the beef tapeworm but its eggs, if released in the upper intestine, can invade the host (autoinfection) (8), setting up the potentially dangerous larval infection known as cysticercosis in muscle, brain or any other site. To date *T. asiatica* has only been identified (by mitochondrial DNA analysis) in Taiwan, Thailand, Korea, China, Malaysia and the Philippines. Its public health significance is still uncertain.

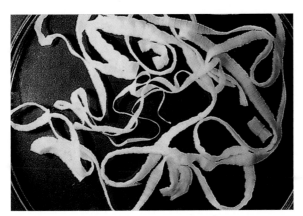

776 Head and part of segments of adult tapeworm
T. solium may reach 2–8 m in length and multiple infections can occur.

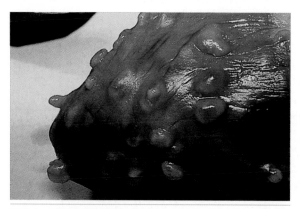

777 Cysticercus in pork
The larval cysticercoid stage occurs in the pig, giving rise to 'measly pork'. Humans are infected by ingesting the meat when it is inadequately cooked. (× 2.0)

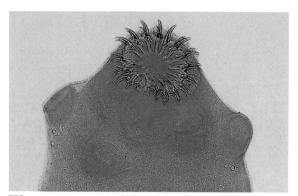

778

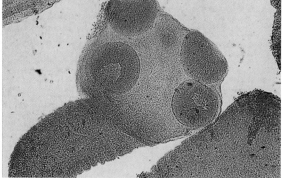

779

778 & 779 Scolices of *Taenia solium* and *Taenia saginata*
The head of *T. solium* (**778**) is armoured with hooks in addition to four suckers. *T. saginata* (**779**) has no hooks. The segments of *T. asiatica* resemble those of *T. saginata*. (× 40)

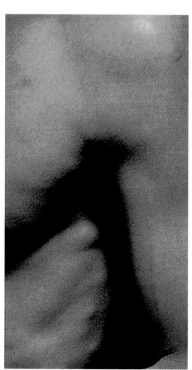

780 *Taenia solium* cysticerci in chest wall
Autoinfection can occur due to the release of eggs following the incorrect use of taeniacidal drugs. If regurgitation of gut contents carries mature segments with eggs into the stomach, the eggs can invade the human tissues, just as they do those of the pig. The cysts (cysticerci cellulosae) may be formed in any tissue. This agricultural student was infected in Thailand.

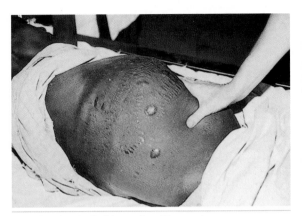

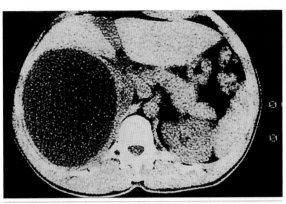

796 Massive hydatid cyst in a Kenyan boy

If humans accidentally ingest eggs, they become the host of the larval (hydatid cyst) stage, with the liver being most commonly affected. Hydatidosis is very common in the Turkana region of northern Kenya, where there is a close association between dogs and humans. A local custom was to use 'nurse dogs' to guard the household, where they were often encouraged to lick small infants clean, so encouraging infection with *E. granulosus* eggs. This young boy's abdomen bears the scars of local treatment aimed at alleviating pain over the grossly enlarged liver.

797 Computed tomography scan of hydatid cyst in liver

The hydatid cyst is usually unilocular, with a double wall comprised of an outer laminated layer and an inner nucleated germinal layer. The figure shows a massive cyst in the right lobe of the liver of a 14-year-old Kuwaiti boy.

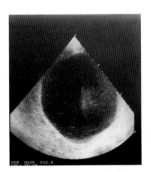

798 Ultrasound scan of hydatid cyst

(Same case as **797**). Diagnostically invaluable scans can be produced in any of the many hospitals equipped with ultrasound imaging technology.

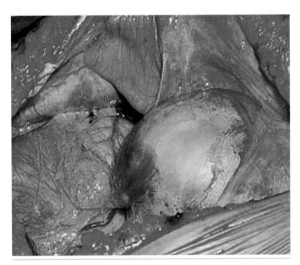

799 Hydatid cyst of the liver

Rupture of such a cyst can result in cardiovascular arrest caused by the sudden, massive release of antigens in the hydatid fluid. (Courtesy of Dr J Main. © Mosby, London.)

800 Gross pathology of liver hydatid

A large number of daughter cysts of various stages of growth is seen here in this postoperative specimen. (Courtesy of Dr R D Goldin.)

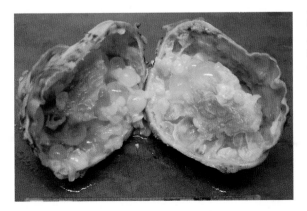

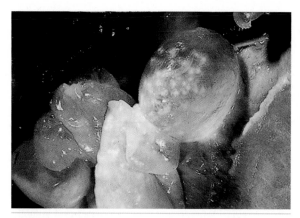

801 Daughter cysts

The germinal layer produces brood capsules inside which grow scolices.

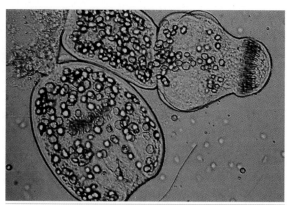

802 'Hydatid sand'

The daughter cysts are attached to the parent-cyst wall or may float free in its milky fluid contents as the so-called 'hydatid sand'. Rupture of a cyst into the tissues results in dissemination and further growth of the scolices. (× 250)

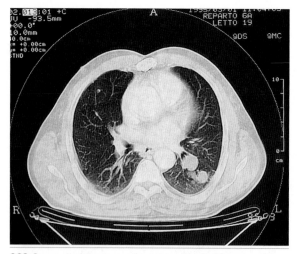

803 Computed tomography scan of hydatid cysts of lungs

Hydatid cysts may occur in 20–30% of infections. This CT scan demonstrates the fluid content of several pulmonary cysts.

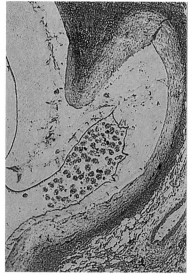

804 Hydatid cyst of lung

Section of cyst removed from a lung, showing the multilayered cyst wall and numerous daughter cysts produced by the germinal layer. (H&E × 40)

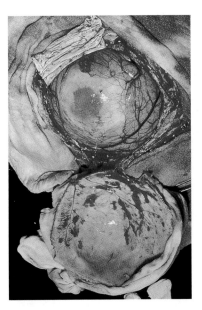

805 Hydatid cyst in brain

This cyst was found in the brain of a 4-year-old girl.

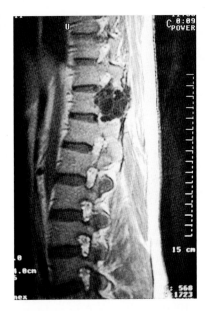

806 Medullary hydatidosis

In this MRI scan of the spine taken in the longitudinal axis the relationship between the medulla and a hydatid cyst that caused hemiplegia is clearly seen. Serology in such cases is often negative.

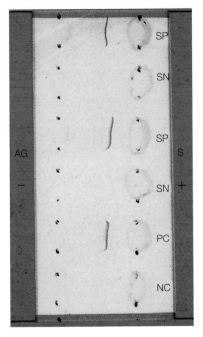

807 Immuno-diagnosis of hydatidosis

The Casoni skin test employed formerly used crude hydatid fluid as antigen. This has been largely replaced by purified antigens such as 'arc 5', which is employed in counter immuno-electrophoresis. SP, positive sera; SN, negative sera; PC, positive controls; NC, negative controls; AG, antigen at cathodic; S, serum at anodic ends.

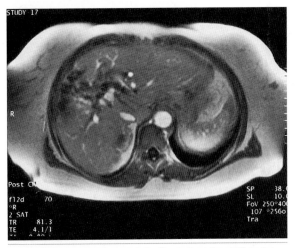

808 Magnetic resonance imagine scan of multilocular (alveolar) echinococcosis

Multilocular or alveolar cysts are caused by infection with *E. multilocularis*. The adult of this species is found in wild canines, especially foxes, and the usual larval hosts are rodents. The parasite is widely distributed in the Palaearctic region and human infection is especially common in areas where domestic dogs also consume rodents. Between 2% and 5% of certain communities in China have been found to be infected, while the disease is reported to be hyperendemic in a number of Inuit villages in North America. Treatment of this life-threatening condition is very difficult, although prolonged therapy with anthelminthic drugs is usually of benefit.

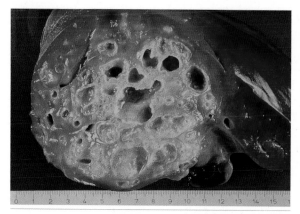

809 Multilocular hydatidosis in human liver
Prior to the use of modern imaging techniques, alveolar cysts in the human liver which may mimic hepatic carcinoma, were usually discovered only, as in this case, at post-mortem.

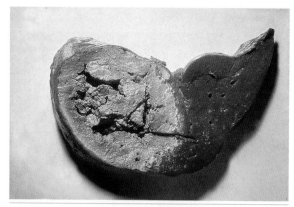

810 Massive multilocular hydatidosis of the liver
The cyst occupied about half the volume of the liver in this post-mortem specimen. (Courtesy Professor B Gottstein.)

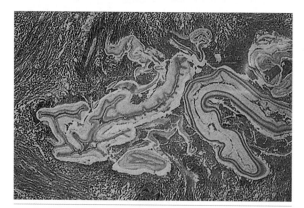

811 Section of alveolar hydatid cyst
Unlike *E. granulosus*, cysts of *E. multilocularis* in humans do not contain daughter cysts with scolices. (× *40*) (cf **804**.)

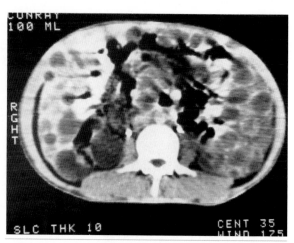

812 *Echinococcus vogeli*
This intestinal cestode of the bush dog (*Speothos venaticus*), and possibly domestic dogs in humid, tropical forest areas of South America normally produces polycystic hydatidosis in pacas, agoutis and spiny rats, but zoonotic infection occasionally occurs in humans. The cysts are found most commonly in the abdominal or thoracic organs. This CT scan of a 20-year-old rubber tapper from Acre State, Brazil, shows large numbers of cystic masses in the abdominal cavity. The infection was probably acquired from his dogs, which were fed on the meat of infected pacas (*Cuniculus paca*). He was cured eventually with a combination of chemotherapy and surgery.

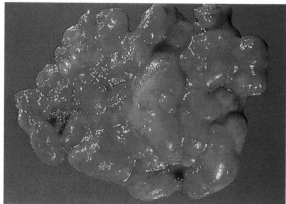

813 Polycystic mass of *Echinococcus vogeli*
This mass was removed surgically from a 22-year-old black Colombian complaining of repeated episodes of fever and purulent cough. At first suspected from a CT scan of having a neoplasm, he was found at laparotomy to have polycystic masses on the surface of the liver. Subsequently, at thoracotomy, groups of cysts were removed from various sites, including the one shown here, which was in the pericardium. (*Natural size*)

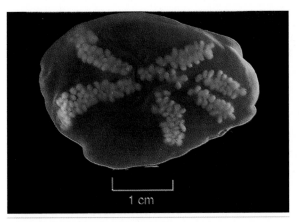

814 Coenurus cerebralis of sheep
This is the larval stage of *Multiceps multiceps*. The adult lives in the intestine of the dog and the 'bladder worm' larva is usually found in the brain of sheep. Fortunately, infection of humans is rare.

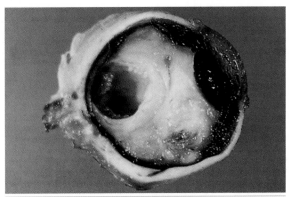

815 Coenurus in human eye
This infection necessitated enucleation of the eye.

PENTASTOMIASIS

Linguatula serrata (tongue worm)

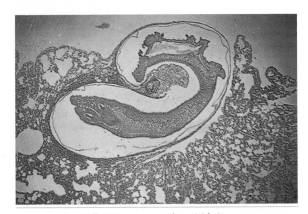

816 Infective third-stage larva in rabbit lung
These endoparasitic and highly specialised parasites have embryonic and ultrastructural affinities to the Arthropoda. Humans may be infected by eating inadequately cooked food containing third-stage larvae. Other carnivores are also infected. The adults of this genus are parasitic in the nasal cavities of carnivores such as domestic and feral dogs and other canids. When the eggs are expelled in nasal secretions or through the gut after being swallowed, they are ingested by herbivores such as goats, sheep, cattle or rabbits, in the intestines of which they hatch. The prevalence of infection in the definitive host may be very high. For example as many as 43% of dogs surveyed in Beirut and up to 72% of cattle in England were found to harbour infective nymphs in the lymph nodes, liver and kidneys. (*H&E × 20*)

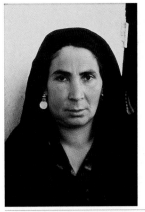

817 'Halzoun syndrome' in a Lebanese woman
Human zoonotic infection with *L. serrata* is fairly common in Lebanon among people whose diet sometimes includes a dish containing raw goat or sheep liver. The excysted nymphs migrate to the nasopharynx, where they can cause severe nasal congestion, deafness, sneezing, cough and other symptoms. Their presence is often associated with facial oedema. In the Sudan a similar syndrome known as *marrara* is seen in people who consume raw offal of various domestic animals, including camel. Visceral zoonotic infection with nymphal stages may occur in people who ingest food contaminated with eggs that have been voided or sneezed out in nasal secretions by dogs. Eggs are passed in the nasal secretions.

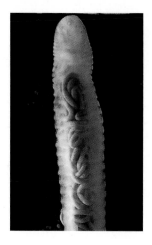

818 Adult *Linguatula serrata*
Cephalic third of a typical adult tongue worm. Note the oral opening and four hooks. The adults reach 3–10 cm in length. ($\times$ 3)

Other pentastomids

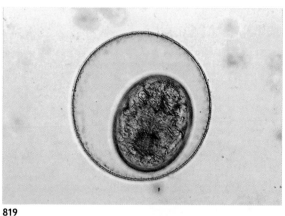

819

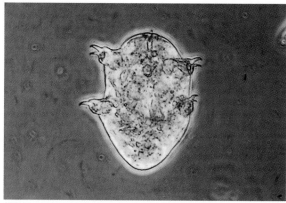

820

819 & 820 Eggs and first-stage larva of *Porocephalus*
The eggs and primary larvae with their four bifurcate legs point to the arthropod origin of this parasite of North American snakes (*Porocephalus crotali*). (**819**, left $\times$ *130*; **820**, right $\times$ *160*)

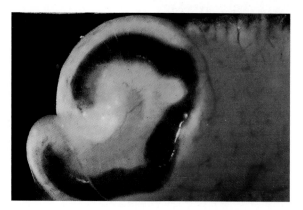

821 *Porocephalus crotali* third-stage larva
After ingestion of eggs in food or water by a secondary host (usually a rodent), primary larvae emerge in the gut. They penetrate the gut wall and encyst in various tissues. This infective third-stage larva lies subperitoneally in a rodent, the normal intermediate host. ($\times$ 4.5)

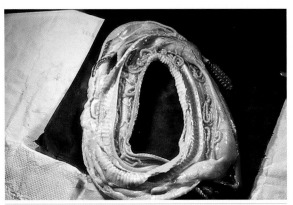

822 Adult *Porocephalus crotali* in rattlesnake lung
Eggs of this 'lungworm' are passed in saliva or in faeces. The parasite is common in snakes, which acquire infection by eating rodents containing third-stage larvae. (× 1/8)

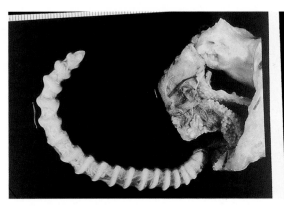

823 Adult males and a female *Armillifer armillatus*
This lungworm is a common parasite of several species of African snakes. The usual intermediate hosts are rodents, but humans are quite commonly infected with the larvae. (× 0.7) (AFIP No. 72–881)

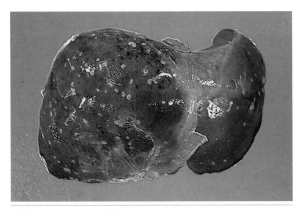

824 Larvae of *Armillifer armillatus*
Third-stage larvae are seen under the capsule of the liver of a Nigerian at post-mortem.

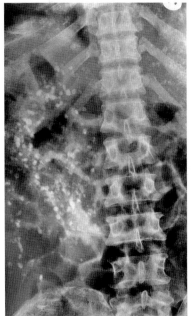

825 Radiograph of calcified nymphal cysts of *Armillifer armillatus* in humans
The C-shaped, encysted nymphs of pentastomids are frequently detected in diagnostic X-rays taken for unrelated symptoms. The heaviness of this widely disseminated infection is remarkable.

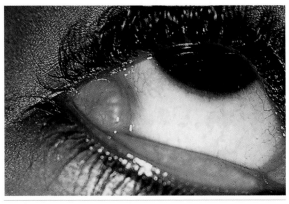

826 Pentastomid larva in eye
The eye is a rare site for pentastomid larvae, the abdomen being mainly affected in humans.

5. Airborne infections

Infections of the upper respiratory tract are acquired mainly by the inhalation of pathogenic organisms for many of which humans are the reservoir. Carriers play an important role and may represent the major part of the reservoir (e.g. in meningococcal meningitis). The three main media for the transmission of airborne infections are droplets, droplet nuclei and dust. Mass vaccination campaigns have reduced the incidence of some of these diseases, which previously caused a very high toll in infant and child morbidity and mortality. On the other side of the coin, two new major threats have surfaced in the past few years. A newly identified coronavirus causing atypical pneumonia that first appeared in southern China late in November 2002 spread rapidly, giving rise to a major epidemic of a severe acute respiratory syndrome (SARS). The infection, which is probably spread by close contact leading to the inhalation of droplets, threatened to develop into a pandemic because of the ease of dissemination through international air travel (see **Frontispiece**). Cases were soon identified as far away as parts of Europe and North America. It has been estimated that about 8000 cases occurred, with a mortality of approximately 10%, before national and international quarantine measures interrupted transmission of the virus, at least temporarily.

The second and, in every way more alarming threat, is the development of a pandemic of avian influenza. This has been most severe in south-east Asia, in parts of which it has long been enzootic and in which, between 1957 and 1958, a pandemic was caused by the H2N2 strain. Although the highly virulent virus responsible for the current infection of domestic and wild birds, influenza H5N1, has at present only a low infectivity to humans, it has killed a high proportion of the few who have so far contracted the infection from domestic poultry. The fear is that, when many people are coincidentally infected by a 'human' strain of influenza, the two could hybridise to produce an exceptionally virulent pathogen that could be spread rapidly worldwide, resulting in the next, long-awaited lethal human influenza pandemic. By April 2006, infection with avian influenza had appeared as far away as the British Isles in western Europe and since there are major migratory routes for several species from both east and west Europe to the African continent, there were fears that H5N1 could become established in areas such as the Rift Valley and sub Sahelian regions of west and central Africa. In the event, the infection had become firmly established in domestic poultry stocks in Nigeria, Niger, Burkina Faso and Cameroon by this date. H5N1 itself might also mutate to a form with an enhanced human-to-human infectivity. A further danger lies in the observation that H5N1 may be disseminated not only via aerosol but also by direct oral contamination from infected body fluids or tissues. For the time being national and international control measures have been based on quarantine (where possible), the mass culling of domestic poultry and, in limited situations, the vaccination of threatened flocks, but the natural or deliberate loss of at least 140 million birds even by early 2005 had already exerted a considerable economic toll (estimated at US$10 billion by early 2005) in the affected countries of south-east Asia. It has now been shown that domestic dogs and cats, as well as large feline species, can also be infected by influenza H5N1.

Other new viral enzootic infections have spread to equines and humans in recent years. The newly named genus *Henipavirus* (in the family Paramyxoviridae) so far contains two viruses, the first recognised being the Hendra virus, which was identified in Queensland, Australia in 1994/95. Fourteen horses were infected (of which 13 died) and three humans who had been in contact with sick horses. Of these people, two died in the first outbreaks. The reservoir has been shown to be species of fruit bat (flying foxes) in that area. The second is the Nipah virus, which occurs especially among pig farmers over a wide area from west Bengal and Bangladesh through Malaysia and Singapore, the reservoir also being species of fruit bats in the genus *Pteropus*. In humans this virus causes an acute form of encephalitis that has a mortality rate of about 50%. First recognised in Malaysia in 1998, by 2001 nearly half of the 265 people with proven Nipah virus infection in that country had died. Fruit bats, which appear to be asymptomatic, excrete virus in their urine and saliva. Pigs are believed to acquire infection by eating contaminated fruit dropped by scavenging bats but humans may be infected by virus in aerosol from bat urine or by eating contaminated fruit. They may acquire virus particles in droplets from infected pigs with pulmonary infection. Infected cats and dogs have also been identified but human-to-human transmission has not yet been proved. Another 'Nipah-like' virus in Bangladesh appeared in 2001 and has killed at least 30% of infected humans. Their infection may have been acquired largely by eating contaminated fruit dropped by fruit bats.

Pneumonic plague continues to pose a localised threat and has recently occurred in epidemic fashion in two localities in the north-east of the Democratic Republic of Congo (see **77**).

Measles is another paramyxovirus that tends to produce severe disease in malnourished children and, in some epidemics in the rural tropics, the mortality rate has been as high as 50%. The infection not infrequently precipitates kwashiorkor. Whooping cough is another important cause of infantile mortality in some areas of the tropics.

Massive pandemics of meningococcal meningitis due to *Neisseria meningitidis* continue to occur periodically in the so-called 'meningitis belt' of tropical Africa (see **840**). In this zone, the pandemics come in waves followed by periods of respite. Over 300 000 cases were reported between 1996 and 2000 and this figure was almost certainly an underestimate. Overall, at least 1.2 million cases of bacterial meningitis occur, of which 0.5 million are due to *N. meningitidis*, with a mortality of about 10%.

Tuberculosis is increasing as a major health problem, not only in many tropical countries, where it is aggravated by poor sanitary conditions and dense overcrowding in urban slums, but also in the Western world, where the problem is aggravated by the development of multiple drug-resistant strains of *Mycobacterium tuberculosis*. The infection presents a wide variety of clinical forms, but pulmonary involvement is the commonest and most important epidemiologically, since it is the form mainly responsible for transmission of the infection. While in the developed countries tuberculosis is seen with increasing frequency in human immunodeficiency virus (HIV)-positive individuals, in Africa it, and pneumococcal pneumonia, are among the commonest causes of death in people with the acquired immunodeficiency syndrome (AIDS) (see **Table 21**). It is estimated that 3 million people die worldwide from tuberculosis each year.

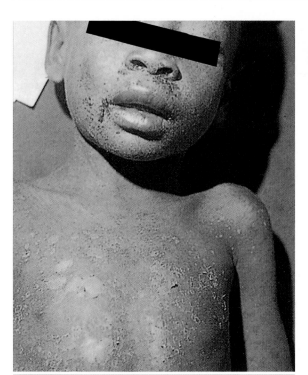

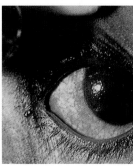

838 Keratoconjunctivitis and xerophthalmia in measles

In malnourished children, these complications are commonly seen.

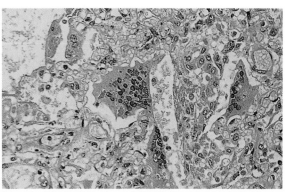

837 Measles in an African child

The desquamating skin rash of measles was accompanied by herpes simplex stomatitis and rhinitis in this child, who died from respiratory complications.

839 Lung in giant-cell pneumonia

Mortality is commonly associated with giant-cell pneumonia during the prodromal stage. This section was from a 10-year-old girl who contracted measles while receiving steroid therapy for treatment of her nephrotic syndrome. (*Haematoxylin and eosin (H&E) × 500*)

MENINGOCOCCAL MENINGITIS

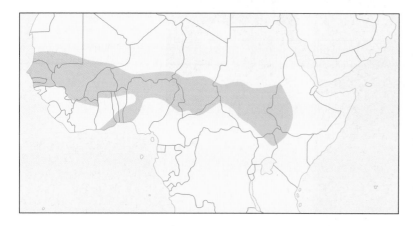

840 Distribution of meningococcal meningitis in Africa

Meningococcal meningitis occurs in epidemic or pandemic form in the 'meningitis belt' of tropical Africa, the zone lying approximately between 5° and 15° North of the Equator, which is characterised by an annual rainfall of between 300 and 1100 mm. In a pandemic of serogroup A *N. meningitidis* infection in this zone, over 300 000 people were affected between 1996 and 2000. The disease, however, is not limited to Africa, and overcrowding enhances the risk of acquiring the infection; nearly 3000 people died from meningitis in two Brazilian cities in 1974. Other epidemics occurred in Nepal in 1983 and 1984 and in Pakistan and India in 1985. Effective vaccines against serogroups A and C are now available.

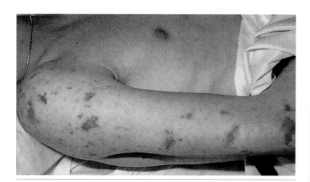

841 Rash of acute meningococcaemia

The rash consists typically of irregular, scattered, nonblanching petechiae, which tend to be peripherally distributed. The lesions, which vary in size, may be macular, papular or clearly purpuric.

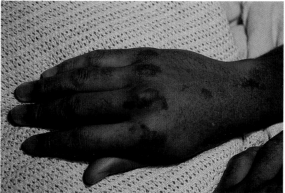

842 Meningococcal septicaemia

Nonblanching and necrotic lesions on the hand of an African patient with meningococcal septicaemia.

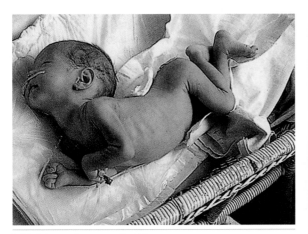

864 Tuberculous meningitis

In infants, miliary tuberculosis and meningitis have a high mortality. This 3-month-old Nepalese infant with tuberculous meningitis and demonstrating pronounced head retraction died despite intensive chemotherapy. Tuberculous meningitis in infants results in permanent neurological sequelae in at least 50% of cases.

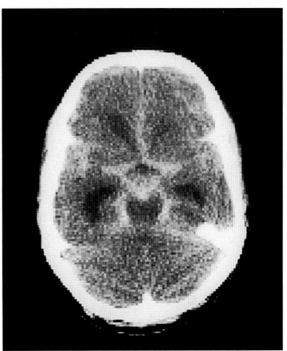

865 Tuberculous meningitis

A CT scan of the brain showing increased uptake of contrast around the vessels at the base of the brain in the circle of Willis in a patient with tuberculous meningitis.

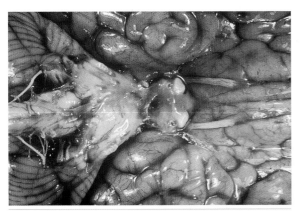

866 Post-mortem appearance of tuberculosis of the base of the brain

This post-mortem specimen shows the gelatinous and fibrinous material that collects particularly at the base of the brain in tuberculous meninigitis.

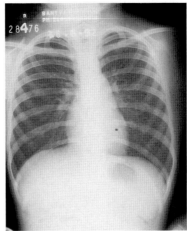

867 Chest radiograph in miliary tuberculosis

Miliary tuberculosis occurs when there is haematogenous spread of mycobacteria leading to bilateral involvement of the lungs.

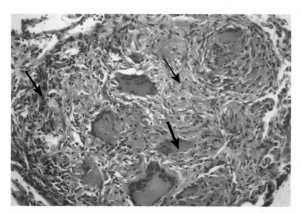

868 Pathology of miliary tuberculosis

The small arrow indicates a focus of caseation in the centre of this figure. Between the granolomas are lymphocytes and plasma cells (indicated by the medium-sized arrow). The Langhans giant cells (large arrow), derived from the fusion of epithelioid cells have multiple nuclei arranged in the shape of a horseshoe. (*H&E × 300*)

WHOOPING COUGH

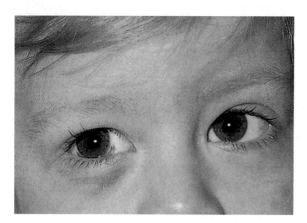

869 Child with whooping cough

Whooping cough is an important cause of infantile mortality in the tropics. Subconjunctival haemorrhages are a common accompaniment of the severe coughing spasms. The haemorrhages resolve rapidly once the child recovers.

PSITTACOSIS

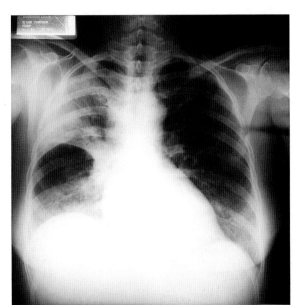

870 Radiograph of patient with psittacosis (ornithosis)
Infection with *Chlamydia psittaci* is usually acquired from pet birds, e.g. parrots, but also occurs widely throughout the animal kingdom. The organism is closely related to *Chlamydia pneumoniae*, which is responsible for a high proportion of respiratory infections, especially in children living in poor urban communities in tropical countries. This radiograph shows dense consolidation of the right upper lobe in a patient who presented with pneumonia due to *C. psittaci*. She was an avid tropical bird collector and had recently taken possession of a new acquisition.

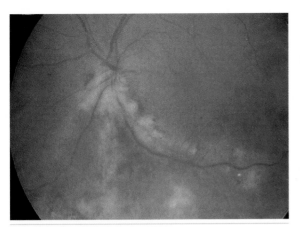

875 Cytomegalovirus chorioretinitis in AIDS

Extensive pathological changes caused by cytomegalovirus, such as those seen here, are relatively common in Caucasians. The retinal swelling, haemorrhages and necrosis that follow viral-induced retinal vasculitis are typical of this condition.

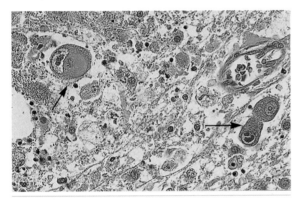

876 Cytomegalovirus encephalitis

Large numbers of viral particles accumulating in the nuclei of enlarged, infected cells give rise to these dense, usually single 'owl's eye' inclusions. (*Haematoxylin and eosin (H&E) × 200*)

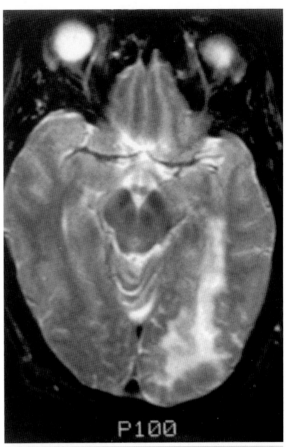

877 Magnetic resonance image of progressive multifocal leukoencephalopathy

Progressive multifocal leukoencephalopathy can occur in the terminal stages of HIV infection. It is due to a virus ('JC', named after the patient in whom it was first found) and results in a demyelinating condition (often periventricular) of the white matter. The magnetic resonance imaging (MRI) findings shown here are fairly typical and the virus from cerebrospinal fluid can be detected by polymerase chain reaction (PCR).

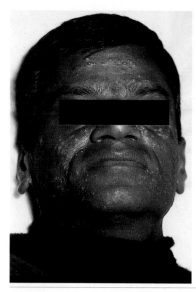

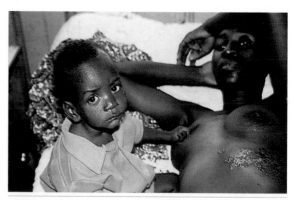

879 Perinatal transmission of AIDS

The virus in African communities, unlike the usual situation in other areas, is transmitted mainly by heterosexual contact, perinatally from infected mothers and by parenteral infection from contaminated blood in transfusions or dirty syringes. This woman with advanced AIDS had severe herpes zoster lesions. Her infant was also HIV-positive.

878 Molluscum contagiosum in a patient with AIDS

The numerous lesions with the classical, umbilicated appearance seen here bear a superficial resemblance to those caused by smallpox. The condition is caused by infection with a DNA poxvirus that is spread by direct person-to-person contact and by fomites. Molluscum contagiosum can be extensive, as shown in this patient who is immunosuppressed with HIV infection.

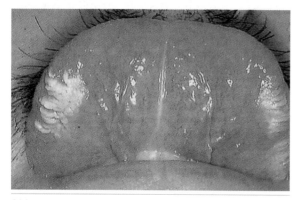

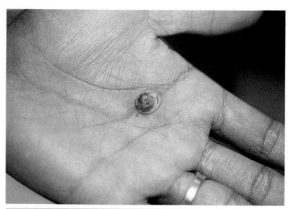

881 Bacillary angiomatosis on the hand of a patient with AIDS

This infection is caused by infection with *Bartonella henselae*, the organism that is also associated with 'cat scratch disease' in individuals with a normal immune system (see **64**). This unusual condition may also be caused by *Bartonella quintana*. (Courtesy of Ciro Martins, MD. From Maenza JR and Chaisson RE. Bacterial Infections in HIV Disease. In: Cohen J and Powderly W, eds. Infectious Diseases, 2nd edn. Edinburgh: Mosby 2004; 1297–1302.)

880 Hairy leukoplakia

This condition, which is possibly due to Epstein–Barr virus infection, consists of hairy projections of keratinised squamous epithelium along the sides of the tongue. It is commonly seen in AIDS.

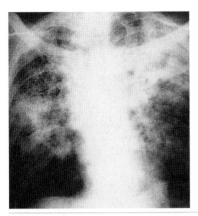

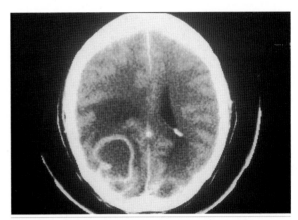

882 Advanced tuberculosis in AIDS

The HIV pandemic is responsible for a serious resurgence of tuberculosis in the Western world, as well as in the tropics and subtropics. Severe postprimary pulmonary tuberculosis, such as that seen here, is common in AIDS patients, particularly in Africa.

883 Computed tomography scan of a tuberculoma of the right occiput

This HIV-positive patient presented with tuberculous meningitis. During the course of treatment he complained of increasing visual difficulty with a left homonymous hemianopia that was originally thought to be due to the ethambutol. However, a computed tomography (CT) scan with contrast showed a large ring enhancing lesion in his right occiput.

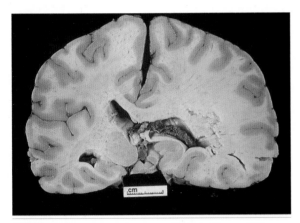

884 Post-mortem appearance of tuberculoma of the right occiput

The figure shows a section of the brain of the patient seen in **883**, who succumbed to his infection. A large area of caseous necrosis was associated with *Mycobacterium tuberculosis*.

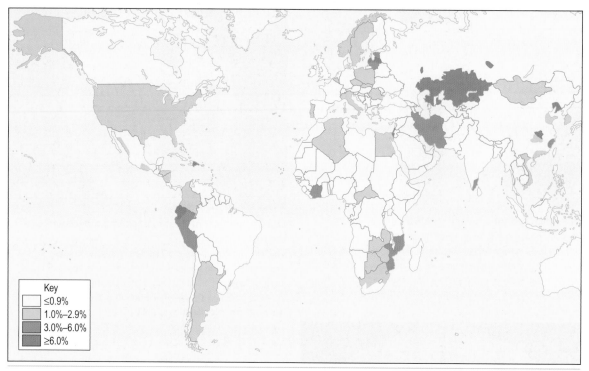

Key
☐ ≤0.9%
☐ 1.0%–2.9%
☐ 3.0%–6.0%
☐ ≥6.0%

885 Estimated prevalence of multidrug resistance among new cases of tuberculosis 1994–2002
This map indicates the estimated prevalence of multi-drug-resistant tuberculosis (MDR-TB) in newly diagnosed cases. Although some of the worst affected areas are those, such as parts of Africa, where tuberculosis is associated with AIDS, MDR-TB is also common and increasing in other areas such as eastern Europe. The major differences between this figure and that showing the global incidence of tuberculosis (see **846**) partly reflect the dichotomy between the availability of appropriate medication and its correct administration. Failure of compliance is a major factor in the exponential increase of MDR TB. (Adapted from WHO 2004 Anti-tuberculosis drug resistance in the world. Report no.3. WHO/HTM/TB/2004.343. Geneva, World Health Organization.)

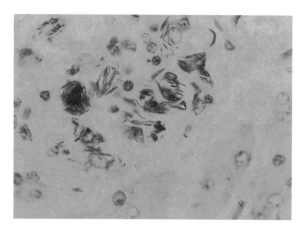

886 Hepatic infection with *Mycobacterium avium–intracellulare*
Foamy histiocytes filled with acid-fast bacilli are seen in a hepatic granuloma. Chronic inflammatory infection with this 'atypical' *Mycobacterium*, and infection of various organs (e.g. the gastrointestinal tract) with other organisms in this group, is particularly common in the terminal phase of the AIDS illness. Paradoxically, no clear interaction has been detected so far between *Mycobacterium leprae* and HIV infection. (*Kinyoun* × *1800*)

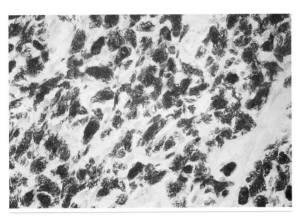

887 Atypical mycobacterial infection of the small bowel of a patient with HIV

The auramine stain shows masses of acid-fast bacilli that, on culture, were shown to be of the *M. avium* complex, in this case *M. intracellulare*. (*Auramine* × 750)

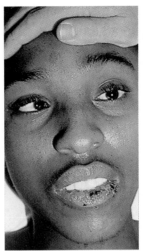

889 Cryptococcal meningitis in AIDS

Cryptococcus neoformans is an increasingly important concomitant pathogen in patients with AIDS in tropical areas. This HIV-positive Zimbabwean man with cryptococcal meningitis has a left-sided cranial nerve paralysis. (© D A Warrell)

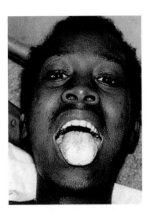

888 Oral candidiasis in an African with AIDS

This patient with 'slim disease' (see **903**) had a very heavy *C. albicans* infection of his buccal cavity.

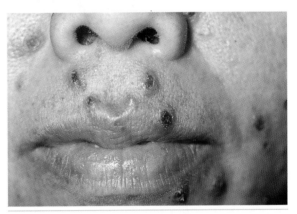

890 Penicilliosis in a man with AIDS

Penicillium marneffei is a facultative invader of human macrophages in immunocompromised individuals. Lesions resembling those of molluscum contagiosum seen in this patient are indicative of the presence of disseminated infection. (From Hoepelman AIM. Opportunistic Fungi. In: Cohen J and Powderly W, eds. Infectious Diseases, 2nd edn. Edinburgh: Mosby 2004; 2341–2362.)

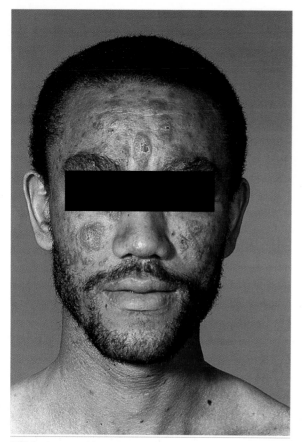

891 Cutaneous histoplasmosis

The typical lesions of cutaneous histoplasmosis are shown in this individual with HIV infection who came from the Caribbean. *Histoplasma capsulatum* is a dimorphic fungus existing as a mould in organic matter and as a yeast in tissue. Disseminated infection occurs especially in the immunosuppressed.

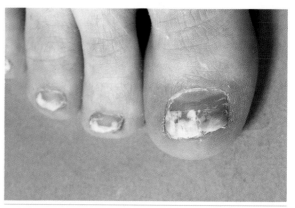

892 Onychomycosis (tinea unguium) in an HIV-positive patient

Fungal infection of the toe nails is most commonly caused by *Trichophyton rubrum*. In this individual who had been treated with zidovudine but no antifungal for four weeks, some clearing of the infection in the proximal toe nail with residual distal infection may be seen.

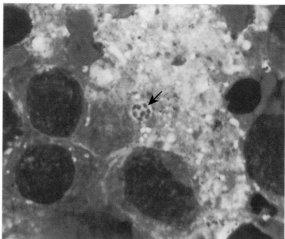

893 *Pneumocystis jiroveci* in lung smear

This organism, which is present as a commensal in many animals, is an opportunistic parasite in humans. It produces eight-nucleated cysts that can be seen in smears of pulmonary aspirates. (*Giemsa × 2500*) (See also **1026**.)

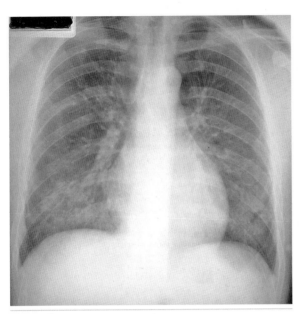

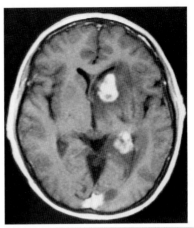

896 Magnetic resonance image in advanced cerebral toxoplasmosis

Encephalitis and brain abscess are common in AIDS. Typical changes with central necrotic areas surrounded by swollen, oedematous brain tissue are clearly visible here. MRI scanning is even more sensitive than CT scanning for the detection of very early lesions.

894 *Pneumocystis* pneumonia

Before the use of a highly active antiretroviral treatment (HAART) in the Western world, but also in Africa, one of the commonest presenting opportunistic infections was *Pneumocystis* pneumonia in patients with AIDS. The above radiograph shows typical features of bilateral, symmetrical, so-called 'ground glass' shadowing, which often spares the apices and costophrenic angles and most commonly radiates from the hila.

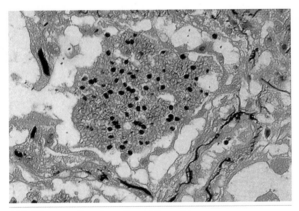

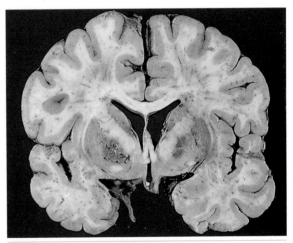

897 Gross autopsy appearance in cerebral toxoplasmosis

Brain from a 33-year-old male with *Pneumocystis* pneumonia who died 2 months after manifesting neurological symptoms. This coronal section shows haemorrhagic foci in the white matter of the frontal gyrus, nucleus caudatum and putamen.

895 Silver stain of section of lung biopsy

The encysted *P. jiroveci* is seen as black objects in the foamy exudate that fills the alveoli. (*Grocott stain × 200*)

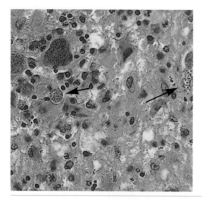

898 Toxoplasmal encephalitis

Several cysts are seen in this section of brain from an AIDS victim dying with acute encephalitis due to toxoplasmosis. This coccidian infection contributes to death in 15% or more of HIV-infected individuals worldwide. (*H&E × 250*)

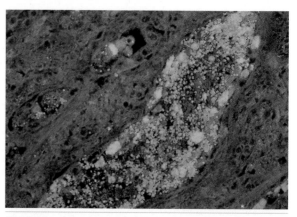

900 *Enterocytozoon hellem* in a kidney

Disseminated infection with this microsporidian in patients with AIDS can involve organs such as the kidneys, eyes or lungs. This section of kidney shows heavy infestation with *E. hellem* in a patient whose urine also contained numerous spores. (*Indirect fluorescent antibody (IFA) × 400*)

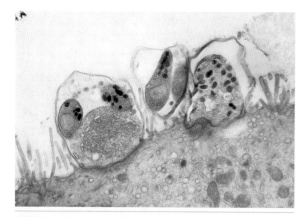

899 Ultrastructure of *Cryptosporidium*

In individuals with HIV infection, the existence of large numbers of *Cryptosporidium* on the surface of the intestinal mucosa can cause intractable, profuse, watery diarrhoea and weight loss. This coccidial infection is a major contributor to death in about 7% of AIDS sufferers in Western countries. The organisms in different stages of schizogony are seen surrounded by a membrane of host-cell origin in this electron micrograph, giving the parasites the false appearance of being extracellular. The section is from a biopsy of rectal mucosa from one of the earliest known victims of AIDS, who had lived in Zaire. The parasites can colonise any part of the intestine from the pharynx to the rectum. The source of infection and the species of *Cryptosporidium* responsible for human infection are still unknown. (*Electron microscopy (EM) × 7,500*)

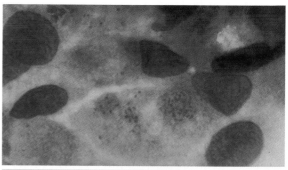

901 *Enterocytozoon bieneusi* in enterocytes

Three groups of encapsulated spores are present in this smear from a duodenal biopsy from a 35-year-old male AIDS patient with chronic diarrhoea. He subsequently developed generalised Kaposi's sarcoma, from which he died. (*Giemsa × 1300*)

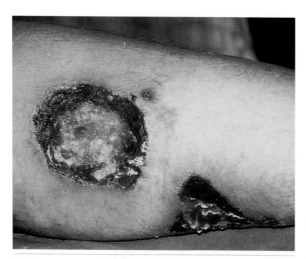

902 *Acanthamoeba castellanii* infection of the skin
Chronic ulceration with species of these facultatively
pathogenic amoebae is seen in some patients with severe
immunodeficiency such as that associated with AIDS. This
35-year-old man, who presented with wasting and fever due
to *Escherichia coli* septicaemia, had a previous history of
episodes of *P. jiroveci* pneumonia and toxoplasmal encephalitis.
During hospitalisation, two skin lesions appeared on the right
arm and the left leg. Four months later, when the patient died
of primary brain lymphoma, cutaneous lesions were present
on all parts of his body. (See also **997**.)

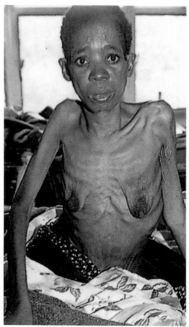

903 'Slim disease' in a 25-year-old African woman
This condition, the result of chronic diarrhoea, which may be caused by *Cryptosporidium hominis* or other opportunistic intestinal parasites, is now recognised to be associated also with fulminating tuberculosis. Gross weight loss and a severe, itchy skin rash are characteristic of the condition, which is usually preterminal.

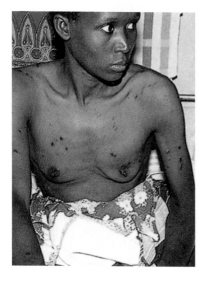

904 Kaposi's sarcoma in an African
Many patients with AIDS develop disseminated Kaposi's sarcoma, thought to be due to human herpesvirus 8. In most AIDS sufferers, the terminal stages are accompanied by a plethora of different infections. (See also **1203**.)

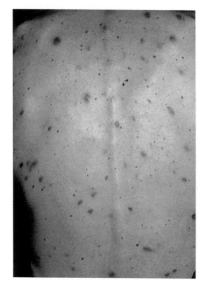

905 Generalised cutaneous Kaposi's sarcoma
This condition is common in patients of all racial origins. Unlike classic Kaposi's previously seen in Africa, it is not restricted to the lower limb and may involve the internal organs, especially the gastrointestinal tract and lungs. It is often accompanied by lesions of the mucous membranes.

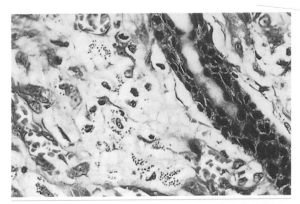

906 Biopsy of Kaposi's sarcoma in association with *Leishmania*

Large numbers of amastigotes were found in this section of a Kaposi's sarcoma lesion removed from the leg of a 35-year-old HIV-positive male. The leishmanial infection, which was probably acquired in Greece, was identified as *Leishmania infantum*. The man, who was afebrile, had an enlarged liver and spleen. Cryptic infection with this protozoan parasite frequently becomes activated in immunodeficient individuals. (*Giemsa–colophonium × 350*)

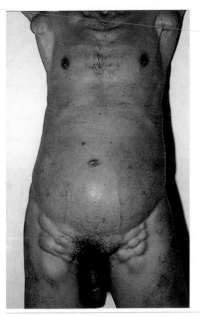

907 Non-Hodgkin's lymphoma

Visceral and cerebral lymphomas of this type are a fairly common feature in AIDS. This man had massive axillary and inguinal lymphadenopathy with gross hepatosplenomegaly and ascites.

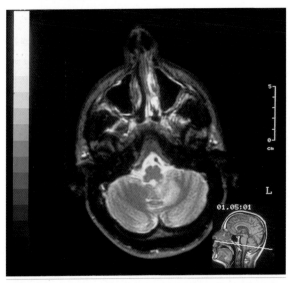

908 Primary central nervous system lymphoma in a patient with AIDS

This patient presented with left-sided cerebellar symptoms and signs. The MRI shows a T2-weighted image with an enhancing lesion in the left cerebellar hemisphere that was found at post-mortem to be a cerebellar lymphoma.

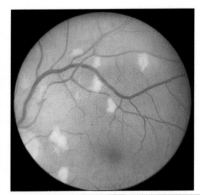

909 HIV-induced retinopathy

Any organism, such as cytomegalovirus, *Toxoplasma gondii*, herpes simplex and varicella zoster virus, can affect the eye of the HIV-infected individual. This particular view shows the retinopathy caused by the HIV virus itself.

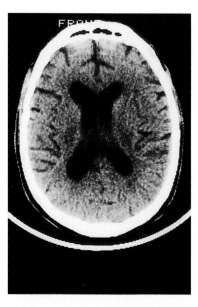

910 Cerebral atrophy in HIV infection

Numerous infections of the central nervous system can occur in HIV, such as toxoplasmosis, cryptococcosis and progressive multifocal leukoencephalopathy. This CT scan shows cerebral atrophy in a patient who presented with dementia that was shown at post-mortem to be due to the HIV virus itself. (See **Table 21**.)

BACTERIAL INFECTIONS

Lymphogranuloma venereum (lymphogranuloma inguinale, climactic bubo, esthiomène)

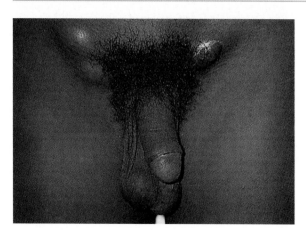

911 Inguinal adenitis in a man

Lymphogranuloma venereum (LGV) is a venereally transmitted infection due to L1, L2 and L3 serovars of *Chlamydia trachomatis*. It is particularly common in tropical countries but, although rare elsewhere, LGV is being encountered increasingly in more temperate countries. The organisms enter the body through epithelial abrasions and are passed to the draining lymphatics. Thus inguinal lymphadenitis is a common feature, resulting in large, sausage-shaped masses such as those seen here, over which the skin is shiny and purplish in colour. Urethritis may develop in males or females. The intracytoplasmic elementary bodies can be identified in cultures made from the lesions (if necessary by aspiration of the buboes) and stained by Giemsa or monoclonal antibodies (see **944**). Serious genitoanorectal lesions can result from this infection. Formerly, the Frei test (a delayed hypersensitivity skin reaction) was of value in the diagnosis. Unfortunately, it is used rarely now, as the antigen is no longer marketed; this renders an accurate diagnosis difficult other than on clinical grounds since an enzyme-linked immunosorbent assay (ELISA) test based on the use of a specific monoclonal antibody is not yet available and other laboratory diagnostic techniques are expensive. The complement fixation test is the most widely used at the present time.

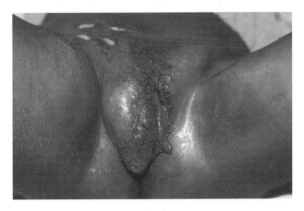

912 Lymphogranuloma in a female adult
The patient seen here had unilateral vulval oedema and inguinal buboes. (From Roth VR and Cameron DW. Lymphagranuloma venereum, chancroid and granuloma inguinale. In: Cohen J and Powderly W, eds. Infectious Diseases, 2nd edn. Edinburgh: Mosby 2004; 839–846.)

Chancroid (soft chancre, ulcus molle)

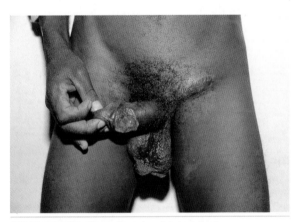

913 Chancroid ulcer of penis with inguinal lymphadenopathy
Chancroid (soft chancre, 'ulcus molle') is a venereal condition caused by *Haemophilus ducreyi*. It occurs most commonly among the poorer populations of developing countries, in whom it is the commonest cause of genital ulcers. Although it occurs in both sexes it is most commonly observed in males. Papule formation commences after a short incubation period (often 4–10 days) after exposure, the papule developing into a deep, very painful ulcer associated with inguinal lymphadenopathy. This also is painful and may be bilateral. The buboes may suppurate, as seen here. In the female, the lesions, usually on the vulva or cervix, are frequently asymptomatic. The severe pain helps to differentiate chancroid from lymphogranuloma venereum, granuloma inguinale and syphilis.

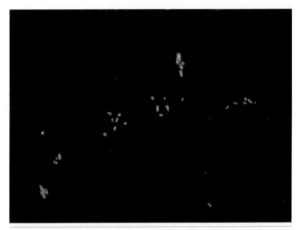

914 Indirect fluorescent antibody test of *Haemophilus ducreyi*
The small, Gram negative bacteria may be seen on a smear or after cultivation on specialised media. They may also be identified by staining smears with a fluorescein-labelled, specific monoclonal antibody as seen here. (*Indirect fluorescent antibody test (IFAT)* × *300*)

Donovanosis (granuloma inguinale, granuloma venereum)

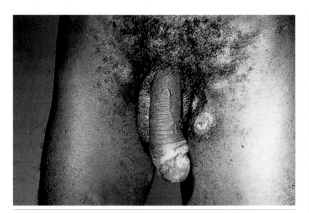

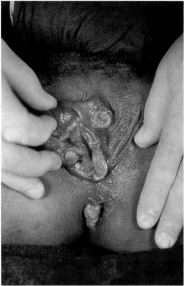

916 Donovanosis of female genitalia
The disease runs a very chronic course. As in lymphogranuloma venereum, mutilating ulceration of the genitalia may occur and anorectal involvement is common. In comparison with lymphogranuloma venereum, the lymphatics are not primarily involved.

915 Donovanosis of penis and adjacent skin of leg
This venereal infection, which occurs mainly in the tropics and subtropics, is caused by a Gram-negative coccobacillus, *Calymmatobacterium granulomatis*. In the male it produces deep, punched-out ulcers of the penis. These are clean and painless initially but, with secondary bacterial infection, may become covered with a thick, offensive, purulent exudate and develop a marked granulomatous reaction; such lesions are painful. As seen here, secondary ulceration may appear on adjacent skin.

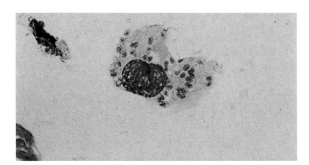

917 Donovan bodies in exudate
The encapsulated coccobacilli of *C. granulomatosis* can be seen in Romanowsky-stained smears within the cytoplasm of macrophages. These are the so-called 'Donovan bodies' in which the bipolar staining gives the appearance of a closed safety pin. (*Wright–Giemsa* × 650)

Gonorrhoea

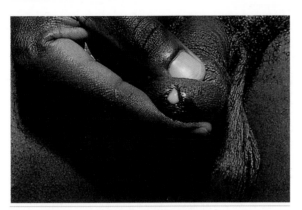

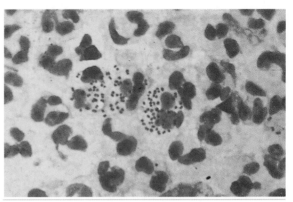

918 Urethral discharge in gonorrhoea
Although gonorrhoea is prevalent worldwide, it is especially widespread in the tropics, where between 4% and 10% of the population may be infected. Chronic gonococcal salpingitis is a common cause of infertility in women. Gonorrhoeal urethral strictures are often seen in men.

919 *Neisseria gonorrhoeae* in urethral exudate
The Gram-negative diplococci are readily seen in smears of the purulent exudate in the cytoplasm of polymorphs. (*Gram × 900*)

Syphilis

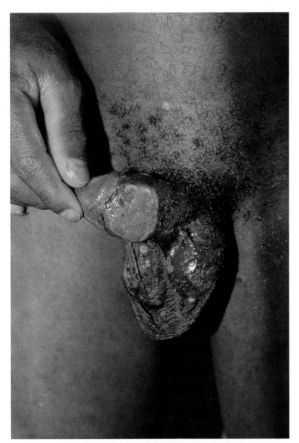

920 Primary syphilitic chancre and secondary rash
Syphilis, the venereally transmitted treponematosis caused by *Treponema pallidum*, is widespread in many parts of the tropics but did not occur where yaws was endemic. The figure shows a typical primary chancre with associated secondary rash on the scrotal and abdominal skin. In contrast to chancroid, the primary chancre is painless, and usually has a clean base and a rolled edge.

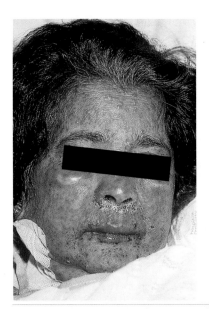

933 Fulminating varicella (chicken pox) with encephalopathy

Although the pock-like lesions of varicella bear some resemblance to those of smallpox and monkey pox, the varicella zoster virus belongs to the alpha subfamily of Herpesviridae. Severe infections, especially in adults such as the Sri Lankan patient seen here, may be complicated by encephalitis, pneumonitis and hepatitis. Herpes zoster (shingles) is usually seen in adults and may be especially severe in patients with human immunodeficiency virus (HIV) infection (see **879**)

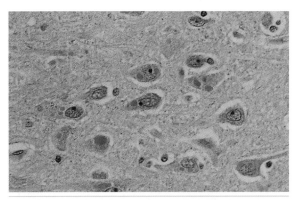

934 Negri bodies in hippocampus cells of rabid dog

Rabies is a zoonotic disease of the nervous system caused by infection with a bullet-shaped RNA rhabdovirus. Although the dog, and to a lesser extent the cat, is the main urban transmitter of infection, foxes and other feline species, as well as vampire bats, are natural hosts and may also transmit the disease to humans. Intracytoplasmic inclusion bodies (Negri bodies) in brain cells are pathognomonic of rabies. Rabies can be prevented by pre-exposure or rapid postexposure vaccination. However, the established clinical condition is invariably fatal. (*Haematoxylin and eosin (H&E) × 200*)

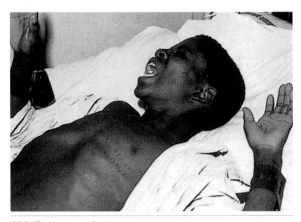

935 'Furious rabies'

A 14-year-old Nigerian boy with hydrophobia following dog bites on the wrist and knee. Inspiratory spasms occurred spontaneously or were induced by the sight of water. The condition developed in spite of his receiving a 14-day course of antirabies vaccine. (© D A Warrell.)

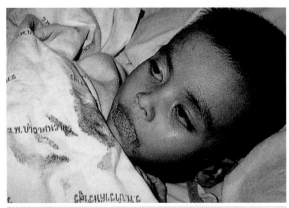

936 Autonomic nervous disorders in rabies

Hypersalivation, profuse sweating due to autonomic nervous system lesions and haematemesis characterised the infection in this Thai boy. (© D A Warrell.)

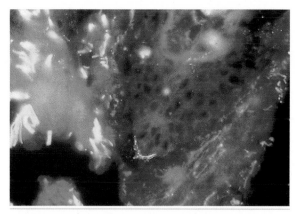

937 Fluorescent antibody staining of rabies virus
The presence of virus may sometimes be detected with the aid of a fluorescent antibody in a biopsy of the corneal epithelium during the incubation period. Here, a nerve is seen fluorescing bright green in such a specimen. (× 440)

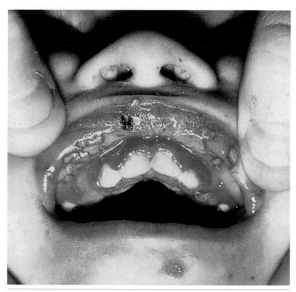

938 Acute herpetic ulcerative gingivostomatitis
This condition, due to herpes simplex virus in children with severe protein–calorie malnutrition, causes a serious illness seen only uncommonly in the developed world.

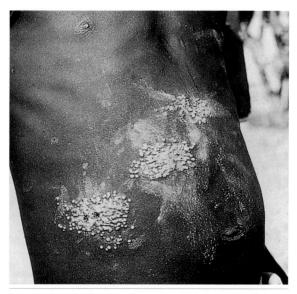

939 Herpes simplex of skin following meningitis
Any debilitating illness that causes a depression of immunity may be followed by an extensive herpetic rash as in this boy who had recovered from meningococcal meningitis.

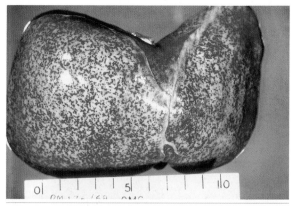

940 Liver in disseminated herpes simplex infection
Disseminated infection may affect the internal organs (e.g. liver, brain, heart, etc.). This complication, which is usually fatal, occurs in patients with AIDS.

BACTERIAL INFECTIONS

Chlamydia trachomatis infections

The genus *Chlamydia* contains three species, one of which, *Chlamydia trachomatis*, includes several distinctive groups of serovars. Serovars A, B, Ba and C cause endemic trachoma, B and D–K cause genitourinary disease and L1, L2 and L3 cause lymphogranuloma venereum. *Chlamydia psittaci* is the agent of avian (and occasionally human) ornithosis, while *Chlamydia pneumoniae* is a respiratory pathogen. The pathogens invade host cells as infectious elementary bodies that develop within phagosomes into reticulate bodies. These, in turn, replicate and then condense into the familiar elementary bodies, which eventually erupt to release a new generation of infective elementary bodies.

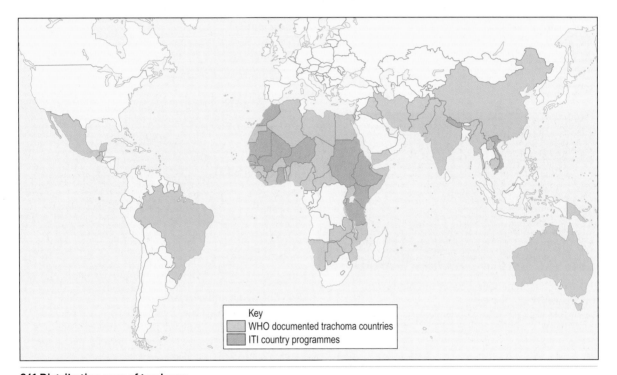

941 Distribution map of trachoma
Trachoma which is endemic in 49 countries, mainly in the Middle East and Africa, as well as in other parts of the tropics, affects over 150 million people, of whom over 5.6 million have been blinded or otherwise visually impaired. Some 500 million people are at risk. The infection is spread both by contact with infective material via soiled hands, clothing, etc. and by flies that feed on lachrymal fluids. Prevention must include improved health education and the use of appropriate antibiotics. The map indicates countries that are documented as trachoma-endemic by WHO and those in which programmes are being supported under the International Trachoma Initiative. (Further country programmes are foreseen for other areas marked in the map, e.g., Brazil.) (Adapted from WHO, 2005, NMH/CHP/CPM-PBD and International Trachoma Initiative, ITI Programs 2006 http://www.trachoma.org/cpro.php)

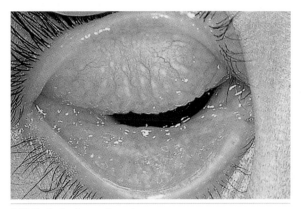

942 Early lesions of trachoma
Small, pinhead-sized, pale follicles beneath the epithelium over the tarsal plates, especially in the upper lid, are a characteristic feature of the disease. The infective agents may be identified in epithelial scrapings at this stage and up to the time scarring commences.

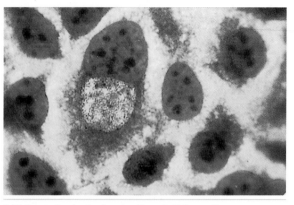

943 Granular inclusion bodies of *Chlamydia trachomatis*
Giemsa-staining demonstrates the typical granular appearance of groups of elementary bodies in this cell monolayer. (*Giemsa* × *660*)

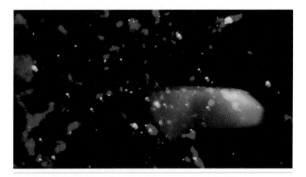

944 Direct immunofluorescence of *Chlamydia trachomatis*
The use of a specific monoclonal antibody facilitates the demonstration of the elementary bodies in tissue smears. (× *590*)

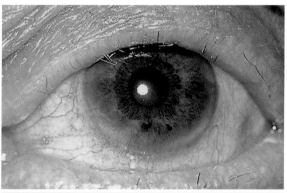

945 Entropion and trichiasis
Scarring of the tarsal plates may be extensive and result in entropion of the edge of the lid. The eyelashes point inwards and rub against the cornea (trichiasis), adding to the damage already done by this pathogen.

946 Late corneal scarring and trichiasis
The end point of trachoma is frequently blindness due to corneal scarring and other complications.

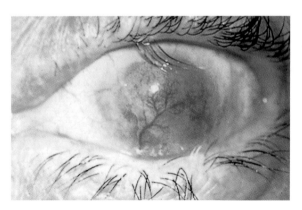

Gonorrhoea

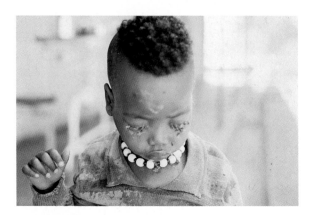

947 Severe gonococcal conjunctivitis in an Ethiopian boy

This child was seen during an epidemic of gonococcal conjunctivitis associated with a massive population growth of a muscid fly, probably *Musca sorbens*. A great reduction in the fly population associated with heavy rains coincided with a spontaneous decline in the epidemic of conjunctivitis. (Courtesy of Dr T.-H. Henriksen.)

Leprosy

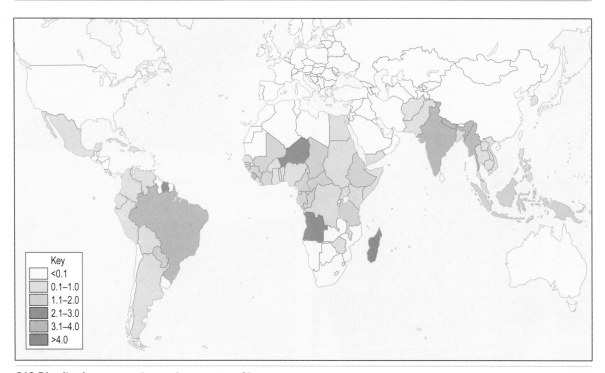

Key
<0.1
0.1–1.0
1.1–2.0
2.1–3.0
3.1–4.0
>4.0

948 Distribution map and prevalence rates of leprosy

By early 2005 prevalence rates between 2.0 and 4.1 per 10 000 population were recorded from nine countries, 1–2 per 10 000 in three countries and between 0 and 1 per 10 000 in 73 countries. Global registered cases had fallen to 286 063 and new cases were 407 791. The greatest concentrations of infected people were still in south-east Asia, parts of Africa and Brazil; Europe, the eastern Mediterranean and western Pacific represented less than 2.8% of the world total of patients. Hopes are high for the eventual elimination of this disease with the aid of early detection, multiple drug treatment and the prevention of disabilities, but vaccination remains an elusive target. The introduction of multiple drug treatment is estimated to have cured more than 12 million patients since 1981. (Adapted from WHO, 2005, http://www.who.int.lep/)

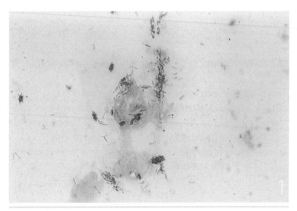

949 *Mycobacterium leprae*
The acid-fast and alcohol-fast bacterial agent of leprosy in a smear preparation. (*Ziehl–Neelsen* × *770*)

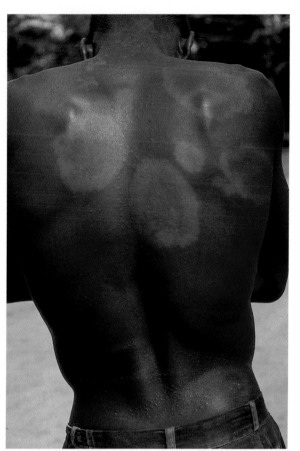

951 Tuberculoid leprosy
The early tuberculoid lesion is characterised by macules showing loss of sensation and hypopigmentation.

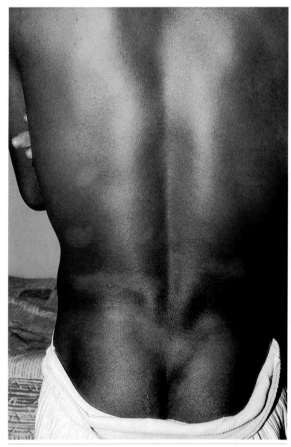

950 Early macules
The disease shows a broad spectrum depending on the patient's immune response, from healing tuberculoid leprosy at one pole to nonresolving lepromatous leprosy at the other. These responses are reflected in the histopathological picture (see **967–969**). An early sign of leprosy, the indeterminate macule, is slightly hypopigmented and ill-defined. It retains tactile sensitivity, sweating function and hair growth.

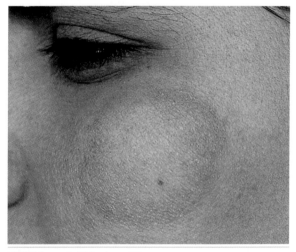

952 Tuberculoid lesion of face
The cooler, peripheral parts of the body are common sites for tuberculoid skin lesions. This patient's face had a large, dry, annular patch, which was anaesthetic.

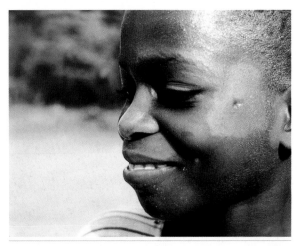

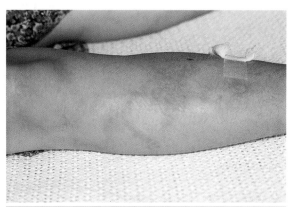

954 Borderline (dimorphous) leprosy
The skin lesions on the right shin of a patient who presented with a depigmented hypoanaesthetic patch with an erythematous periphery.

953 Tuberculoid macules of face
A large, depigmented macule with a small necrotic centre and a smaller, preauricular lesion are seen on this west African boy.

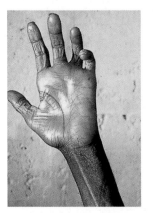

955 Bilateral ulnar nerve lesions
Damage to the ulnar nerve in tuberculoid leprosy leads to weakness and wasting, followed by complete paralysis and atrophy of the ulnar-innervated hand muscles, resulting in the characteristic picture of the *'main de prédicateur'*.

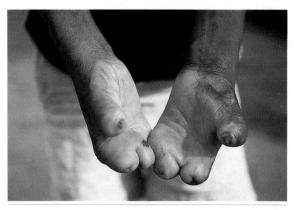

956 Loss of extremities in late tuberculoid leprosy
Neurotrophic atrophy eventually leads to the loss of phalanges, especially following trauma resulting from the anaesthesia. The hands, as seen in this Liberian man, or feet may be affected.

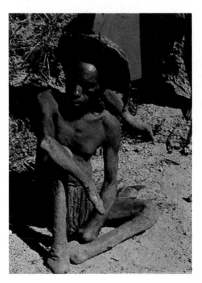

957 Total deformity in late tuberculoid leprosy
This New Guinea highlander suffered complete loss of hands and feet and was totally incapacitated.

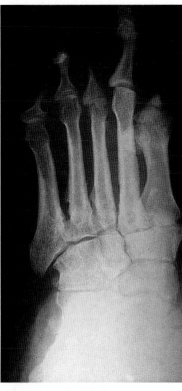

958 Atrophy of toes in tuberculoid leprosy
The partial or complete loss of the bony structures of the toes can be seen in this radiograph of a Costa Rican patient with advanced tuberculoid lesions.

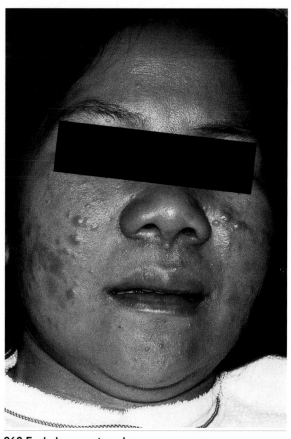

960 Early lepromatous leprosy
This adult female patient has numerous, small, lepromatous nodules on the face.

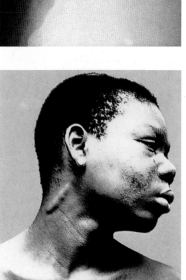

959 Nerve thickening
Thickening of the great auricular nerve is a common feature in tuberculoid leprosy.

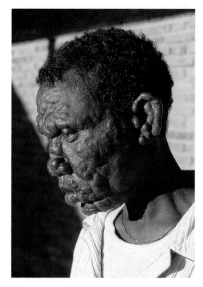

961 Advanced lepromatous leprosy
Lepromatous leprosy, showing extensive infiltration, oedema and corrugation causing 'leonine facies'. Note depilation of eyebrows and face, and thickening of the ear in this Ethiopian patient.

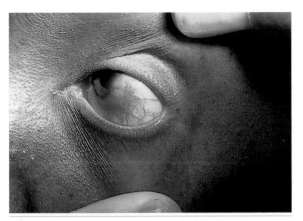

962 Lepromatous nodule in eye
Leprosy is a common cause of blindness in the tropics.

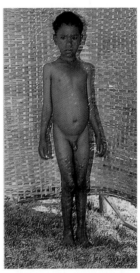

963 Young boy with lepromatous leprosy
This Ethiopian youngster had multiple nodules on the face and extremities, including the penis, but his trunk was clear.

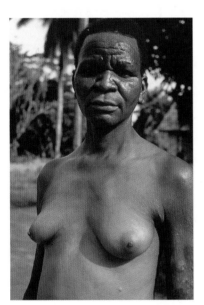

964 Gynaecomastia in leprosy
This condition, which is relatively common in adult males with long-standing lepromatous leprosy, follows testicular atrophy.

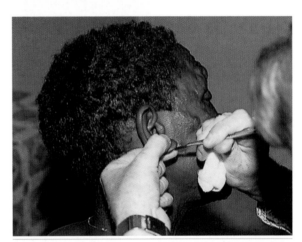

965 Preparation of skin smear
A biopsy is taken from a nodule and smeared for staining with Ziehl–Neelsen stain (see **949**). In the context of the current strategy for the elimination of leprosy and the potential risks inherent in the procedure, it is no longer considered essential to take skin smears to monitor the progress of treatment, reliance being placed on clinical findings.

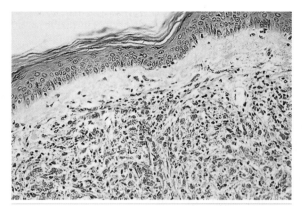

966 Organisms in skin biopsy stained by TRIFF method
M. leprae is readily seen, staining deep red in skin sections
stained by this method. In dubious cases, the application of
PCR can be useful in confirming the presence of bacterial DNA.
(*TRIFF × 150*)

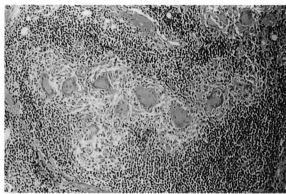

967 Histopathology of active tuberculoid leprosy
The presence in this biopsy of granulomata containing
numerous epithelioid cells and Langhans giant cells is
characteristic of the healing response in cases of tuberculoid
leprosy. No bacilli are visible. (*H&E × 30*)

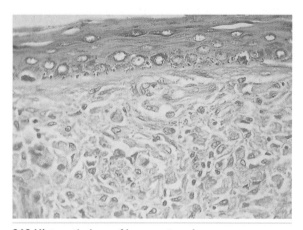

968 Histopathology of lepromatous leprosy
Very large numbers of acid-fast bacilli in vacuolated
macrophages are present in this skin biopsy of a nodule from a
patient with lepromatous leprosy. The infiltrate does not extend
to the basal layer of the skin. (*H&E × 200*) (AFIP No. 74–2725.)

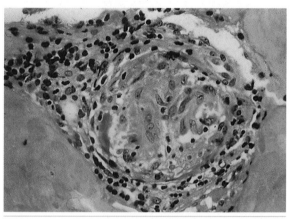

969 Biopsy of nerve in tuberculoid leprosy
Cellular infiltration of the neural sheath leads to destruction of
the nerve fibres, resulting in sensory and motor loss in the
areas affected. This slide shows an epithelioid granuloma of a
nerve. (*H&E × 200*)

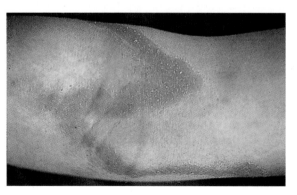

970 Lepromin test
The Mitsuda reaction, which usually attains its maximum in
4–5 weeks, indicates the sensitivity of the patient to the mixture
of antigens (prepared from leprosy bacilli) that have been
injected. The reaction is expressed in millimetres, with or
without ulceration, and is read on about the 21st day after
injection. In patients with lepromatous leprosy, the reaction is
completely negative. In patients with tuberculoid leprosy, it is
variably positive.

Mycobacterium ulcerans and *Mycobacterium marinum*

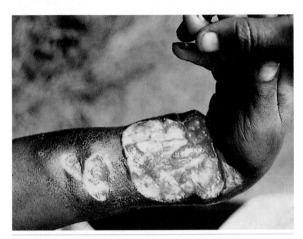

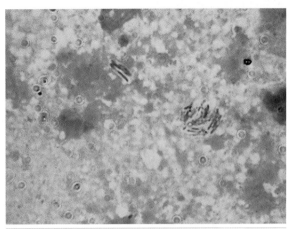

971 Typical Buruli ulcer in a Nigerian child
The condition is characterised by gross, necrotising skin ulcers in which numerous acid-fast bacilli are present (*M. ulcerans*). The disease occurs in localised tropical areas in all continents. While the mode of transmission remains unknown, there is a clear association with moist vegetation and infection by aquatic insects has been postulated. Some cross-protection against multiple lesions in children appears to be affected by vaccination with bacille Calmette–Guèrin (BCG) as used against tuberculosis.

972 *Mycobacterium ulcerans* in section of ulcer
Acellular necrosis occurs involving the dermal layers and subcutaneous fat. Acid-fast bacilli are found in the necrotic material. Application of the PCR procedure greatly improves the ease and speed of diagnosis in material from exudates and biopsies when organisms are difficult to find with classical staining. (*Ziehl-Neelsen* × *1,000*)

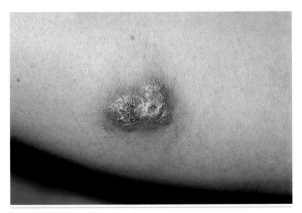

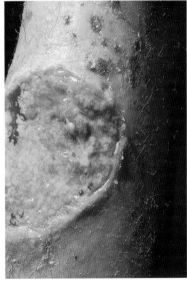

974 Tropical (phagedaenic) ulcer
Chronic necrotising ulcers involving the skin and subcutaneous tissues are common in country areas in the humid tropics. They contain a mixed bacterial flora including *Bacillus fusiformis* and *Treponema vincenti.*

973 'Fishtank granuloma'
The purplish lesion of a patient who kept tropical fish as a hobby. *Mycobacterium marinum* was grown from a biopsy of the chronic, nodular lesion.

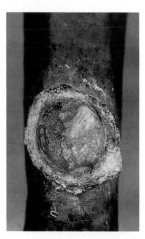

975 Bone involvement in tropical ulcer

Sequestra result when bone involvement occurs, as is seen here.

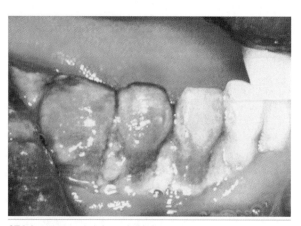

976 Acute necrotising gingivitis

Associated with malnutrition and other diseases, this condition, which has been recorded in over 70% of African children seen in some surveys, is a consequence of poor dental hygiene, often aggravated by reduced immunoreactivity. If inadequately treated it can lead to alveolar bone resorption or, in more severe cases, the destructive facial condition known as 'noma'. (Courtesy of Professor D Pittet and colleagues. Reprinted with permission from *Lancet Infectious Diseases* 2003; 3:419–431.)

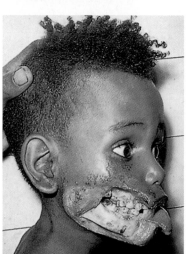

977 Cancrum oris (noma)

This gangrenous condition of the facial region commences with necrotising stomatitis, which can evolve very rapidly (within 24–48 hours). Soft and hard tissues of the cheek can be destroyed, leading to gross disfigurement, as well as death in a significant proportion of patients in spite of intensive antibiotic and local treatment. An association with measles was commonly noted and concomitant AIDS now undoubtedly plays a role in the pathogenesis. A number of bacterial species are believed to play a role in the pathogenesis of noma, including *Prevotella intermedia* and *Fusobacterium necrophorum*. Cytomegalovirus is also commonly present. Gross disfigurement usually results. Some 770 000 individuals are believed to be affected by the sequelae of noma.

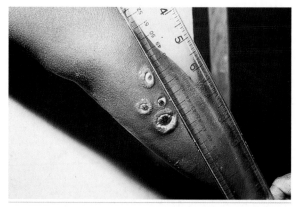

978 Cutaneous anthrax

Four discrete lesions on the arm of an African patient infected with *Bacillus anthracis*. The black eschars are associated with direct inoculation through a break in the skin after contact with infected animal material or from transmission by biting flies such as tabanids. The lesion is painless without pus but is often surrounded by an arc of oedema and ultimately heals, leaving a scar. Anthrax-infected game or domestic animals that are eaten have also been recorded as the source of human infection, for example in Namibia in 2004.

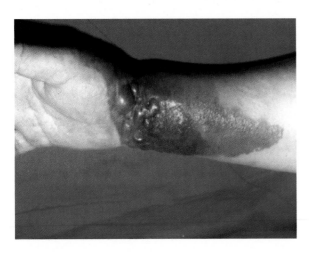

979 Extensive erythema and haemorrhagic bullae in cutaneous anthrax

This condition may be seen 2–4 days after the initial infection. People who work with potentially contaminated animals or animal skins are especially liable to this type of infection by anthrax spores. Although about 95% of all human anthrax lesions are located in the skin, infection acquired by the ingestion or inhalation of spores may cause life-threatening disease of the internal organs.

Tropical pyomyositis

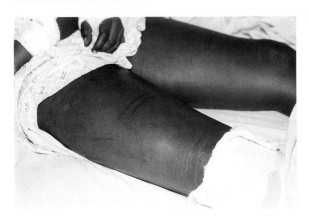

980 Tropical pyomyositis

The right thigh is swollen with infection by *Staphylococcus aureus*. Such infections are common in tropical Africa but uncommon in temperate climates. It is not understood why the organism selects muscle rather than any other tissue in which to multiply. This suppurative muscle infection may occur in as many as 1 per 1000 individuals in tropical countries.

Tetanus

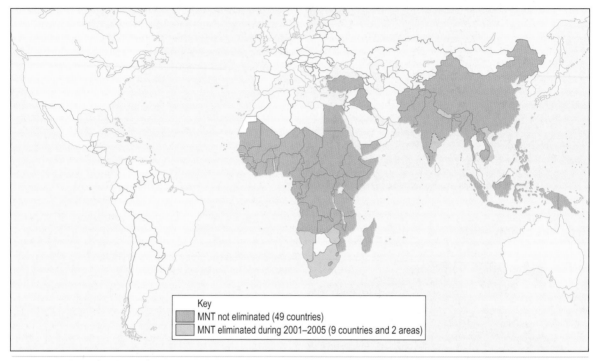

Key
MNT not eliminated (49 countries)
MNT eliminated during 2001–2005 (9 countries and 2 areas)

981 The status of the elimination of maternal and neonatal tetanus
The map shows the countries from which maternal and neonatal tetanus (MNT) had been eliminated by the end of 2005 and the situation in the rest of the world. It will be seen that the countries still most severely affected are in Africa and parts of Asia as well as the western Pacific. MNT remains an especially important infection in several tropical countries where the basic health service infrastructure is still unable to implement the simple measures (vaccination of pregnant women and clean delivery services) on an adequate scale. By the end of 2005 MNT had been eliminated from nine countries and two areas but remained in 49 countries as indicated here. (After data from WHO in http://www.who.int/immunization_monitoring/diseases/MNTE_status_progress.jpg)

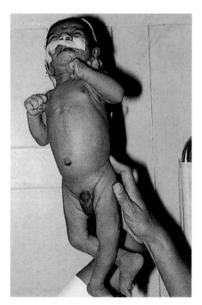

982 Tetanus neonatorum
Infection through the umbilical cord with *Clostridium tetani* is common where poor facilities for childbirth are available. One of the characteristic features is the 'risus sardonicus' resulting from spasms of the facial muscles.

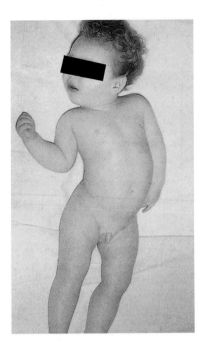

983 Opisthotonos in neonatal tetanus

The generalised muscle contraction leads to arching of the back and limb rigidity; in the conscious patient it is extremely painful and distressing. Urgent treatment with antitetanus immunoglobulin, appropriate muscle relaxants and, if indicated, positive pressure ventilation are essential. Prevention by the immunisation of mothers and improved delivery services have greatly diminished the incidence of neonatal tetanus in developing countries. For example, the number of cases prevented in 1997 was estimated to have been in the order of 1.2 million.

Nonvenereal trepanomatoses See also **Table 4**.

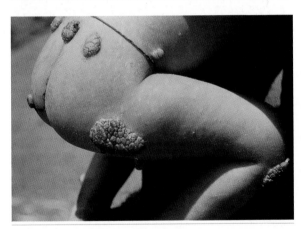

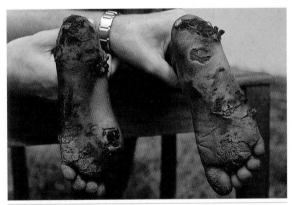

985 Plantar hyperkeratosis

Hyperkeratosis of feet and hands is a common secondary phenomenon in yaws. This man's feet were seriously eroded.

984 Secondary framboesiform yaws

Thanks to the mass, penicillin-based eradication campaign of the 1950s, yaws is now a relatively rare disease in the humid tropics, although a new outbreak was recently recorded in Ghana. This Papuan child shows classic framboesiform lesions, caused by *Treponema pertenue*. Secondary lesions are frequent also at mucocutaneous junctions.

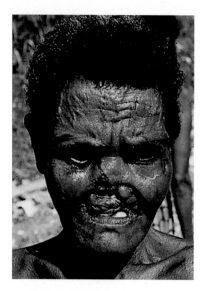

986 Gangosa
The most advanced and destructive lesions affect the maxillary bones and hard palate, resulting in a condition known as 'gangosa'.

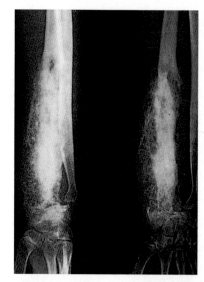

987 Radiograph of forearm with yaws osteitis
Focal cortical rarefaction and periosteal changes are seen, especially in the tibia ('sabre tibia') but also in other long bones.

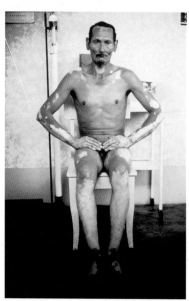

988 Depigmented lesions of pinta
Pinta is endemic in the New World from Mexico to the Amazon. 'Pintids' start as small papules and develop into plaques with actively growing edges that become confluent. In the late stages the pintids become depigmented. The causative organism of pinta, *Treponema carateum*, is morphologically indistinguishable from that of syphilis and bejel.

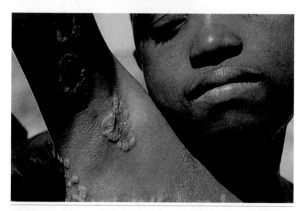

989 Secondary rash in endemic syphilis
These nonvenereal spirochaetoses ('endemic syphilis') occur mainly in dry parts of Africa, the Balkans and Australia. A florid, secondary, maculopapular eruption and associated adenitis is usually the first sign. Tertiary complications, including gangosa, may develop. In the Middle East the condition is known as bejel. Other forms of nonvenereal 'endemic syphilis' are njovera (Zimbabwe), skerlievo (Borneo), dichuchwa (Botswana) and siti (Gambia).

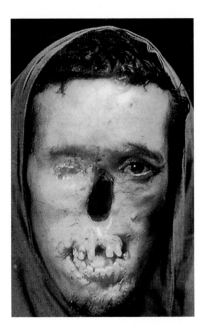

990 Gummatous lesions in bejel
If left untreated, bejel can produce severe, gummatous changes of the bone, cartilage and skin as seen in this unfortunate sufferer from the Middle East.

PROTOZOAL INFECTIONS See also **Table 17.**

Infection with 'free-living' amoebae See **Table 17.**

A number of free-living amoebae that are widely distributed in soil and water are also facultative parasites in humans. They are responsible for three disease syndromes: primary amoebic meningo-encephalitis (PAM), granulomatous amoebic encephalitis (GAE) and chronic amoebic keratitis (CAK). GAE is seen in immunocompromised individuals.

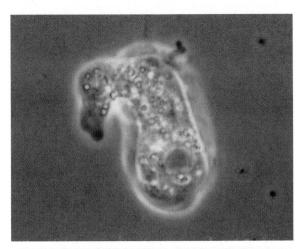

991 Living trophozoite of *Naegleria fowleri*
Several species of *Naegleria* (Vahlkampfiidae) have been incriminated as the causative pathogens of amoebic meningoencephalitis, a condition with a high fatality rate that is usually acquired from bathing in warm water. *N. fowleri* has been isolated from such water in various swimming places, including thermal baths. Infection appears to be acquired through the cribriform plate of the nasal cavity following immersion in contaminated water. As its cysts are susceptible to desiccation, its dispersal may be more restricted than that of *Acanthamoeba* species. *N. fowleri* develops a biflagellate form in water. (*Phase contrast × 1200*)

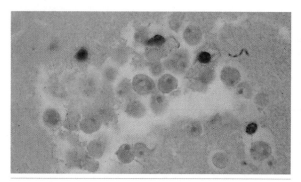

992 *N. fowleri* in the brain of a patient with primary amoebic meningoencephalitis
Numerous trophozoites are seen in this brain section taken at autopsy from a patient who died of PAM in Texas. (*H&E × 100*)

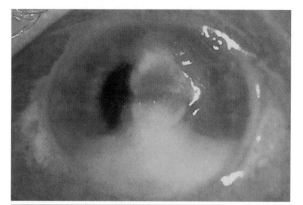

994 Corneal infection with *Acanthamoeba* species
This condition, previously rare, is increasing with the more frequent use of 'soft' contact lenses. A recent study of contact lens infections revealed *Acanthamoeba polyphaga* in 15 cases and one each of *Acanthamoeba hatchetti* and *A. castellanii* in the series. Over 200 such cases have been reported in the past two decades.

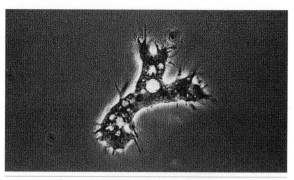

993 Living trophozoite of *Acanthamoeba castellanii*
The 'prickly' appearance of the surface membrane from which these organisms acquire their name is seen clearly; a large vacuole is also present. Various species have been incriminated as the causative agents of granulomatous amoebic encephalitis and infections of the eye (see **972**), with *Acanthamoeba culbertsoni* being the most notorious. The cysts, which are resistant to desiccation, are probably airborne (see also **902**). (*Phase contrast × 1000*)

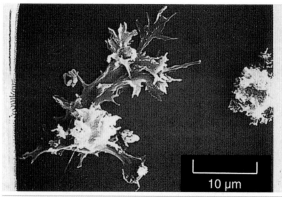

995 Trophozoite of *Balamuthia mandrillaris*
This leptomyxid amoeba was first isolated from a baboon and has since been found in a number of cases of GAE in humans. The patients are usually immunodeficient in some way (e.g. through extremes of age or with HIV infection). However, cerebral infection can result from the amoebae migrating from wounds caused by facial injury. The living trophozoites in culture are extremely irregular in shape and readily distinguished from those of *Naegleria* or *Acanthamoeba*. (*Scanning electron microscopy (SEM)*)

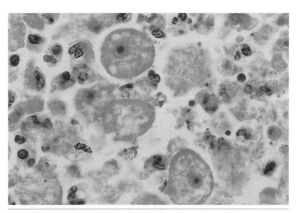

997 Section of brain with granulomatous amoebic encephalitis

This section is from a Zambian patient who died from AIDS. The parasites, which were first believed to be an *Acanthamoeba* species, failed to react with a specific antiserum and are probably attributable to *B. mandrillaris*. In this section, the nuclear structure of the invasive trophozoites is clearly seen. The amoebae of both *B. mandrillaris* and *Acanthamoeba* species are also quite frequently found in skin abscesses in patients with AIDS. (*H&E × 260*) (See also **902.**)

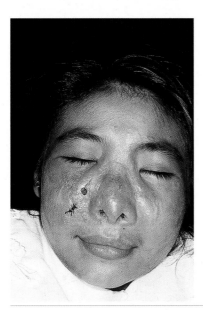

996 *Balamuthia mandrillaris* infection in a Peruvian girl

This girl was believed to have become infected from swimming in ponds in northern Peru. The organism causes a necrotising, granulomatous encephalitis in humans and animals in the New World, as well as in Europe, Australia and possibly Africa (see **997**). Parasites were recovered from the biopsy site seen on the right cheek. A bilateral, granulomatous lesion was present on the face and computed tomography revealed extensive, intracranial masses, which were presumed also to be caused by this pathogen. (© D A Warrell.)

THE SUPERFICIAL MYCOSES See Table 22.

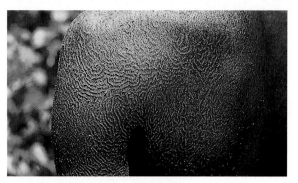

998 Tinea imbricata

Trichophyton concentricum produces characteristic, superficial, scaly lesions in parallel lines and concentric circles. While it is common in the south Pacific and parts of the Far East, it is occasionally seen in other hot, humid areas.

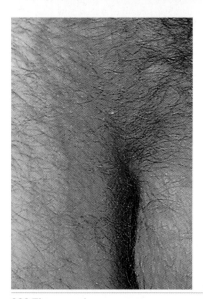

999 Tinea cruris

This infection, which is very common in young males in hot, humid areas, is usually caused by *Epidermophyton floccosum*, *Trichophyton rubrum* or *Trichophyton mentagrophytes* var. *interdigitale*. The red, slightly raised margin of the lesion in this patient can be seen to be advancing down the inner thigh.

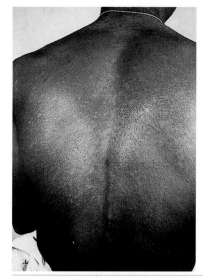

1000 Pityriasis versicolor

Infection with *Malassezia furfur* is a common cause of hypopigmentation in dark-skinned young adults. Fluorescence of the patches in Wood's light helps to differentiate the condition from vitiligo and other depigmenting lesions.

THE SYSTEMIC MYCOSES See Table 22.

Table 22 Superficial and systemic mycoses

Group	Clinical syndrome	Causative agents
Superficial (dermatomycoses)	Mainly hair affected	
	Black piedra	*Piedraia hortae*
	White piedra	*Trichosporon beigelii*
	Favus	*Trichophyton schoenleinii*
	Tinea barbae	*Trichophyton* spp.
	Tinea capitis	*Microsporon* spp.
	Hair not affected	
	Tinea cruris	*Epidermophyton* spp.
	Tinea pedis	*Trichophyton* spp.
	Tinea unguium	*Trichophyton* spp.
	Tinea corporis	*Microsporum* spp.
	Pityriasis versicolor	*Malassezia furfur*
	Tinea imbricata	*Trichophyton concentricum*
	Otomycosis	Various genera
	Superficial candidiasis	*Candida albicans**
Systemic	Actinomycosis	*Actinomyces israelii*
	Madura foot (mycetoma)	Wide variety of organisms, including *Nocardia* spp., *Streptomyces* spp., *Pseudallescheria* spp., etc.
	Chromomycosis	*Phialophora* spp., *Cladosporium carrionii*
	Keloidal blastomycosis (Lôbo's disease)	*Lôboa lôboi*
	Blastomycosis	*Blastomyces dermatitidis*
	Paracoccidioidomycosis	*Paracoccidioides brasiliensis*
	Coccidioidomycosis	*Coccidioides immitis*
	Cryptococcosis (torulosis)	*Cryptococcus neoformans**
	Systemic candidiasis	*Candida* spp.*
	Sporotrichosis	*Sporothrix schenckii*
	Histoplasmosis	*Histoplasma capsulatum**
	African histoplasmosis	*H. duboisii*
	Zygomycosis	various genera
	Rhinosporidiosis	*Rhinosporidium seeberi*
	Aspergillosis	*Aspergillus fumigatus*
	Pneumocystosis	*Pneumocystis jiroveci*** [†]
	Penicillosis	*Penicillium marneffei*

* Mycotic infections can become fulminant in immunocompromised subjects. Those marked * are especially associated with AIDS. [†] Formerly called *Pneumocystis carinii* or *P. carinii hominis*.

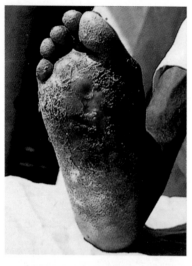

1001 Mycetoma ('Madura foot')
This chronic and disabling condition may be caused by a wide variety of organisms ranging from *Actinomycetes* to various Fungi Imperfecti. This patient was seen in the Sudan, where mycetoma is common.

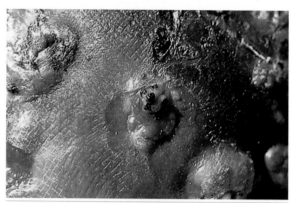

1002 Fungal grains discharging
Close-up of **1001** showing the coloured fungal grains being discharged from multiple sinuses.

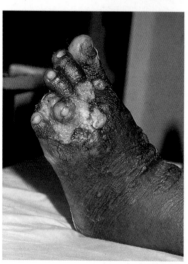

1003 Dorsum of Madura foot in an African patient
Discharging sinuses and distortion of some of the toes are seen in this patient's left foot.

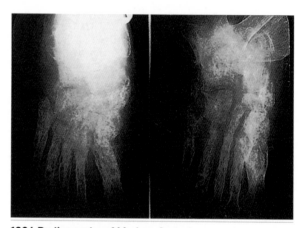

1004 Radiographs of Madura foot
Infiltration of the tarsals and metatarsals occurs in late cases.

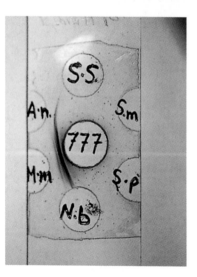

1005 Serological diagnosis
Fungal species identification can be made serologically. This serum contains antibodies to *Madurella mycetomae*.

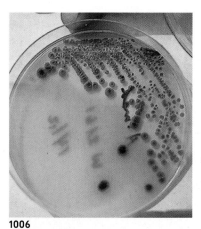

1006

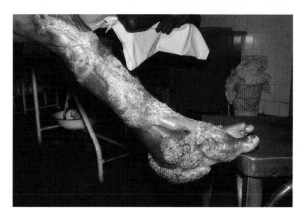

1007

1006 & 1007 Culture diagnosis
M. mycetomae (**1006,** left) and
Streptomyces pellietieri (**1007,** right) on
Sabouraud medium show typically
shaped and pigmented colonies.

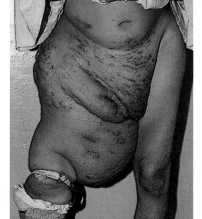

1008 Chronic maduromycosis due to *Streptomyces somaliensis* infection
Extensive sinus formation and osteitis have led to gross disfigurement in this Sudanese man.

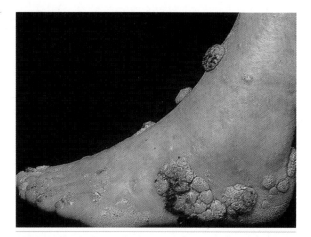

1009 Early chromomycosis
The early lesions show a violet discoloration. The primary ulcer spreads slowly and is followed by verrucous lesions. This condition is seen in many tropical areas, including Queensland, where this man was infected.

1010 Verrucous dermatitis
This is the late stage of chromomycosis. The lesions are very chronic, and are usually painless but irritating. Lymphoedema follows lymphatic stasis.

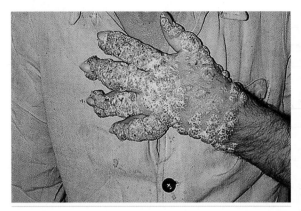

1011 Chromomycosis of the hand
The infection can also cause severe but usually superficial lesions on the hands, as in this man from the north-east of Brazil.

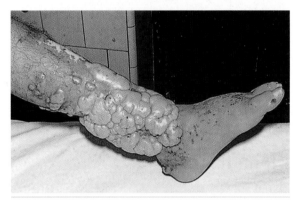

1012 Lôbo's disease
This condition, usually presenting with shiny, keloid-like lesions, produces a general picture similar to late chromoblastomycosis and occurs in the north-east of Brazil. It is caused by *Lôboa lôboi*.

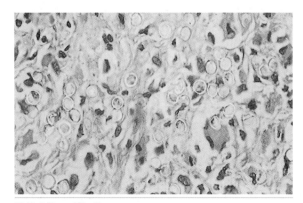

1013 *Lôboa lôboi*
The typical spores of this fungus are seen in this biopsy specimen from the keloidal lesions. (*H&E × 350*)

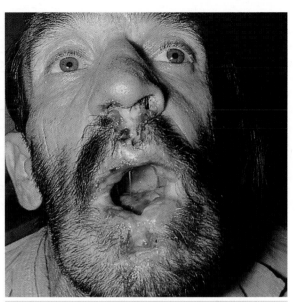

1014 Mucocutaneous lesions in paracoccidioidomycosis
In adults, gross infiltration of mucocutaneous and mucous surfaces by *Paracoccidioides brasiliensis* may spread to the pharynx and larynx. The diagnosis is made by demonstrating the fungi in smear or biopsy preparations, or by serological testing.

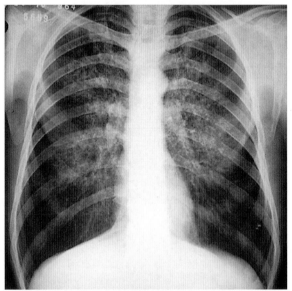

1015 Radiograph of chest in paracoccidioidomycosis
Chronic pulmonary infiltration may result in fibrosis and eventual death from respiratory insufficiency in infections with *P. brasiliensis*.

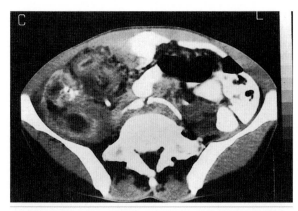

1016 Pseudotumoural form of paracoccidioidomycosis
Computed tomography (CT) scan of the abdomen of a 57-year-old Brazilian man who presented with right lumbar pain and massive weight loss 15 years after having oropharyngeal infection. Physical examination suggested the presence of a colonic carcinoma but radiography and a CT scan revealed the presence of abscesses involving the psoas muscle as well as calcification and thickening of the ileocaecal region of the intestine. Material removed during radical surgery confirmed that the lesions were caused by infection with *P. brasiliensis*.

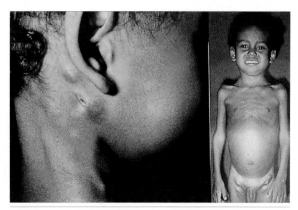

1017 Paracoccidioidomycosis in a Brazilian child
In children, *P. brasiliensis* infection is a widely disseminated disease affecting macrophages and causing generalised lymphadenopathy and hepatosplenomegaly. Although it is uncommon prior to adolescence, this boy was aged only 4¹/₂ years. Ultrasound may help to locate intra-abdominal lymphadenopathy, which was present in this case. Infection of the macrophages results in a state of immunodeficiency, which was reflected here by a negative skin test. Note the general emaciation associated with an enlarged abdomen, generalised lymphadenopathy and ulcerating cervical lymph nodes. In this boy, a titre of 1/1 280 against *P. brasiliensis* was recorded.

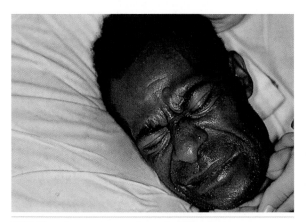

1018 Chronic cryptococcal meningitis
Infection with *Cryptococcus neoformans* or its tropical subspecies, *C. neoformans gattii*, is most often manifested as a chronic meningitis but may localise in the lungs or disseminate to other organs, especially in individuals who are immunocompromised and is seen especially in HIV-positive individuals in Africa. This Papuan man with chronic meningitis shows marked meningism. In disseminated disease, cutaneous and lytic bone lesions are common. Surprisingly, *C. n. gattii* has recently become established in the temperate climate of Vancouver Island, British Columbia, where it occurs in soil and on trees. It can also survive in sea water. The organism has evolved into a far more virulent one than that normally encountered in tropical areas and has killed humans, horses and porpoises. (See also **889** and **Table 21**.) (© D A Warrell.)

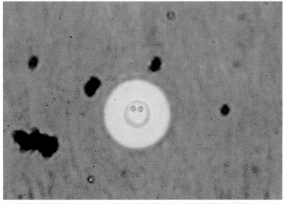

1019 *Cryptococcus neoformans* in cerebrospinal fluid
The organisms are readily visualised in Indian-ink preparations of infected cerebrospinal fluid (CSF) from patients with meningitic infection. They may also be cultured from CSF, blood or urine in some cases. The prostate gland is believed to be an important reservoir for the organisms, which may lead to reactivation of the disease after therapy in some patients. (× 500)

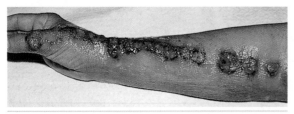

1020 Lesions of sporotrichosis

The primary lesion on the thumb, and the lymphatic spread (with ulceration) of secondary nodules on the arm, seen here in a Brazilian woman in São Paulo, are characteristic of this mycotic infection.

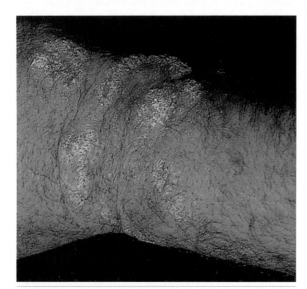

1021 Sporotrichosis of the wrist

This patient was infected in Queensland. Like other deep mycoses, infection with *Sporothrix schenckii* occurs in a number of tropical regions.

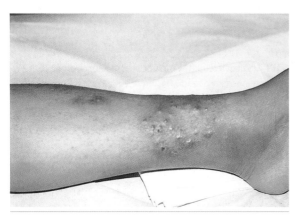

1022 Early lesions of sporotrichosis

Characteristic nodular lesions caused by *S. schenckii* on the lower leg of a patient from Mauritius.

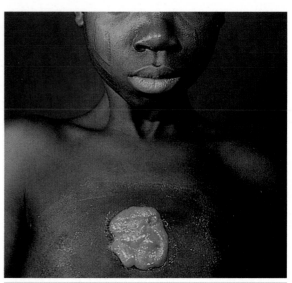

1023 African histoplasmosis

Histoplasmosis caused by *Histoplasma duboisii* commonly produces large destructive lesions of the skin and subcutaneous tissues. Bones are often involved in the invasive process. Histoplasmosis has been reported as an opportunistic infection in AIDS sufferers in the Caribbean.

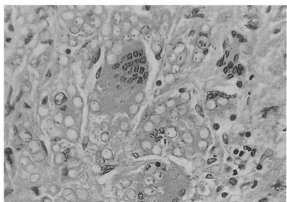

1024 *Histoplasma duboisii* in biopsy

The typical giant-cell reaction to the presence of *H. duboisii* spores is seen in this figure. (*H&E* × *350*)

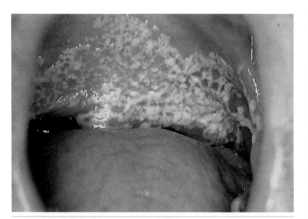

1025 *Candida albicans* of the palate
Severe candidiasis of the mouth and gastrointestinal tract is commonly seen in AIDS patients.

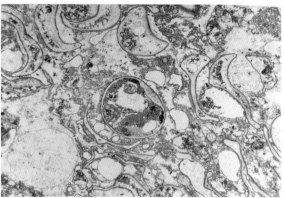

1026 Ultrastructure of *Pneumocystis jiroveci*
Comparison of the DNA and ribosomal RNA of *P. jiroveci*, which is an opportunistic parasite commonly found in immunocompromised individuals (see **893–895**), with that of a wide range of protozoa and fungi, has confirmed that it is one of the group of ustomycetous red yeast fungi. The recent finding by molecular techniques that *Pneumocystis* DNA was a transient occupant of the respiratory tracts of 20% of a sample of 50 healthy, immunocompetent adults raises the possibility that such individuals may serve as carriers of this fungus within the community. The ultrastructure of the organisms is shown here. (× *26 500*)

ECTOPARASITIC ARTHROPODS

Parasitic mites See **Table 23**.

Table 23 Acari (ticks and mites) of medical importance

Order	Family	Genus and species	Notes
Tetrastigmata (red mites) Metastigmata (ticks – see **Tables 1, 2, 3**)		*Holothyrus* spp.	May be toxic if ingested
Mesostigmata (gamasid mites)	Dermanyssidae	*Dermanyssus gallinae*	Poultry red mite, infests humans
		Liponyssoides sanguineus	Carries *Rickettsia akari*
		Ornithonyssus bacoti	Tropical rat mite
		Ornithonyssus sylviarum	Northern fowl mite
		Ornithonyssus bursa	Tropical fowl mite
		Androlaelaps casalis	In nests of birds and small mammals, may carry Q fever
Astigmata	Acaridae (sensu lato)	*Tyrophagus putrescentiae*	Causes 'copra itch'
		Suidasia nesbitti	Causes 'wheat-pollard itch'
		Acarus siro	Causes 'baker's itch'
		Carpoglyphus lactis	Causes dried-fruit dermatitis
		Glycyphagus domesticus	Causes 'grocer's itch'
		Glycyphagus destructor	Common in hay, causes allergy
		Goheria fusca	In flour, causes allergy
	Pyroglyphidae	*Dermatophagoides* spp.	Feed on skin detritus, birds, mammals, Common in house dust
		Dermatophagoides pteronyssinus	Main house dust allergen
		Dermatophagoides farinae	Common house dust allergen
		Euroglyphus maynei	Common house dust mite
	Sarcoptidae	*Sarcoptes scabiei*	Scabies, Norwegian scabies
Prostigmata	Pyemotidae	*Pyemotes ventricosus*	Grain, straw mite, causes dermatitis
	Cheyletidae	*Cheyletiella parasitovorax*	In dog fur, causes dermatitis
		Cheyletiella blakey	Mainly in dog fur
		Cheyletiella yasguri	In dog, cat, rabbit fur
		Cheyletus eruditus	Predator of grain mites etc.
	Demodicidae	*Demodex folliculorum*	In human hair follicles
		Demodex brevis	In sebaceous glands
	Trombiculiidae	*Eutrombicula* spp.	Causes 'scrub-itch'
		Schoengastia spp.	Causes 'scrub-itch'
		Neotrombicula autumnalis	'Harvest mite'
		Leptotrombidium akamushi	Vector of *Orientia tsutsugamushi* (scrub typhus)
		Leptotrombidium deliense	Vector of scrub typhus
	Anystidae	*Anystis* spp.	'Whirligig mites'

Adapted from Alexander JO'D 1984 Arthropods and human skin. Springer-Verlag, Berlin and Lane RP, Crosskey RW (eds) 1993 Medical insecta and arachnids. Chapman & Hall, London.

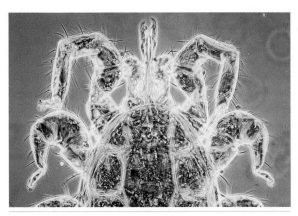

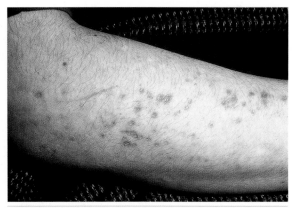

1027 *Ornithonyssus bacoti*, the tropical rat mite
Gamasid mites of the family Dermanyssidae are ectoparasites of birds and small mammals. Humans are an accidental host but a number of gamasid species transmit human pathogens (see **Tables 1, 23**), as well as causing severe cutaneous reactions. In spite of its name, *O. bacoti* is a cosmopolitan species found commonly in seaports. It frequently bites humans and produces large, irritating, papular lesions. Most species feed nocturnally and all those that affect humans tend to produce a similar response consisting firstly of itching, the onset of which may be delayed by some hours, followed by a rash. This varies in character from simple macules, papules or wheals to a varicelliform reaction. The history of exposure, which may be related to the individual's occupation, gives a clue to the diagnosis of the condition. The mites are relatively large (many about 1 mm long) compared with Astigmata (including sarcoptid and trombiculid mites) and Prostigmata.

1028 Varicelliform reaction to bites of *Dermanyssus gallinae*
Note the scratch marks due to the intense irritation on the skin of this man, who was bitten by the red poultry mite, another of the gamasid mites, while plucking turkeys.

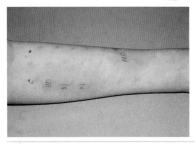

1029 Skin test for hypersensitivity in a patient with urticaria and hay fever
The reaction can be seen to allergens derived from house dust (HD), house dust mites (M) and pollen (CP), compared with the control (C). *Dermatophagoides pteronyssinus* and *Dermatophagoides farinae* are commonly found in house dust and have been associated in recent years with the common 'stuffy nose' syndrome that afflicts many people at night. They feed mainly on dead epithelial scales and other organic matter in house dust. The presence of protein from dead mites, which is probably responsible for allergic reactions to these mites, can also precipitate paroxysms of asthma in sensitised individuals and may cause atopic skin eruptions, including eczema, in others. Over 100 mites/g of dust have been recovered from the house dust of some asthmatic individuals, whose condition may improve if they can be moved to a mite-free environment.

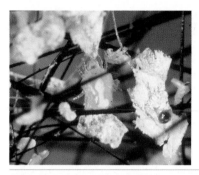

1030 *Cheyletiella parasitivorax*
The Cheyletidae are parasitic on small mammals, living in their fur and feeding mainly on dead epidermis, on hair and on other fur mites. Humans are affected by handling infested dogs or cats. This figure shows hair combings from a puppy. Three species in this genus are now recognised to cause lesions in humans. (× 25)

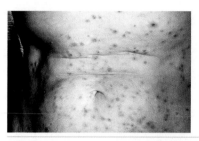

1031 Rash caused by *Cheyletiella parasitivorax*
The lesions developed in a woman who had recently acquired a puppy. The lesions consisted of small, erythematous papules with haemorrhagic, vesicular centres, which were intensely irritating. They may become pustular and may be excoriated by scratching. Management of cases should include the use of acaricides to rid pet animals and their bedding of the mites.

Scabies

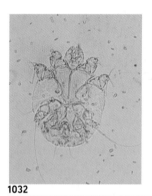

1032

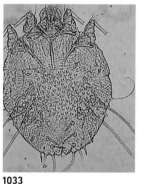

1033

1032 & 1033 Male and female scabies mites
The gravid female *Sarcoptes scabiei* (**1033**, right) burrows into the epidermis, lays its eggs and dies at the end of the tunnel. It is cosmopolitan in distribution. (**1032** left, ventral view × 115; **1033** dorsal view × 85)

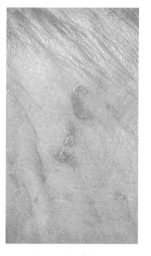

1034 Scabies burrows
These are seen here on the instep of the foot of an infant. The foot is the second commonest site of early infection at this age, with the axillae and neck also being invaded in some cases. The darker colouring represents the inflammatory reaction to the mites and their detritus.

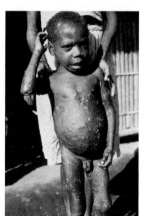

1035 Infected scabies in a Papuan boy
Intense local pruritus and dermatitis appear within a few days of infection. The tortuous tunnels may extend for several centimetres.

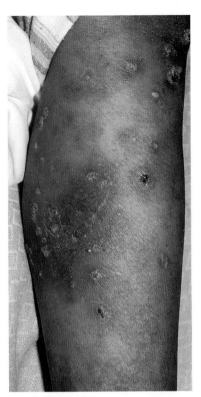

1036 Secondary erythema in scabies
Secondary infection is common, and erythema may be associated with bacterial invasion of the sarcoptic tracks.

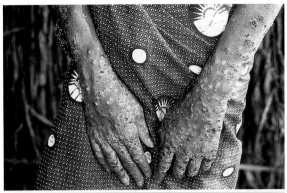

1037 Chronic eczematous scabies in a Gambian woman
The backs of the hands and arms are heavily infested in this woman. Constant scratching due to the intense itching may result in lichenification of the dry skin. The condition would need to be differentiated from onchocerciasis where both conditions are present.

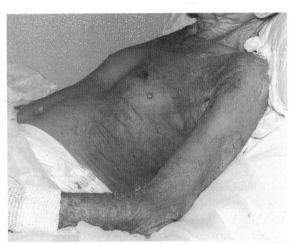

1039 Norwegian scabies in an old man
This 91-year-old man had had pruritus with crusty skin lesions, some over 1 cm thick, for 6 months prior to admission to hospital. In addition to the discovery of a heavy scabies infection he was found to have carcinoma of the bladder. The skin condition improved rapidly following anti-mite treatment. (Courtesy of A Biglino, D Casabianca and A Mastinu.)

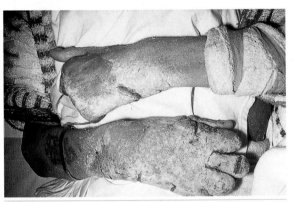

1038 Hyperkeratotic ('Norwegian') scabies in a patient who had suffered a 70% burns injury
This condition is often associated with immunosuppression, which may result, among other causes, from severe burns and includes HIV infection. The dorsum of the hands and fingers are most affected in this patient.

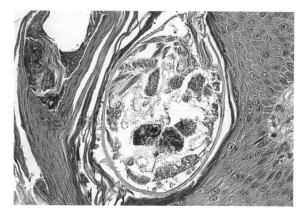

1040 Section of biopsy from patient with Norwegian scabies
This skin section shows some of the cuticular spines and internal organs of a female mite which lies within a subepidermal pocket under a thick layer of dead epidermis. The mites can be present in such patients in vast numbers. (*H&E* × *40*)

Other mite infestations

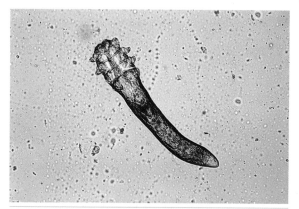

1041 Ventral view of *Demodex folliculorum*
This species inhabits human hair follicles, especially on the head and ears. It is believed that the mites can be found if carefully looked for in most healthy adults, in whom they cause no pathological changes. The follicles of the nose, nasolabial folds and malar prominences are most commonly infested, while the eyelashes often shelter numerous mites. Details of their life cycle are still obscure but they seem to undergo several moults in rather rapid succession. Infection is probably acquired during infancy from close physical contact with the infected mother. The mites are especially common in sebaceous skins and may cause a condition on the head of some individuals known as pityriasis folliculorum. The condition is confirmed by expressing the mites from individual nodulopapules or pustules. In recent years a second species has been identified in human sebaceous glands, *Demodex brevis*. (*Phase contrast* × *25*)

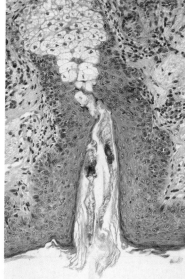

1042 Section of biopsy with *Demodex folliculorum*
Part of the body of the mite is seen in section within a hair follicle. (*H&E* × *100*)

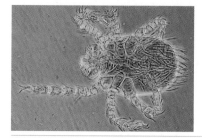

1043 Larval *Trombicula autumnalis*
These 'harvest mites' are common in grassland in temperate climates. The larvae, which normally feed on small mammals and birds, also attack humans, causing intense irritation. (× *75*). (*See also* **49**.)

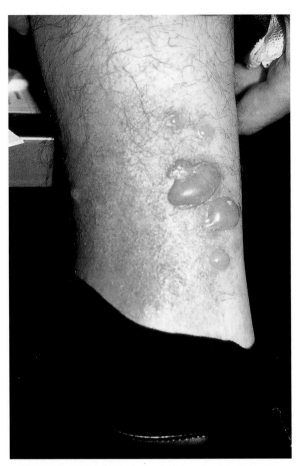

1044 Bullous lesions following 'chigger' bites
The larvae do not ingest blood but feed through the 'stylostome' on host tissue that has been dissolved by salivary secretions. After feeding the larvae develop into free-living, predatory nymphs.

Louse infestation

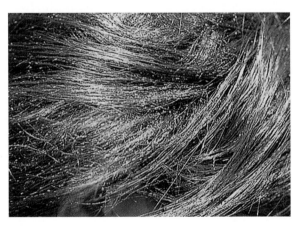

1045 *Pediculus capitis*
The head louse, *P. capitis*, is very common, and heavy infestations such as that seen here in an Indian girl can cause severe irritation. The eggs ('nits') are attached to the hairs and appear as masses of white dots. Unlike *Pediculus corporis*, *P. capitis* is not known to be a disease vector. DNA fingerprinting has recently confirmed the specific identity of head and body lice. The evolutionary origin of the two species and that of their hosts are still being debated by geneticists.

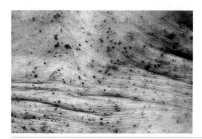

1046 Severe pediculosis corporis

Heavy infestation is common where people live in unhygienic conditions. Body lice spread rapidly wherever suitable ecological conditions prevail and are common in soldiers and refugees during wartime, in institutions for the mentally subnormal, prisons, etc. Formerly known also as 'vagabond's disease', severe dermatitis due to the presence of heavy louse populations and the scratching that the bites stimulate, especially at night, is often accompanied by pigmentation of the affected areas, restlessness causing loss of sleep and, in chronic cases, lichenification and eczema. As in this patient, thousands of lice may be present on the patient's body and in his clothes.

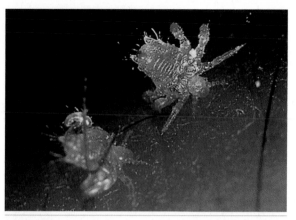

1047 *Phthirus pubis*

The pubic or 'crab' louse is commonly spread during sexual intercourse. Sites infected other than the pubic area include the eyelashes. (× 7)

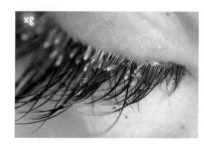

1048 Eggs of *Phthirus pubis* attached to the bases of eyelashes

As seen here, the infection can be severe in this location.

Bed bugs

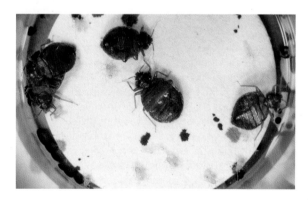

1049 *Cimex lectularus*

This species and the tropical bed bug, *Cimex hemipterus*, frequent houses, where they feed on the blood of the inhabitants at night. Multiple bites are very common and may be due to interrupted feeding by a single bug. Blood is actively sucked up by pumping action of the hypopharynx once the stylets have pierced a small blood vessel, from 10–20 minutes being required for the bug to become fully engorged. The bite itself is not painful but erythema and itching develop later. Bedbugs are a considerable pest but probably of no major importance in disease transmission. It is believed that their numbers are increasing in some Western countries because of their unobserved importation with the possessions of returning 'backpacker' tourists who sleep in insanitary accommodation, especially in tropical areas. (× 3)

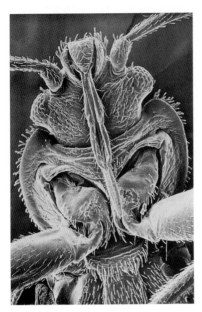

1050 Ventral surface of head of *Cimex hemipterus* showing proboscis
Scanning electron micrograph showing the biting mouth parts of the bedbug. They are contained in the proboscis, which is held under the body when not in use. This is the tropical bedbug, *C. hemipterus*. (× *150*)

Flea infestations

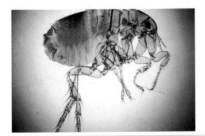

1051 Female *Pulex irritans*
The 'human flea' is a cosmopolitan species that is becoming uncommon in houses in many temperate countries. Under especially favourable climatic and environmental conditions, fleas may appear in almost epidemic proportions. Humans are most commonly bitten by cat and dog fleas of the genus *Ctenocephalides*. (× *20*)

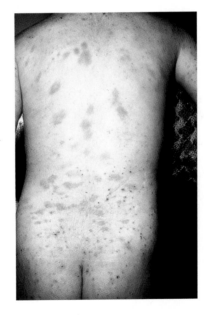

1052 Extensive papular urticaria caused by massive flea infestation
The intense irritation in the lumbar region caused this man to scratch incessantly, producing marked excoriation of lesions that were accessible.

Tungiasis

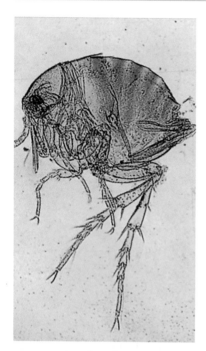

1053 Male *Tunga penetrans*

The 'jigger' or 'chigoe' flea, which is common in tropical areas of South America and Africa, is only 1 mm long and the smallest flea known. The male, which has a characteristically angular head, is free-living. (× 28)

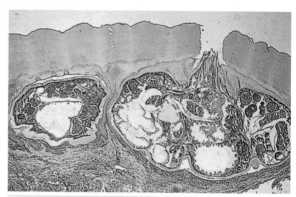

1055 Section of female *Tunga penetrans* in the skin

Having buried itself in the skin, often under the toenails, the female swells up to the size of a small pea within 8–10 days as its eggs mature. (*H&E* × 75)

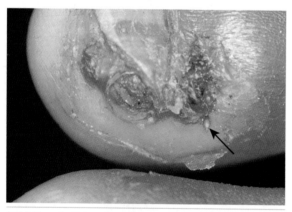

1054 Female jigger flea penetrating the skin of a toe

The gravid female (arrow) burrows into the epidermis, where it settles with its posterior end facing the entrance hole. The periungual region is a favoured site of entry. Here two lesions are visible near the rim of the nail. There is inflammation and desquamation of the adjacent skin. Secondary infection is common when pathogenic microorganisms enter through the entry hole. (Courtesy of Professor H Feldmeier and Dr M Eisele.)

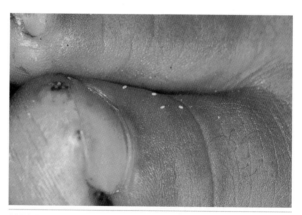

1056 Female *Tunga penetrans* laying eggs

Some 150–200 eggs per day are actively ejected through the entry hole as seen in this photograph showing a line of recently projected eggs. Oviposition continues over a period of about 5 weeks, after which the flea dies. The eggs mature in 3–4 days in the dust and dirt covering the floors of dwellings. (Courtesy Professor H Feldmeier and Dr M Eisele. Reproduced by permission of Springer-Verlag from Eisele M, Heukelbach J, Van Marck E et al 2003 Investigations on the biology, epidemiology, pathology and control of *Tunga penetrans* in Brazil: I Natural history of tungiasis in humans. Parasitology Research 90: 94, Fig. 15).

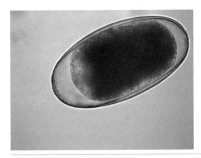

1057 Living egg of *Tunga penetrans*

The oval egg, which is readily seen macroscopically as a tiny pearly object (see **1056**), is about 0.5 mm long and 0.3 mm in diameter. (× *70*)

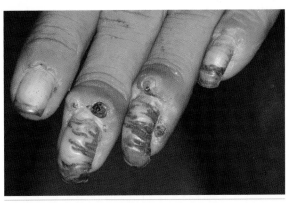

1058 Heavy infection with *Tunga penetrans* in the fingers of a Brazilian patient

Although the feet are most commonly infected, other parts of the body may also be implicated in tungiasis. Two of this individual's fingernails are badly distorted. A large survey covering 1184 residents of a Brazilian 'favela' showed that 33.6% had tungiasis. About 5.5% of them had lesions on the hands, others on the elbows, thighs and gluteal areas. (Courtesy of Professor H Feldmeier and Dr M Eisele.)

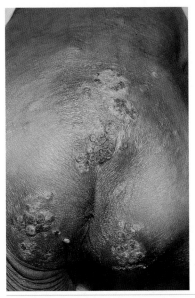

1059 Massive infection with *Tunga penetrans* in an Amerindian

This patient in Cayenne had about 1000 female *T. penetrans* embedded in his hands, feet, buttocks, elbows and knees. He made an uneventful recovery after removal of the insects with forceps following the local application of salicylated Vaseline. (It is important to protect such a patient with antitetanus vaccine before and a topical antibiotic after such treatment.) (Courtesy of Dr Emmanuel Clyti, Institut Guyanais de Dermatologie Tropical.)

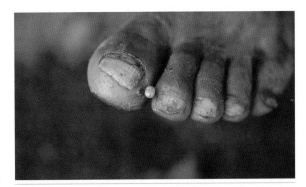

1060 *Tunga trimamillata* gravid female

A second species of chigger flea, *T.trimamillata*, has been described in patients with tungiasis in Ecuador where it was first observed in pigs, goats and cattle. This species co-exists with *T.penetrans* in some localities. Here the gravid female has been extracted from a site at the corner of the patient's left big toe. Although only 10 species of *Tunga* have been recognised to date it seems quite likely that others remain unidentified up to now. (Courtesy of Dr M L Fioravanti.)

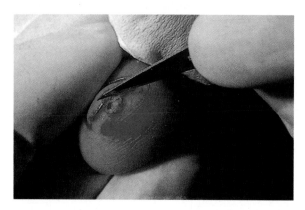

1061 Jigger flea being removed from toe
Habitual sufferers shell the gravid females out of the skin with a pin or sliver of bamboo, usually scattering eggs in the process. Tetanus is a common sequel to this type of self-treatment. The larvae that are usually scattered in the process of extraction mature to adulthood on the ground. In heavy infections the application of salicylated Vaseline leads to the death of the embedded fleas with minimal trauma to the host. Some lotions based on coconut oil, in addition to promoting healing, are of value in prophylaxis.

Myiasis See **Table 24**.

Table 24 Myiasis-producing diptera of medical importance

Family/subfamily	Genus and species	Other names	Notes
Calliphoridae			
Calliphorinae			
'Metallic group'	Chrysomya bezziana	Old World screw worm ⎫	Feed on living tissue in wounds
	Cochliomyia hominivorax	New World screw worm ⎭	
	Lucilia spp.	Greenbottles ⎫	Feed on dead tissue in wounds
	Calliphora spp.	Bluebottles, blow flies ⎭	
	Phormia regina	'Black blow fly'	Can cause dermal, enteric myiasis
	Cynomopsis cadaverina		Invades wounds
'Nonmetallic group'	Auchmeromyia senegalensis*	Congo floor maggot	Sucks blood from skin
	Cordylobia anthropophaga	Tumbu, mango fly	Causes subcutaneous boils
Sarcophaginae	Wohlfahrtia spp.	Flesh flies	Invade wounds or normal tissue, especially on head
	Wohlfahrtia magnifica		Commonest species in humans
	Sarcophaga haemorrhoidalis		May occur in gut
Cuterebridae	Dermatobia hominis	Human bot fly	Causes subcutaneous boils
	Cuterebra spp.	North American bot flies	Skin and eye lesions
Gasterophilidae	Gasterophilus spp.	Stomach bot flies	Invade skin and may migrate to eye
Hypodermatidae	Hypoderma spp.	Warble flies ⎫	Cause dermal, eye or nasopharyngeal lesions
	Hypoderma lineatum	Lesser cattle warble ⎭	
	Hypoderma tarandi	Reindeer warble	Ophthalmomyiasis
	Cephenemyia ulrichii	Moose throat bot fly	
Oestridae	Oestrus ovis	Sheep nasal bot fly	Invades nasopharynx and eye

This table does not include facultative parasites such as larvae of the family Syrphidae, which may be found in the lower intestine or urogenital tract, faeces or urine. Species of Muscidae, genera *Fannia*, *Musca* and *Muscina*, may also be found in faeces.

* Formerly known as *Auchmeromyia luteola*.
Modified from Zumpt F 1965 Myiasis in man and animals in the Old World. Butterworths, London and Lane RP, Crosskey RW (eds) 1993 Medical insecta and arachnids. Chapman & Hall, London.

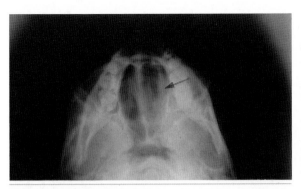

1062 Radiograph of nasal sinuses invaded by larvae of Chrysomya bezziana

The patient was a 14-year-old girl from the eastern province of Saudi Arabia who complained of recurrent nose bleeding and pain of 5 days' duration. Radiography showed that the lateral wall of her left nasal cavity (indicated by the arrow) had been destroyed. More than 80 larvae were removed surgically from the sinuses and the patient recovered.

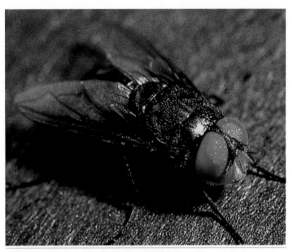

1063 Male Cochliomyia hominivorax

The family Calliphoridae contains six metallic-coloured flies in the subfamily Calliphorinae of which two species, the screw-worms, have carnivorous larvae that are obligatory feeders on living flesh and four species are essentially scavengers of decaying flesh. The New World screw-worm is a notorious parasite of domestic livestock and its depravations in the 1950s and 1960s caused huge economic losses in North, Central and South America amounting to over US$100 million. Humans are frequently infected. Fortunately the female only mates once and this has made possible a control campaign using mass-reared, irradiation-sterilised males that has pushed the frontier southwards from the USA towards Mexico. The fly was discovered for the first time in Africa in Libya in the 1980s, (probably having been imported with cattle from South America), where it infected over 2000 cattle and 200 people before its presence was exposed. Since adult females can fly over 200 km, it was feared that the species could spread across north Africa and perhaps south across the Saharan trade routes. However, a mass international campaign using sterilised males (reared and imported from the USA), was successful in eradicating it. The larvae also attack open wounds on humans, feeding on living as well as dead tissue. (× 8.2)

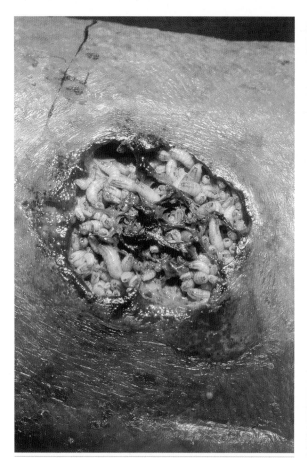

1064 Massive screw-worm infection of the leg

A large mass of larvae of *C. hominivorax* can be seen in a gaping wound in the right leg of this 72-year-old man in Cayenne. The local application of a solution of 10% ivermectin in propylene glycol rapidly paralysed the larvae so that, within 24 hours, over 150 dead larvae could be removed easily. A heavy infection with *C. hominovorax* can kill a large animal such as a cow in 10 days. (Courtesy of Professor R Pradinaud, Institut Guyanais de Dermatologie Tropicale.)

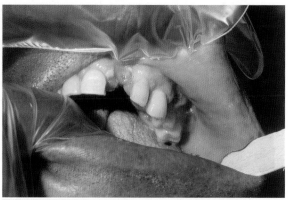

1065 Buccal infection with *Cochliomyia hominovorax*

This 70-year old man in Cayenne complained of feeling a number of foreign bodies between his teeth. Examination revealed the presence of larvae within cavities in the mucosa. An hour after the application of ivermectin five immobilised screw-worm larvae were removed with forceps. (Courtesy of Professor R Pradinaud, Institut Guyanais de Dermatologie Tropicale.)

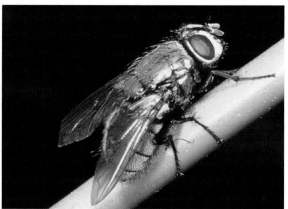

1066 Adult female *Lucilia sericata*

'Greenbottles', the larvae of which are opportunistic feeders on carrion and other dead organic matter, sometimes invade wounds but there feed only on dead tissue. Another species that sometimes invades wounds is *Lucilia cuprina*. (× 5)

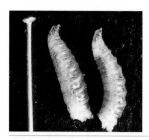

1067 Third instar larvae of *Lucilia sericata*

Note the fleshy posterior appendages known as 'anal lobes'. Because they do not invade healthy tissue, the larvae of this calliphorid fly have been used to help in the debridement of infected wounds, for example under occlusive plaster of Paris splints in patients with osteomyelitis. This practice is currently becoming more popular especially in the presence of antibiotic resistance. The larval stages, however, last only about 1 week, after which the insects pupate. The adults hatch in about 7–10 days. (× 5)

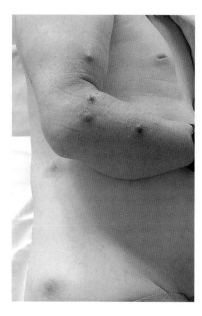

1068 Tumbu fly lesions

Multiple infections with larvae of *Cordylobia anthropophaga* caused painful boils on the body and arm of this 53-year-old man who had been infested in Zimbabwe about 2 weeks earlier with newly emerged larvae, probably from clothing left on the ground to dry after it was washed.

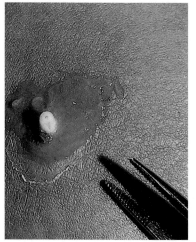

1069 Extracting a larva

The larva leaves the skin if it is covered in oil, which blocks the spiracles. It can then be removed easily with forceps.

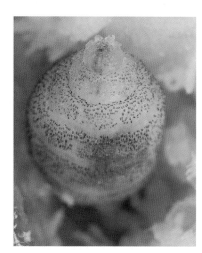

1070 Larva of Tumbu fly

The figure shows the powerful hooks with which the larvae feed inside the skin. (× 20)

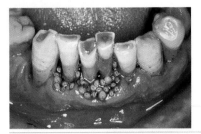

1071 Mouth of an old man infected with larvae of an unidentified *Wohlfahrtia* species

The larvae of this genus of 'flesh flies' of the subfamily Sarcophaginae are essentially scavengers in decaying flesh, faeces, rotting food, etc. but are occasionally found in wounds and sores. The females are larvivorous, producing batches of 20–40 first instar larvae, which develop rapidly, the third instars burrowing in soil to pupate. This man was infected while asleep under a tree in a Middle East country. The spiracles of the numerous larvae are very obvious in this view. Normally they are not easily seen, since they are situated within a larval pit.

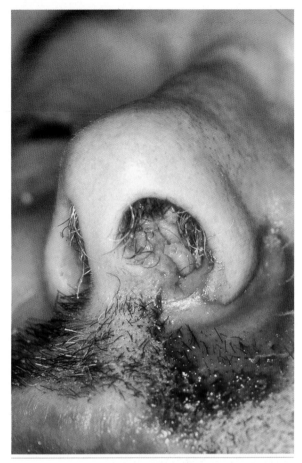

1072 Larvae of *Sarcophaga* in the nose of a man with a nasal tumour

The spiracles, concealed in the spiracular pits, are not visible in this figure. Like *Wohlfahrtia*, the larvae of flies in this closely related genus are normally found in decaying organic matter but may be laid in malodorous wounds or tumours, as in this case. The species may be *Sarcophaga carnaria*.

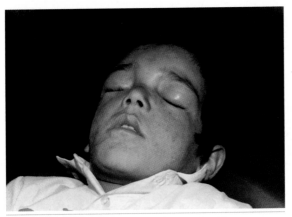

1096 Facial oedema due to cardiac dysfunction following the sting of *Hemiscorpius lepturus*
If a sufficiently high concentration of the venom of this scorpion reaches the circulation, it can exert serious changes in the central nervous and cardiovascular systems, as well as causing acute haemolysis, which may necessitate blood transfusion, and depression of the circulating lymphocytes in the blood. This Iranian boy is one of 54 who showed systemic effects among 2534 patients stung by *H. lepturus*.

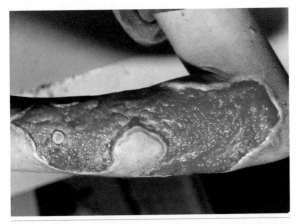

1098 Extensive sloughing of skin and epidermis of arm
The figure shows complete sloughing of the skin of the arm in the child seen in **1097**, necessitating extensive skin grafting.

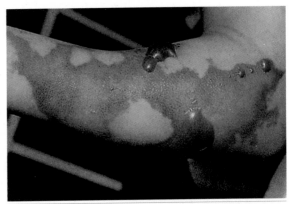

1097 Lesions following sting of *Hemiscorpius lepturus*
The venom of chactid scorpions is mainly haemolytic and proteolytic. This child's arm shows an early stage of skin necrosis following the sting of *H. lepturus*, a species that occurs in Iran and Iraq.

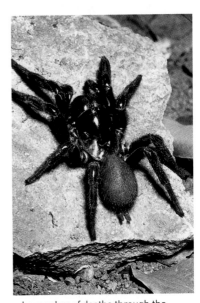

1099 Female *Atrax robustus*
This large Australian arthropod (the 'Sydney funnel web spider', female body length up to 4 cm), one of several species of *Atrax* on that continent, is a large, nocturnal spider that frequently enters houses in New South Wales. Its bite is extremely painful and it has caused a number of deaths through the injection, by means of its large fangs, of atrotoxin, to which humans are peculiarly susceptible. This neurotoxin induces spontaneous action potentials in nerves supplying skeletal muscle as well as the autonomic nerve system. The clinical picture in severe envenomation is a mixture of signs starting with severe muscular twitching, profuse salivation and lacrimation, nausea and vomiting, abdominal pain and diarrhoea, followed by acute hypertension, extreme restlessness, dyspnoea possibly leading to asphyxia, confusion and finally coma and death. The initial treatment should be to apply a strong pressure bandage and immobilise the affected limb to slow the absorption of the venom, followed by the administration of specific antivenom.

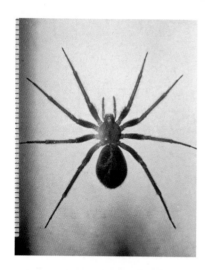

1100 Female *Loxosceles laeta* (Scytodidae)

This genus, which is widely distributed throughout much of the world, contains well over 60 species of which four, *L. laeta*, *Loxosceles reclusa*, *Loxosceles gaucho* and *Loxosceles rufescens*, are especially poisonous to humans, although envenomation has also been recorded from bites of other species. These spiders are also called 'violin spiders' because of the characteristic violin-like marking on the dorsal surface of the cephalothorax in many species, or 'brown spiders' because of their dull brown coloration. *Loxosceles* spin an irregular web and feed mainly on small arthropods that they ensnare. However, they are mainly nocturnal and, since they seek dark places to shelter, they are commonly attracted to human habitations. If accidentally handled, they bite with their inwardly pointing fangs, at the same time actively ejecting venom. This is essentially cytolytic, since it is normally used to partially digest the bodies of their prey, which can then be ingested through the mouth. However, in mammals it can also be haemolytic. This species is found over much of South America except the extreme northern parts and is responsible for hundreds of severe injuries, with up to about 10% of fatalities. (× 2.3)

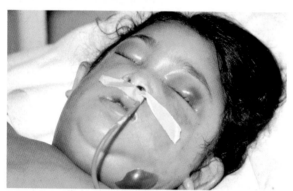

1101 Girl bitten by *Loxosceles laeta*

Loxoscelism presents in two forms, the first limited to the skin and subcutaneous tissues and the second systemic due to the haemolytic effects of the venom when absorbed. This Chilean child who was bitten on the right cheek shows the effects of severe intravascular haemolysis, as well as the beginning of blistering and necrosis of the skin. The massive facial oedema is evident and she is comatose. This type of response to envenomation occurs in about 13% of the victims of *L. laeta* bites. Up to a third of such cases die with haematuria, anuria and other evidence of haemolysis unless treated urgently with antivenom and general supportive therapy.

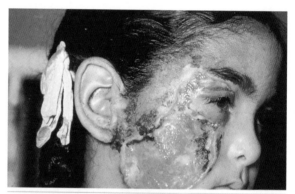

1102 Sloughing of skin following spider bite

This Chilean child was bitten by *L. laeta*. Necrosis and sloughing followed severe blistering at the site of the bite and generalised facial oedema.

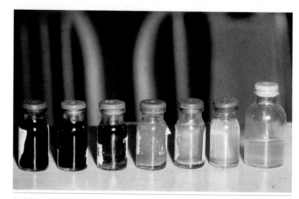

1103 Urinary changes following a bite by *Loxosceles laeta*

These urine samples were taken 2, 3, 5, 6, 7, 8 and 9 days following a bite that was treated by the administration of antivenom followed by corrective surgery in a Chilean patient.

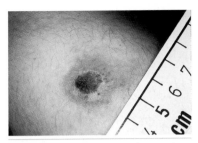

1104 *Loxosceles gaucho* bite on the thigh after 48 hours
Initially the site of the bite, which is very painful, shows an area of oedema with a central violaceous plaque. After a while the centre becomes necrotic and is surrounded by an area of ischaemia, beyond which is an erythematous halo. (© D A Warrell.)

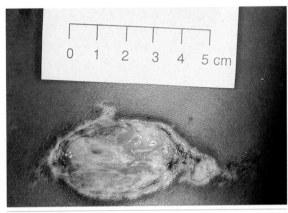

1105 Lesion caused by *Loxosceles gaucho* 25 days after the bite
The affected skin was removed surgically as the area surrounding the bite is now known to have a high content of venom. Debridement can assist by removing this material, although skin grafting is often required later to promote healing. Antibiotics to control secondary bacterial infection are indicated, and sometimes corticosteroids. (© D A Warrell.)

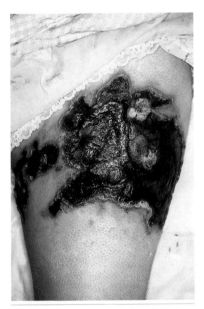

1106 Severe necrosis following the bite of *Loxosceles reclusa* in the western USA

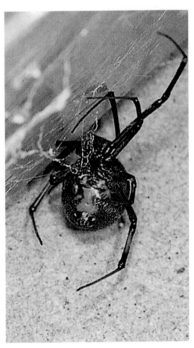

1107 Female 'black widow' spider
Among the best known poisonous spiders is the 'black widow', *Latrodectus mactans*. Humans are bitten only by the females, which produce α_t-atrotoxin, a venom that causes the rapid release of acetylcholine at neuromuscular junctions. Noradrenaline (norepinephrine) is also released, causing signs of overstimulation of the sympathetic nervous system. A transient acute psychosis may follow, but most victims make a full recovery. (× *1*)

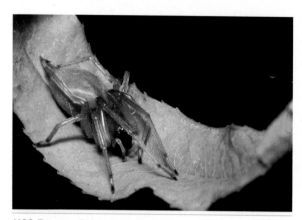

1108 Female *Chiracanthium lawrencei* (Clubionidae)
The 'sac spiders' are cosmopolitan and some frequent houses. Envenomation causes severe pain, which radiates proximally and is followed by sweating, nausea and sometimes vomiting. The site of the bite can become necrotic. This aggressive species, which has widely separated fangs, is responsible for about 75% of all poisonous spider bites in the more humid parts of South Africa. (Courtesy of Dr G Newlands.)

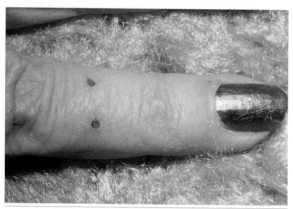

1109 Bite marks caused by *Chiracanthium lawrencei*
The fang marks are distinctive and sometimes have a greenish tinge that is the colour of the venom, against which no antivenom is yet available. This woman was bitten 1 week prior to being photographed. (Courtesy of Dr G Newlands.)

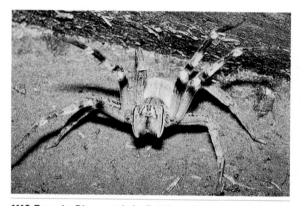

1110 Female *Phoneutria* in fighting stance
The chelicerae and fangs are very clear in this picture of a specimen seen in Cayenne. These species inhabit the Amazonian part of Brazil and neighbouring countries. The banana spiders are aggressive creatures and will attack their attacker, moving very rapidly and climbing anything available to reach them. (× 0.75)

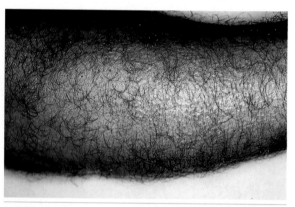

1111 Bite by *Phoneutria nigriventer*
One of the bite marks is visible. The venom is neurotoxic and functions in a similar manner to atrotoxin by causing the release of acetylcholine and catecholamines that stimulate the parasympathetic and sympathetic nervous systems. About 2 hours after the bite there is marked local swelling, sweating and piloerection due to the release of catecholamines. The associated signs are similar to those described for poisoning by atrotoxin but, in addition, priapism often occurs in male children. Death caused by *Phoneutria* occurs rarely. In Brazil a polyvalent antivenom is available against *Phoneutria*, *Lycosa* and *Loxosceles*. (© D A Warrell.)

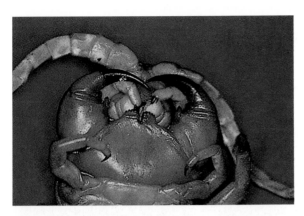

1112 Head of a venomous centipede

A few of the large species of tropical centipedes are capable of inflicting an intensely painful but probably nonlethal sting. The venom is passed through the piercing forcicules seen on the ventral surface of the head of this large *Scolopendra* species from Singapore. (× *2*)

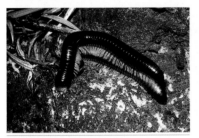

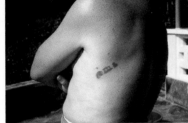

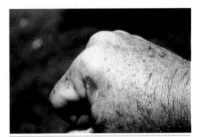

1113 *Epibolus pulchripes* (Spirobolida)

These giant millipedes from east Africa are harmless unless provoked, preferring to hide in moist earth or humus, where they feed on vegetable matter. The glossy male is readily distinguished from the female, which has a comparatively matt surface. The pairs of orange legs on each segment and the bright orange, jointed antennae of the male are well illustrated here. Some tropical species, such as the African *Graphidostreptus gigas*, can exceed 28 cm in length.

1114 'Burn' caused by contact with *Epibolus pulchripes*

The victim unwittingly slept on the millipede, which had entered his bed. Within an hour he noted itching and discomfort and the following morning the site was erythematous. It subsequently turned purple. Five days later the hardened skin cracked and peeled, leaving a raw patch that eventually healed, leaving no residual pigmentation.

1115 'Burn' caused by fluid droplets squirted by *Polyconoceras alokistus*

This giant streptobolid is endemic in Papua New Guinea, the child shown here being attacked at Lae on the north coast. Like that of *Epibolus pulchripes*, the liquid that this species can eject for some 25 cm causes immediate pain and brown staining on contact with the skin, followed by erythema and oedema, which may remain visible for a week or more. If the fluid reaches the conjunctiva or cornea it can cause serious and very painful conjunctivitis with subsequent ulceration of the conjunctiva and cornea.

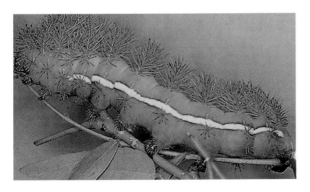

1116 Poisonous spines on a caterpillar

The larvae of many species of moths are protected with venomous spines. The toxin of many species (including the saturniid species, *Automeris liberia*, from Cayenne, seen here) contains histamine. (× *0.7*)

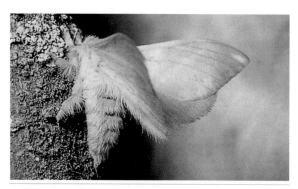

1117 Female *Hylesia metabus* (Saturniidae)
The abdomens of adult moths of this genus are covered with strongly barbed, urticating hairs (fléchettes) that are readily shed if the insects are damaged. The presence of large numbers of these moths has caused epidemics of 'lepidopterism' or 'erucism' of sufficient gravity that a number of tropical tourist centres have had to be temporarily abandoned. (× *1.1*)

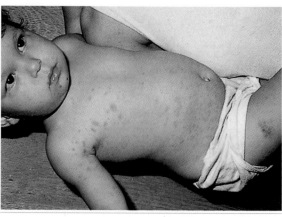

1118 Rash caused by contact with *Hylesia*
This child in São Paulo State, Brazil, was probably affected by *Hylesia paulex*, which is common in that area. The venom of another Brazilian moth, *Lonomia achelous*, contains a fibrinolysin. (© D A Warrell.)

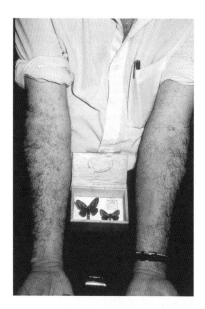

1119 Severe dermatitis caused by *Hylesia* moths
Hairs from female moths gave rise to a severely irritating and oedematous rash on the left arm of this man. He worked as an entomologist in Brazil and the display case shows the offending specimens (? *Hylesia paulex*).

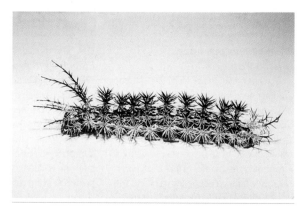

1120 Caterpillar of *Lonomia achelous* (Saturniidae)
This hemileucine species, which occurs in the Amazon region of Brazil, has poison spines that deliver a potent fibrinolytic toxin. Similar toxic responses to saturniid caterpillars have been reported from Venezuela.

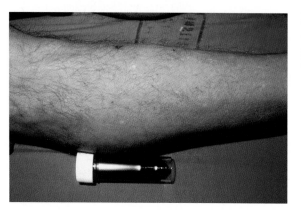

1121 Leg of a Brazilian man stung by *Lonomia achelous*
This man's calf was stung while he was resting on the ground. Later he noticed blood in his urine and bleeding from his gums. The local skin reaction was minimal. (© D A Warrell.)

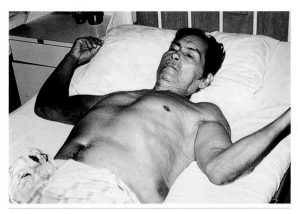

1122 Brazilian adult with severe haemorrhagic syndrome after being stung by a larva of *Lonomia achelous*

Following contact with the insect there is a localised burning sensation, then headache and generalised discomfort. Extensive ecchymoses appear after 8–72 hours in the affected area and then over other parts of the body. There may be profuse bleeding from the orifices.

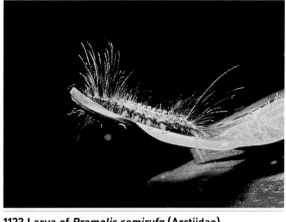

1123 Larva of *Premolis semirufa* (Arctiidae)

Stinging by this Brazilian caterpillar causes a condition known as 'pararama'. The long barbed hairs at both ends of the insect are prominent in this picture, as are the brown dorsal tufts. The latter carry short, venomous hairs that cause a severe inflammatory reaction at the sites of the skin that are penetrated. ($\times 0.9$)

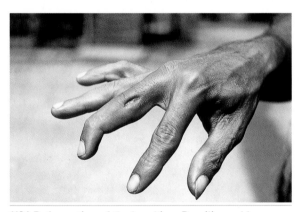

1124 Deformation of the hand in a Brazilian rubber tapper

Premolis semirufa feeds on the leaves of the rubber tree, *Hevea brasiliensis*, and is commonly encountered by plantation workers. The stings cause deep inflammation around the joints that may leave the victim permanently disabled.

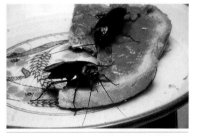

1125 Adult *Periplaneta americana* feeding

Cockroaches such as these and *Blatella germanica*, which frequent houses and feed on rotting organic matter, food, excrement and other debris, can carry pathogens mechanically on their feet, legs and mouthparts. There is increasing evidence that antigens derived from cockroaches such as these are responsible for asthma, especially among people living in highly infested, poor-quality housing. ($\times 0.75$)

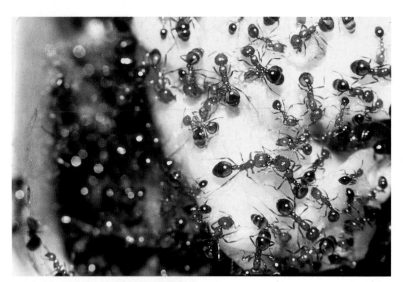

1126 Workers of *Solenopsis* (Myrmicinae)

Two sizes of worker of this unidentified species of 'fire ant' from Cayenne are seen feeding on a piece of meat. *Solenopsis* have gained their name because of the extremely painful stings they inflict. The venom is composed largely of various 2,6-dialkylpiperidines, the exact compounds being species-dependent. They are haemolytic and cytolytic. Some proteinaceous material and a small quantity of phospholipase A and hyaluronidase are also present. Like all Myrmicinae, they also possess mandibular gland venoms that are rich in ethyl ketones. (× 2.4)

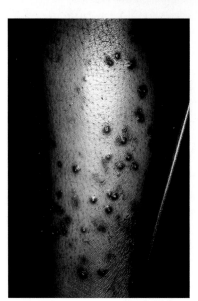

1127 Healing bites of *Solenopsis* in a dark skinned individual

The pustules rupture, leaving a crust that heals in 3–10 days. As with other hymenopterous stings, some individuals become sensitised and repeated stings by *Solenopsis* can lead to severe anaphylactic responses. In the southern USA it has been estimated that 1 million people are stung every year by *Solenopsis geminata*.

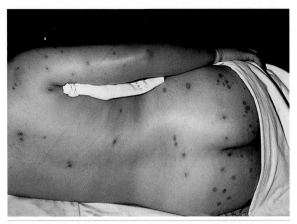

1128 Acute renal failure following multiple stings by *Vespa affinis*

Hornets in this genus occur worldwide and are generally large, very aggressive insects. They often attack in large numbers and are responsible for many deaths. *Vespa orientalis* occurs from north and east Africa through the Middle East and central Asia to south-east Asia. This Thai soldier, who was stung by over 100 hornets, developed intravascular haemolysis associated with frank haemoglobinuria and acute renal tubular necrosis leading to renal failure. He eventually recovered after dialysis. Such serious consequences of multiple hornet stings are not uncommon. Another effect of hornet venom is rhabdomyolysis associated with myoglobinuria and renal failure. Recovery can be achieved with prompt dialysis and other supportive measures. Phospholipase A associated with kinins in the venom is believed to trigger the red cell lysis and may also have a direct toxic effect on the renal tubular epithelium. Wasp venom also contains a mast-cell degranulating peptide called mastoparan. This is also a potent stimulator of endogenous phospholipase activity (comparable to the melittin in bee venom). Such severe responses can be distinguished from hypersensitivity reactions, since the latter are almost immediate and may follow even a single sting. Purely toxic effects may take 24 hours or more to become evident.

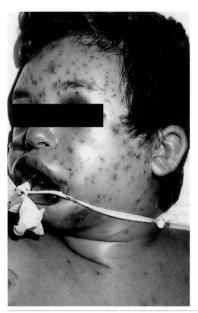

1129 Fatal, multiple bee stings by *Apis mellifera scutellata*, the African 'killer bee'

This highly aggressive bee was introduced into Brazil in 1956 because of its good honey productivity. It has competed with the local subspecies of *Apis mellifera* and is now colonising other countries of both South and North America, where the aggressive behaviour of its swarms has caused many casualties and deaths. As distinct from the stings of wasps, those of bees are barbed and cannot be removed from the site of the attack in skin. Unlike the venom of wasps, that of the Apidae is constituted by melittin (about 50%), phospholipase A (12%), histamine (0.1–1.5%), hyaluronidase (1–3%), apamin (2%) and a mast cell discharging peptide (MCD) (1–2%). Histamine produces the acute pain following bee stings. Melittin is a stimulator of endogenous phospholipase A (like the mastoparan of wasps, which also combines the action of MCD). Apamin has a neurotoxic action. Melittin is actually a mixture of several peptides that appear to be antigenic but not anaphylactogenic. Apamin, which may also contain several small peptides, acts on polysynaptic reflexes at the level of the spinal cord. The figure shows a Brazilian boy, aged 13 years, 48 hours after he was attacked by a swarm of *Apis mellifera scutellata* in São Paulo State, Brazil. He received more than 1500 stings. At first he developed extensive oedema and bruising, his consciousness was impaired and he became oliguric. The remains of many bee stings can still be seen in the skin and hair. Later the boy developed bronchospasm, hypotension, intravascular haemolysis with haemoglobinuria and myoglobinuria. He also had spontaneous bleeding from the mouth and other sites. Soon he became anuric and hypertensive, dying on the third day after being stung. (© D A Warrell.)

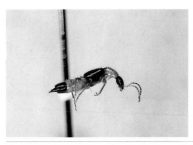

1130 *Paederus fusca* (Staphylinidae)
These small, colourful staphylinids produce vesicating lesions if crushed on the skin due to the release from their bodies of pederin, an extremely toxic alkaloid. *P. fusca* is common in rice fields in Thailand and other countries of south-east Asia and causes blisters in rice pickers during the harvest season. (× 4.5)

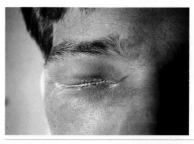

1131 'Nairobi eye', ophthalmia caused by *Paederus sabaeus*
Severe periorbital swelling is seen, associated with a linear vesication of the upper eyelid and adjacent bridge of the nose, as well as a purulent conjunctivitis. The patient was affected by a beetle that flew into his eye 39 hours before this photograph was taken.

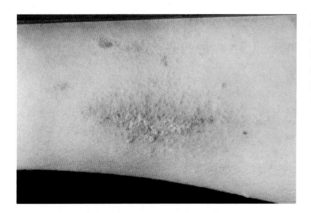

1132 Linear vesication caused by a blister beetle in the Gambia
Fluid from the broken bulla in the centre has contaminated the adjacent skin. Scratching or simple contact with a primary lesion often produces secondary vesication in adjacent or even distant areas of skin. (Courtesy of Mr C Argent.)

MARINE VERTEBRATES

Venomous fish

Poisoning by fish may be direct, through envenomation by various mainly tropical fish that have poison-carrying spines, or indirect, through the ingestion of a number of species inhabiting coral reefs that produce a lipid-soluble substance called ciguatoxin. The latter, which causes gastro-intestinal and neurological symptoms in a syndrome known as 'ciguatera', is common, mainly around tropical coastal areas. Although rarely fatal, it is a public health problem in some regions especially of the Caribbean and south Pacific. In the latter the annual incidence in 1984 was estimated at about 3.6 per 10 000 population. Treatment of ciguatera is essentially symptomatic. Ciguatoxin is synthesised by a number of dinoflagellates and fish are now believed to acquire the substance from them through the food chain.

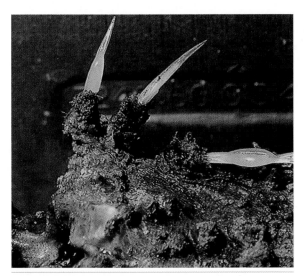

1133 Venomous spines of the stone fish *Synanceja horrida*

Many species of fish, including weever fishes and stone fishes, have venomous spines. The stone fish lies well concealed in the sand of marine shores. Venom produced in glands that emerge at the tips of the dorsal spines causes intense pain if they enter the skin, and severe stings can be fatal. The pain that follows envenomation may be sufficient to cause delirium and can persist for days. This coastal stone fish, one of the most dangerous, occurs around Indo-Pacific coasts as far south as southern Australia. Stone fishes belong to the family Scorpanidae, which also includes scorpion fishes and zebra fishes. Many of the species are found in the eastern Pacific and Atlantic coastal waters, as well as the Indo-Pacific region. As the venom is rapidly denatured by heat, placing the injured part in water as hot as can be tolerated safely can speed the rate of recovery.

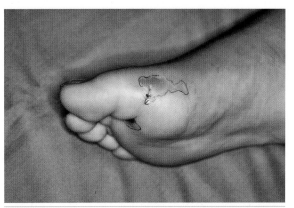

1134 Foot of woman stung by the stone fish *Synanceja verrucosa*

Concentric, necrotising cellulitis spreading from two points of entry by stone fish spines is seen on the medial side of the forefoot of this patient, who was stung by this 'reef stone fish' in Tahiti. Such lesions are commonly secondarily infected by bacteria such as *Pseudomonas* species and heal with difficulty even after the deployment of antibiotics. (Courtesy of Professor E Caumes.)

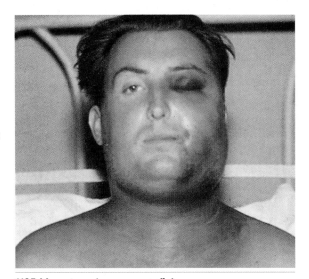

1135 Man stung by a weever fish

Weever fish, which are distributed along north-east Atlantic and Mediterranean coasts, have venomous spines over the gill covers and dorsum. The venom is both neurotoxic and haemotoxic. This man shows the haemorrhagic effects of weever fish venom.

Poisonous amphibians

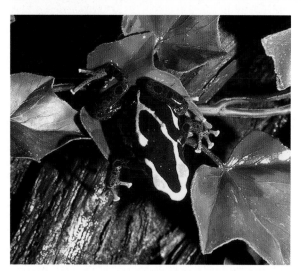

1136 *Dendrobates tinctorius,* a tropical poison dart frog
The skin of many species of frog and toad contains pharmacologically active compounds called batrachotoxins, some of which are extremely poisonous, even more so than curare and strychnine. They contain toxic alkaloids that have selective effects on ion permeability, leading to irreversible depolarisation of nerve and muscle. This small frog, which grows up to about 6 cm in length, lives in the rain forests of Guyana, Surinam, Cayenne and parts of Brazil. The skin secretions were employed by Indian hunters to coat the tips of their arrows. It is possible that some of these toxins are acquired from certain species of beetle that the frogs consume. Accidental poisoning of humans is rare but caution must be exercised by people who keep them as a hobby.

SNAKES (See Table 25.)

Venomous snakes include members of four families: sea snakes (Hydrophiidae); cobras, mambas, kraits and taipans (Elapidae); vipers and rattlesnakes (Viperidae); and the boomslang (Colubridae). Travellers to remote areas where venomous snakes are prevalent should be informed of the steps to be taken in the event of a bite and of antivenins available locally against the main species. Snake bites account for an estimated 50 000–100 000 deaths every year. Some 25 000–35 000 of these occur in Asia, where the Russell's viper, *Daboia russelii*, and the 'saw-scaled' or 'carpet viper', *Echis carinatus*, are the main culprits.

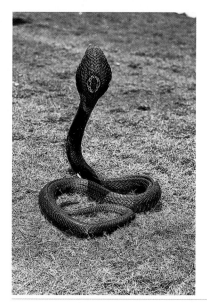

1137 Elapidae: monocellate cobra from Southeast Asia
The venom of Asian cobras (genus *Naja*), such as the *Naja kaouthia* shown here, contains both postsynaptic neurotoxins that cause paralysis and cytotoxic components that produce local tissue necrosis at the site of the bite. (© D A Warrell.)

Table 25 Principal venomous snakes responsible for morbidity and mortality

Family	Subfamily	Genus and species	English name	Distribution
Atractaspididae		*Atractaspis* spp.	Burrowing asps, stiletto snakes	Africa, Middle East
Elapidae		*Naja nigricollis*	Black-necked spitting cobra	Africa
		Naja haje	Egyptian cobra	Africa
		Naja naja	Indian cobra	South-east Asia, Far East
		Naja kaouthia	Asian cobra	South-east Asia
		Dendroaspis spp.	Mambas	Africa
		Bungarus caeruleus	Indian krait	South-east Asia
		Acanthophis spp.	Death adders	Australasia
		Oxyuranus scutellatus	Common taipan	Australasia
		Pseudechis australis	Mulga, king brown snake	Australasia
		Pseudonaja textilis	Eastern brown snake	Australasia
		Notechis scutatus	Eastern tiger snake	Australasia
Hydrophiidae		*Enhydrina schistosa*	Beaked sea snake	South-east Asia
Viperidae	Crotalinae	*Crotalus adamanteus*	Eastern diamondback rattlesnake	North America
		Crotalus atrox	Western diamondback rattlesnake	North America
		Crotalus viridis subspp.	Western rattlesnakes	North America
		Crotalus durissus durissus	Central American rattlesnake	Central America
		Crotalus durissus terrificus	South American rattlesnake	South America
		Bothrops atrox asper	Terciopelo, caissaca	Central America
		Bothrops jararaca	Jararaca	South America
		Calloselasma (Agkistrodon) rhodostoma	Malayan pit viper	South-east Asia
		Trimeresurus spp.	green pit vipers	Southeast Asia
		Trimeresurus flavoviridis	habu	Far East
		Trimeresurus mucrosquamatus	Chinese habu	Far East
	Viperinae	*Vipera berus*	Viper, adder	Europe
		Vipera ammodytes	Long-nosed viper	Europe
		Vipera palaestinae	Palestine viper	Asia, Middle East
		Macrovipera lebetina	Levantine viper	Asia, Middle East, north Africa
		Daboia russelii	Russell's viper	Indian sub continent, south-east Asia
		Echis spp.	'Saw-scaled' or 'carpet' viper	Africa, Middle East, south-east Asia, Indian subcontinent
		Bitis arietans	Puff adder	Africa
Colubridae		*Dispholidus typus*	boomslang	Africa

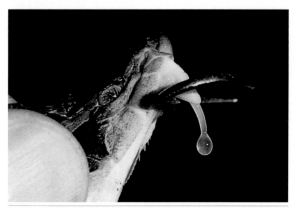

1138 Viperidae: venom being squeezed from the tip of the fang of a Malayan pit viper (*Calloselasma rhodostoma*) by gentle pressure over the venom glands
Venoms of Viperinae and Crotalinae (pit vipers) contain toxins mainly affecting blood coagulation, damaging vascular endothelium and lowering blood pressure. (© D A Warrell.)

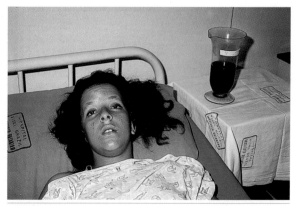

1139 Myoglobinuria following rattlesnake bite
This patient was bitten by a tropical rattlesnake (*Crotalus durissus terrificus*) in Brazil. 18 hours after the bite she had 'myasthenic facies' resulting from paralysis of muscles innervated by the cranial nerves and was passing myoglobin in the urine. Both features are the result of venom phospholipases A$_2$, which damage nerve endings and skeletal muscle. (© D A Warrell.)

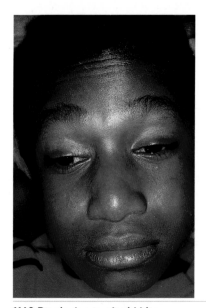

1140 Ptosis due to elapid bite
This boy had been bitten by a Papuan taipan (*Oxyuranus scutellatus canni*) 4^1/$_2$ hours previously. Elapid venom results in neuromuscular block, initially of muscles innervated by the cranial nerves, progressing to bulbar respiratory and, finally, generalised paralysis. This patient shows bilateral ptosis (inability to open the eyes despite contraction of the temporalis muscle puckering the brow), external ophthalmoplegia (divergent squint), paralysis of facial muscles and inability to open the mouth and protrude the tongue. (© D A Warrell.)

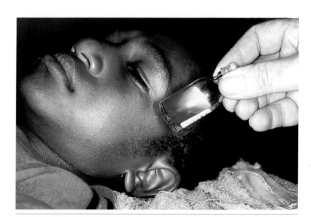

1141 20-minute whole-blood clotting test
This is an invaluable bedside test to detect incoagulable blood resulting from consumption coagulopathy caused by the venom of Viperidae and some species of Colubridae and Australasian Elapidae. Blood taken by venepuncture from the patient shown in **1140** was left undisturbed in a new, clean, dry, glass vessel for 20 minutes. It remained liquid, indicating systemic envenoming. (© D A Warrell.)

KWASHIORKOR AND MARASMUS

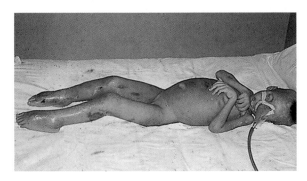

1147 Oedema and hypopigmentation

The presence of oedema may give a false impression that a kwashiorkor infant is well nourished. General hypopigmentation, together with some haemorrhagic skin lesions, is seen in this infant, who died shortly after the photograph was taken. The exact cause of kwashiorkor is still debated. Rather than being due to simple protein–energy malnutrition, it is suggested that it is related to a deficiency in the diet of the trace element selenium, which is essential to glutathione-peroxidase-mediated oxidation–reduction processes in the tissues. Aflatoxins and other so far unidentified factors may also play a role.

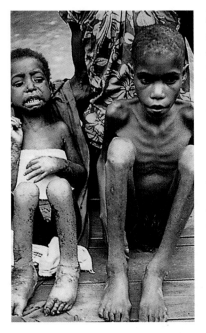

1148 Kwashiorkor and marasmus in brothers

Compare the miserable expression, pale hair, generalised oedema and skin changes in the child on the left, who has kwashiorkor, with the marasmic wasting of his older brother. Kwashiorkor frequently follows acute infection and/or diarrhoea in a child during the weaning period.

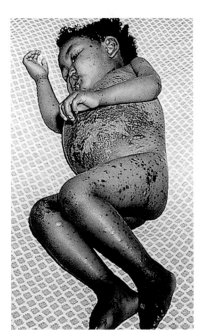

1149 Skin changes in kwashiorkor

Serious skin changes including erythema, followed by hyperpigmentation, 'black enamel skin' and peeling, may terminate in serious ulceration and gangrene. Note the ulceration where desquamation has occurred in this child.

Nutritional marasmus

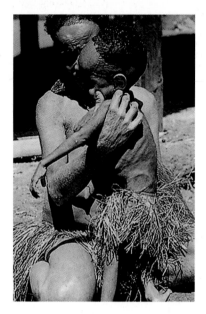

1150 Papuan child with nutritional marasmus
Note the obvious wasting and dehydration in this marasmic infant, an all too common picture in times of famine when the total calorie intake is grossly insufficient. (The mother has tinea imbricata of the skin; see **998**.)

AVITAMINOSES

Vitamin A

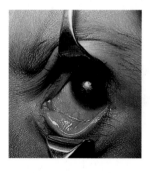

1151 Xerophthalmia
Vitamin A deficiency is a common cause of blindness among preschool children in the tropics, especially in Asia. The dryness of the cornea and conjunctiva (conjunctival xerosis) give the eye a dull, hazy appearance.

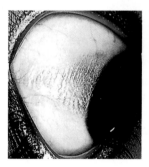

1152 Bitot's spots
These are silver-grey, foamy spots, situated on the conjunctiva usually external to the cornea and often bilateral. They are associated with a mild to moderate decrease in vitamin A intake. In older children they may not disappear with vitamin A treatment.

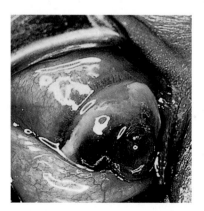

1153 Keratomalacia
A softening or coagulative necrosis of the cornea occurs in chronic, severe vitamin A deficiency. As with kwashiorkor, vitamin A deficiency may be precipitated by acute infections in undernourished children.

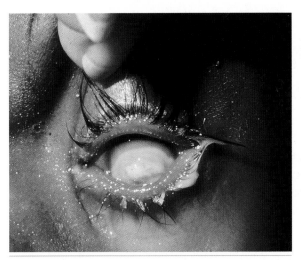

1154 Blindness due to vitamin A deficiency
Complete loss of vision may follow untreated keratomalacia as in this African child.

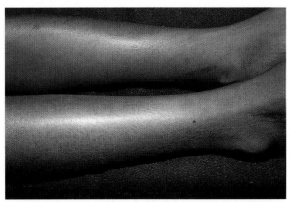

1155 Early skin changes due to vitamin A deficiency
The skin of the legs of this Indian patient show ichthyosiform ('crazy paving') changes associated with a moderate degree of vitamin A deficiency. Later skin changes include the development of phrynoderma, a form of papular, follicular hyperkeratosis.

Vitamin D

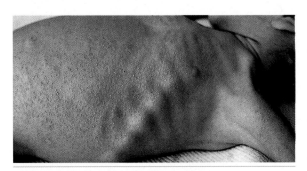

1156 Infantile rickets – 'rickety rosary'
This is a disease of infants and children due to insufficient vitamin D. Infants are sometimes overprotected from the sun by their mothers to avoid too-rapid pigmentation of the skin; rickets occurs in this situation when it could easily be avoided. Rounded swellings that appear over the costochondral junctions near the sternum give rise to the term 'rickety rosary'.

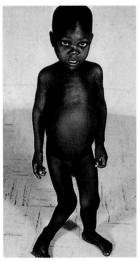

1157 Infantile rickets
Note the gross deformity of the legs and pigeon chest of this boy.

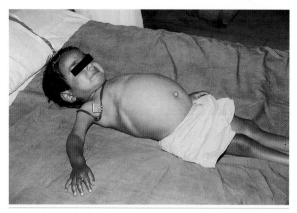

1158 Indian child with rickets
Although this infant appears to be generally well nourished, note the pigeon chest and the swollen joints of the right hand and fingers.

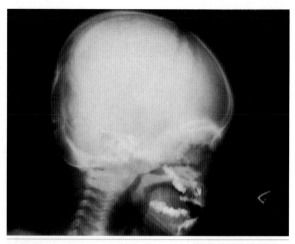

1159 Skull of 2-year-old infant with rickets
The anterior fontanelle remains open and its edges soft.

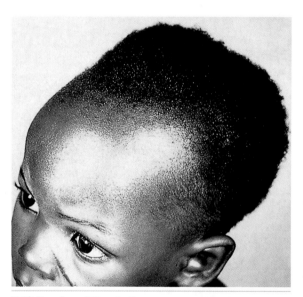

1160 Bossing of the skull
Bossing of the frontal and parietal eminences occurs.

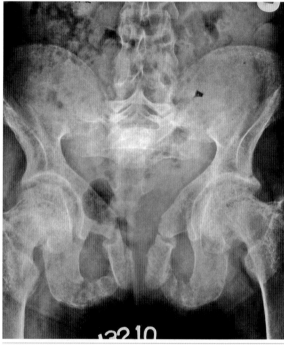

1161 Osteomalacia
The increased demands of pregnancy may result in gross deformity of the pelvis. This occurs, for example, in mothers kept in purdah.

The B vitamins

Thiamine (B₁)

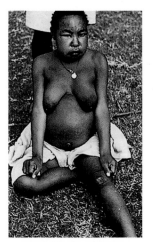

1162 Beri beri oedema
'Wet' beri beri is a disease characterised by generalised oedema, peripheral neuropathy and sometimes heart failure associated with thiamine deficiency.

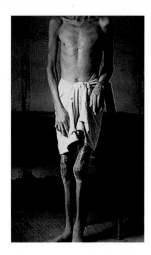

1163 Peripheral neuropathy
Wrist drop and marked wasting of the lower extremities occur in some patients.

Riboflavin (B₂)

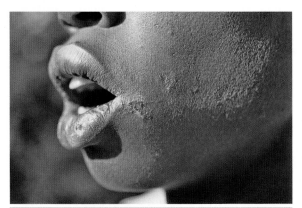

1164 Angular stomatitis
Riboflavin deficiency of a mild degree produces this condition, which consists of grey-white fissures at both angles of the mouth. This African boy also has early signs of sore, cracked lips (cheilosis).

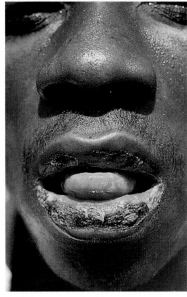

1165 Cheilosis
This cracked condition of the lips seen also in association with riboflavin deficiency is very marked in this African patient.

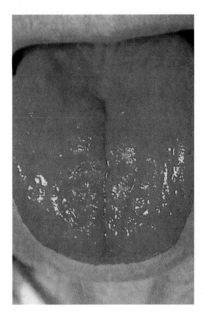

1166 Glossitis
The tongue is sore, smooth and an abnormally deep red colour. This sign may also occur with other nutritional deficiencies.

Folic acid

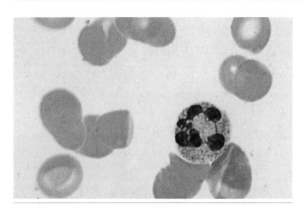

1167 Anaemia of folic acid deficiency
Folic acid deficiency results in a macrocytic megaloblastic anaemia. Shown here is a characteristic, hypersegmented neutrophil. (*Giemsa × 1350*)

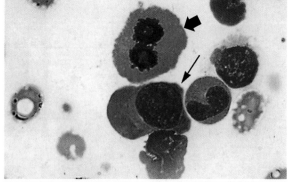

1168 Bone marrow in folic acid deficiency
The appearance in this marrow is characteristic of folic acid deficiency with megaloblastosis of erythroid precursors (large arrow) and large leukocyte precursors (small arrow). (*Giemsa × 900*)

ZOONOTIC VIRAL INFECTIONS

See Table 26.

Congo–Crimea haemorrhagic fever

This condition, caused by a virus of the genus *Nairovirus* in the family Bunyaviridae, occurs in Europe, the Middle East, Asia and Africa, where it is usually acquired from tick bites by people in close contact with cattle, particularly in drier or semi-desert areas where tick infestation levels are high. A number of human–human outbreaks have also been reported among hospital staff and patients. During 2003 in Iran 47 people were confirmed to have been infected out of 137 who were suspected to have Congo–Crimea haemorrhagic fever (CCHF), and five of those died. In Mauritania, which has long been known as a centre of transmission for CCHF, a small epidemic was traced to direct contact with infected goats slaughtered for food, followed by a number of secondary person-to-person cases.

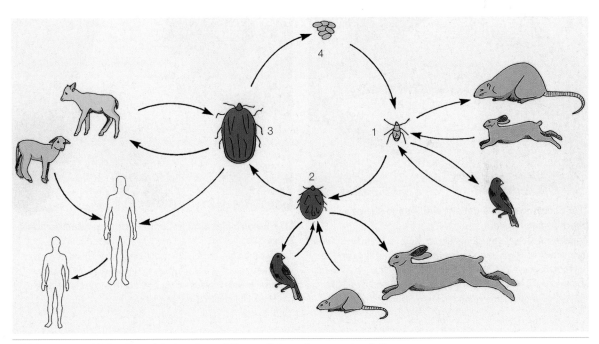

1173 The cycle of infection with the virus of Congo–Crimea haemorrhagic fever
Several species of ixodid ticks transmit this arbovirus, as well as other viruses causing haemorrhagic fevers (**Table 26**). This figure shows how larvae of ticks of the genus *Hyalomma* and related genera (1) acquire the virus from birds, rodents or leporids, transmit it in the nymphal stage (2) to leporids, rodents, birds and, occasionally, humans, then via the adults (3) to humans and domestic animals. Through transovarial transmission (4) the virus can then pass to the next generation of larvae and in them from stage to stage. The ticks thus serve as a reservoir for the virus. The relative sizes of the hosts in the diagram reflect their relative importance as reservoirs at the different stages of the cycle. Neither wild nor domestic ruminants appear to suffer from clinical disease in spite of having heavy virus loads.

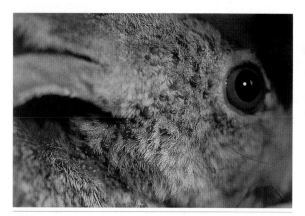

1174 *Hyalomma truncatum* nymphs and adults feeding on a West African hare, *Lepus whytei*

This African lepurid is a common vertebrate reservoir of CCHF virus.

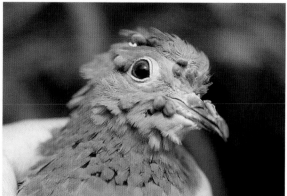

1175 Immature *Hyalomma marginatum rufipes* feeding on an African dove, *Streptopelia senegalensis*

H. marginatum rufipes, which often lives on birds, is another host of this virus. The bird tick is widely distributed from Africa to the former Soviet Union and Asia.

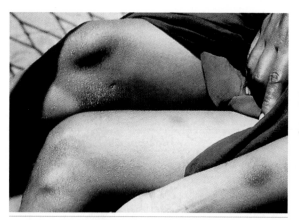

1176 Ecchymoses in a patient with Congo–Crimean haemorrhagic fever

Although this disease is generally an acute, self-limiting infection characterised by a petechial rash and soft palate haemorrhages, it can produce severe haemorrhages, as in this and the next patient, associated with collapse and a 15–70% mortality rate, the latter during epidemics.

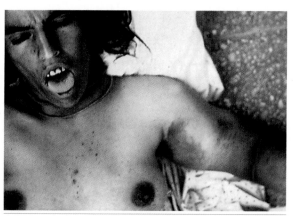

1177 Severe bleeding in Congo–Crimean haemorrhagic fever

This woman has large petechial haemorrhages on her upper chest and massive ecchymoses in the left arm and axilla. Mucosal bleeding also occurs, and death is commonly due to uncontrollable haemorrhage and shock.

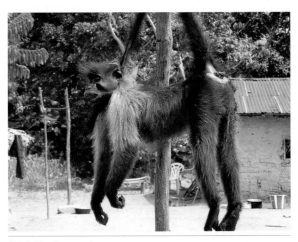

1186 'Bush meat'

Monkeys as well as larger apes, which are killed for food in a number of countries, may be the source of simian and primate viruses that can infect humans. Moreover there exists a large illegal export of 'bush meat' to other countries in spite of importation restrictions, which are often inadequate. In 2004, for example, at least 11 600 tons were estimated to have been brought into the United Kingdom. This grey-cheeked mangabey (*Cercocebus albigena*), a species that is frequently eaten, was seen in a village in Gabon. Bushmeat can also be the source of anthrax infection, as well as newly, described human T-cell lymphotropic viruses (HTLV-3 and HTLV-4), which may have been acquired by cross-species infection from African monkeys. These two viruses were discovered during a survey in 2004 for simian retroviruses in over 900 Cameroonians who had handled or eaten bushmeat. (Courtesy of Dr P Rouquet.)

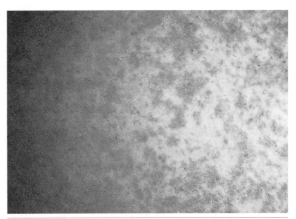

1187 Ebola haemorrhagic fever

Haemorrhagic manifestations in the skin and internal organs are common. However, mild cases, as well as asymptomatic carriers, do also occur. In these a papular rash is seen, usually around the fifth day of the illness. The natural reservoir of the Ebola group of viruses in Africa has not yet been identified although it is suspected that certain bats in the rain forest may play a role in maintaining transmission (see **1184**).

Hantavirus infections

An ever-increasing number of viruses in the genus *Hantavirus* (Family Bunyaviridae) (**Table 26**) are responsible for solitary or epidemic zoonotic infection in countries ranging from the Old World to the neotropics. Although known to Chinese physicians for over 900 years, the first of these viruses to be clearly identified as a cause of serious illness in humans was that found in Korea in 1976. Scandinavian 'nephropathia epidemica' (Puumala virus), the cause of haemorrhagic fever with renal syndrome and Balkan HFRS (Porogia virus) are related viruses, the last of these killing 15–30% of those infected. Various rodents, such as species of *Apodemus* and *Clethrionomys*, act as natural reservoirs, with the virus residing in their lungs; even infected laboratory rats have been found in several countries. Transmission may be direct or airborne via contaminated rodent urine, saliva or faeces or, possibly, through tick bite during epidemics. Other hantaviruses include Prospect Hill virus (which gives rise to asymptomatic infection in humans in the USA), as well as Muerto Canyon (or 'Four Corners') virus – which is enzootic in deer mice (*Peromyscus maniculatus*), causing a severe, acute hantavirus pulmonary syndrome with over 50% mortality in parts of the USA west of the Mississippi river. Several hantaviruses are also enzootic in Latin America. In the south of Argentina, for example, high infection rates have been recorded in up to 5.4% of peridomestic *Oligoryzomys longicaudatus* in association with HPS in rural habitats. The Andean virus appears to be transmitted mainly via the rodent host's saliva, probably in aerosol form.

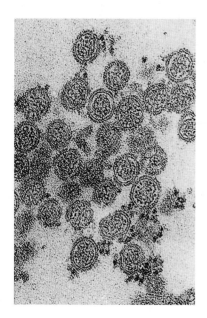

1188 Ultrastructure of a Hantaan virus
This RNA hantavirus of the family Bunyaviridae (see **Table 26**) has been identified as the cause of a widely distributed HFRS that is sometimes associated with acute nephropathy and renal failure. Hantaan viruses infect nearly 150 000 Asians yearly, producing a 5% mortality rate. Korean haemorrhagic fever (Seoul virus) was responsible for thousands of cases in military personnel in that country. The Hantaan virus particles seen here in section were grown in Vero E6 cells. (× *62 000*)

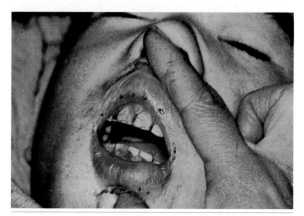

1189 Haemorrhagic fever with renal syndrome in a Chinese patient
Three days after the onset of his illness, severe haemorrhages occurred in the mouth of this 20-year-old man.

PARENTERALLY ACQUIRED ACUTE VIRAL HEPATITIS

See **Table 15**.

Four viruses associated with acute viral hepatitis are acquired by the parenteral route. HBV (a DNA hepadnavirus with affinities to the retroviruses), which can be transmitted from mother to infant at birth, causes the most serious infections and results in a chronic carrier state in over 40% of adults. Over 1 million children die from the acute infection each year. In China, south-east Asia and Africa, 10–20% of the population are HBV carriers; there are probably over 300 million worldwide. Chronic active infection with this oncogenic virus may lead to hepatic cirrhosis and is responsible for up to 80% of all cases of hepatocellular carcinoma, one of the 10 commonest tumours. HDV ('Delta virus') is a 'defective', so-called 'piggy-back' RNA virus that develops only in the presence of HBV antigen. The combined infection can give rise to a fulminating form of hepatitis. HCV (a togavirus) and HFV (a virus that is still incompletely characterised) were formerly confused under the name of HNANB(P) (non-A, non-B virus). HCV, like HBV, can give rise to a chronic carrier state and is common in Japan. A very effective vaccine now available against HBV, which should reduce the incidence of new infections in the future, is particularly indicated for the protection of neonates.

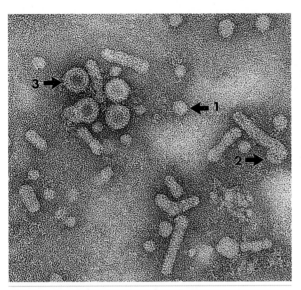

1190 Serum containing hepatitis B antigen
Three distinct morphological entities are seen: Australia antigen surface coat in the form of (1) small, pleomorphic spherical particles measuring 20–22 nm in diameter; (2) tubular forms of varying length with a constant diameter of 20 nm (frequently with a terminal bulbous swelling); (3) double-shelled spheroidal Dane particles of HBV, approximately 42 nm in diameter, with a core measuring 27 nm in diameter surrounded by surface coat. (× *227 000*)

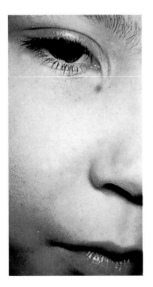

1191 Jaundiced child with hepatitis A
Fever, anorexia and, later, jaundice are characteristic clinical features. The disease is particularly severe in pregnancy. Note deep jaundice and spider naevus on the cheek.

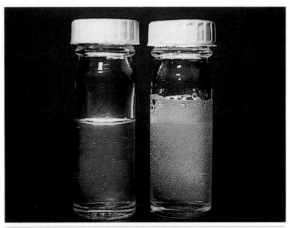

1192 Urine from child with hepatitis
The dark-coloured urine contains bilirubin and urobilinogen, which derive from conjugated bilirubin discharged into the blood from damaged hepatocytes.

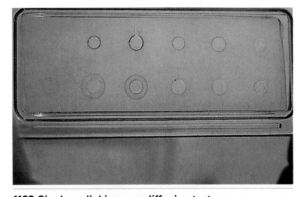

1193 Single radial immunodiffusion test
HBV-antigen-positive serum is readily detected by this simple serological procedure.

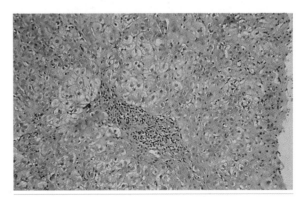

1194 Biopsy of liver in hepatitis
Histologically, the characteristic features are ballooning and a feathery degeneration of the liver parenchymal cells. (× *150*) (See also **609–611**.)

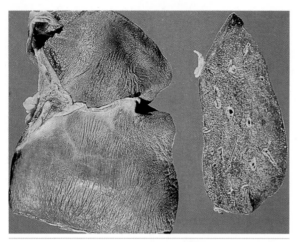

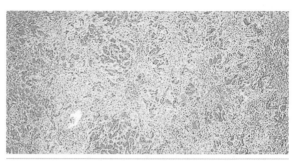

1196 Hepatic parenchyma in massive liver necrosis
Only a few isolated plaques of hepatocytes remain in the liver parenchyma. (*H&E × 100*) (AFIP No. 65–3784)

1195 Massive hepatic necrosis
Gross appearance of a liver with massive necrosis caused by HBV infection. Note the wrinkled capsular surface and the 'nutmeg' appearance of the cut surface, which is due to loss of cells and congestion in the central lobular zones.

NEOPLASTIC CONDITIONS

Burkitt's lymphoma

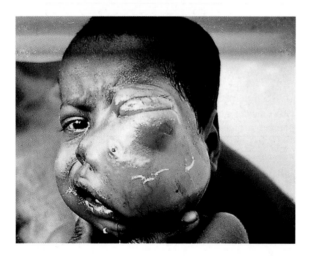

1197 African child with Burkitt's lymphoma of the maxilla
The geographical distribution of Burkitt's lymphoma in high incidence is mainly controlled by two climatic parameters: temperature and humidity. In sub-Saharan Africa, the distribution of Burkitt's tumour is roughly the same as that of malaria. This highly malignant tumour is believed to be caused by the immunodepression associated with chronic malaria in individuals who are carriers of the Epstein–Barr virus and characteristically show a chromosomal translocation that leads to uncontrolled B cell proliferation. One of the most common forms of clinical presentation is facial swelling. The jaws are most frequently affected, one or more quadrants being involved.

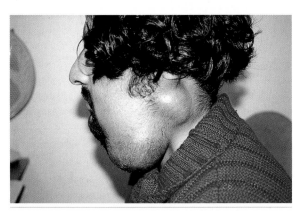

1198 Burkitt's lymphoma in an Asian adult
The photograph shows enormous cervical lymphadenopathy, which was initially suggestive of tuberculous lymphadenitis but which biopsy showed to be due to Burkitt's lymphoma.

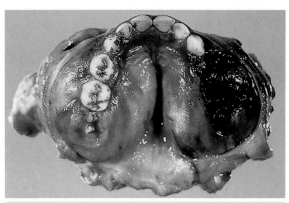

1199 Maxillary tumour at autopsy
The extensive infiltration of both maxillas by Burkitt's lymphoma tissue are evident in this autopsy specimen. This neoplasm, which accounts for at least half of all childhood tumours in tropical Africa, is also found in highly endemic, malarious areas of the New Guinea lowlands.

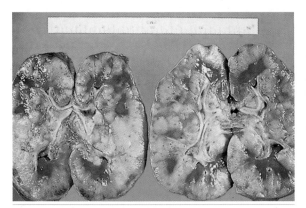

1200 Kidneys with Burkitt's lymphoma
Massive replacement of both kidneys with tumour cells is apparent here. Any organ can be affected.

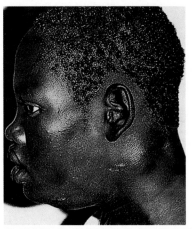

1201 Nasopharyngeal carcinoma
This condition, which is also associated with Epstein–Barr virus, has a high incidence rate in southern China. It also occurs in neighbouring countries such as Malaysia and Singapore, where it is 20 times as common in those of Chinese origin than in those of other races. The tumour is found also in several African countries. Massive cervical lymphadenopathy is seen in this Sudanese patient. The presenting symptoms are very variable and depend upon the precise location of the tumour. Cranial nerve involvement develops in nearly half of cases.

Hepatocellular carcinoma

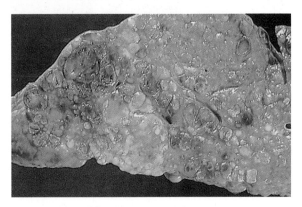

1202 Macroscopic appearance of liver
Primary hepatocellular carcinoma of the liver (of which more than 250 000 arise yearly) is one of the 10 commonest tumours in the world and is especially common in the tropics. Coarse, nodular changes can be seen in this specimen. A clear relationship has been established between HBV (see **Table 15**), HCV and hepatocellular carcinoma, 85% occurring in individuals who have chronic hepatic cirrhosis. Vaccination against HBV should afford protection against hepatoma, and large-scale trials are currently in progress. Aflatoxins in certain diets appear to be an important contributory factor.

Endemic Kaposi's sarcoma in Africa

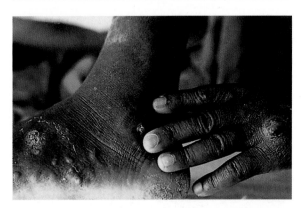

1203 Endemic (non-AIDS) Kaposi's sarcoma of the hand and foot
This malignant tumour was originally described in Austria, with its highest incidence in special ethnic communities such as southern European Jews. Later, it was recognised to be endemic in parts of sub-Saharan Africa, particularly in Nigeria, eastern Zaire and western Uganda. It affects mainly males, with the lesions usually starting as tumour nodules on the extremities. The lesions run a long-term course but sometimes become more aggressive and infiltrative, causing gross lesions. Typical nodular lesions are seen on the hand and foot of this African male from Lesotho. It is now suspected that human herpes virus 8 (in association with chronic immunodepression, especially human immunodeficiency virus, HIV) may cause this tumour. (See also **904–906**.)

Neoplasia due to chronic solar exposure

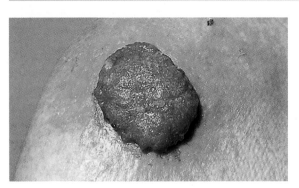

1204 Squamous-cell carcinoma
Chronic exposure to solar radiation, particularly in people with light skin pigmentation, can result in various degenerative or neoplastic changes in the exposed parts of the body. Increasing reduction of the ozone layer is predicted to result in an increased frequency in such conditions as squamous-cell carcinoma, seen here on the shoulder of an albino patient.

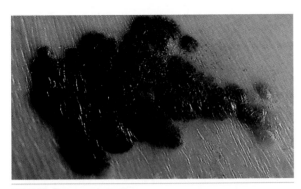

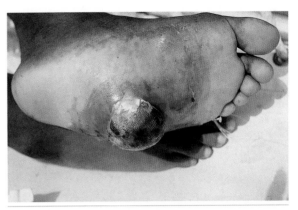

1205 Malignant melanoma

A sudden increase in pigmentation and enlargement of freckles following prolonged exposure to sunlight may be precursors to the development of a malignant melanoma in a fair-skinned individual. The large melanoma seen in this 54-year-old Caucasian woman shows marked local infiltration and carries a very poor prognosis. Her skin also show some generalised elastotic degeneration.

1206 Malignant melanoma of the foot

The primary site of this condition is usually the non-pigmented sole, or occasionally the palmar surface of the hand, in dark-skinned people such as the African patient seen here. In these individuals a malignant melanoma may occasionally occur in an area of vitiligo. (Courtesy of Professor K F Schaller.)

GENETIC BLOOD DYSCRASIAS

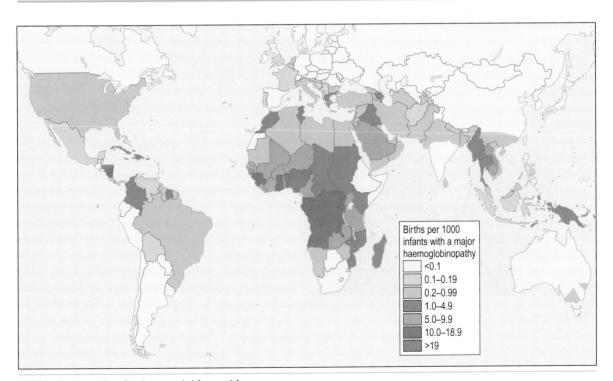

Births per 1000 infants with a major haemoglobinopathy
- <0.1
- 0.1–0.19
- 0.2–0.99
- 1.0–4.9
- 5.0–9.9
- 10.0–18.9
- >19

1207 Incidence of major haemoglobinopathies

The map indicates the estimated numbers per 1000 births of infants with major haemoglobinopathies. This can be compared with **1208**. (Adapted from Christiansen A, Streetly A, and Darr A. BMJ 2004; 329: 1115–1117, quoting map from WHO Genomic Resource Centre.)

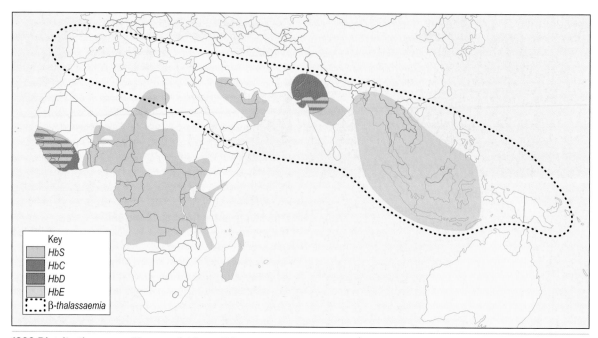

1208 Distribution map of haemoglobinopathies

The most important abnormal haemoglobins (Hb) in the tropics are HbS, HbC and HbE. Thalassaemia, which is the result of decreased synthesis of one of the chains of haemoglobin (α or β), is also widespread. HbD has a limited distribution and is clinically mild. The abnormal haemoglobins also occur in Central and South America, because of migration, and among African-Americans in the USA. The haemoglobin AS phenotype in the same population, which renders the erythrocytes unfavourable to the development of *Plasmodium falciparum*, favours the survival of the gene in tropical Africa, where falciparum malaria is holoendemic, although the SS phenotype increases host mortality. It is likely that the median survival of homozygotes in the African continent is less than 5 years. This is known as 'balanced polymorphism'. α and β thalassaemia, HbE and G6PD deficiency are also believed to afford relative protection against severe *P. falciparum* infection in heterozygotes (see **118**).

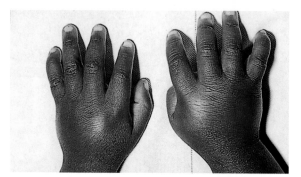

1209 Dactylitis due to sickle-cell disease

Severe bilateral dactylitis is a common presentation of sickle-cell disease in children. It is caused by destructive changes in small bones – the result of multiple infarction complicated by infection.

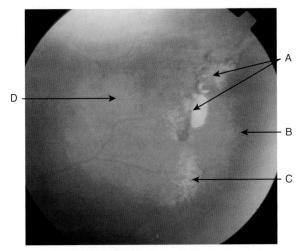

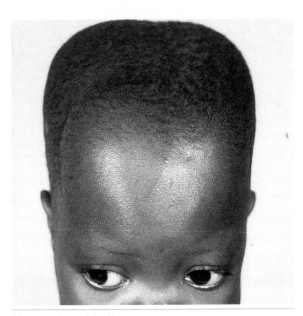

1210 Proliferative retinopathy associated with sickle-cell disease

New vessels develop as a response to vasoproliferative growth factors produced by ischaemic retina – itself a result of occlusion of precapillary arterioles by sickled erythrocytes. The new vessels are friable and often bleed into the vitreous gel, causing floaters and sight loss. Fibrovascular sequelae may cause traction retinal detachment and irreversible blindness. This peripheral retinal photograph shows three new vessels, one of which has autoinfarcted. A, active new vessels with preretinal haemorrhage; B, ischaemic retina; C, autoinfarcted sickle new vessel; D, arteriovenous shunt. (Courtesy of Dr G. Vafidis, Northwest London Hospitals Trust.)

1211 Bossing of skull

Bossing of the skull due to hyperplasia of the marrow is another feature of sickle cell disease. Similar appearances may be seen in thalassaemia and in any other severe, congenital haemolytic anaemia.

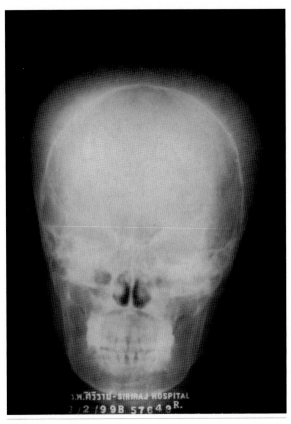

1212 X-ray of skull in thalassaemia

Thalassaemia disease produces this typical 'hair-on-end' appearance of the skull in X-rays.

DISEASES OF UNUSUAL OR UNCERTAIN AETIOLOGY

Endomyocardial fibrosis

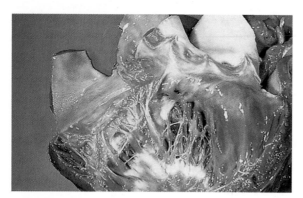

1213 Fibrotic changes in the heart of an African
Endomyocardial fibrosis is a common cause of heart disease in the tropics. It presents in three clinical forms: mainly left-sided, as mitral incompetence; right-sided, with features suggestive of constrictive pericarditis; a form involving both sides of the heart, presenting as congestive cardiac failure.

Ainhum

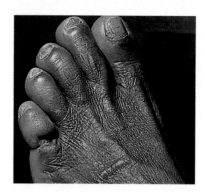

1214 Ainhum of small toe
This condition of unknown aetiology is a progressive encircling fibrosis of a toe, usually the fifth. In this patient, the lesion was bilateral, affecting also the fifth toe of the right foot.

Postinfective malabsorption syndrome (tropical sprue)

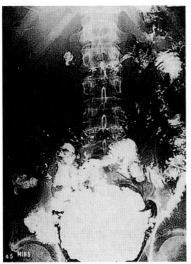

1215

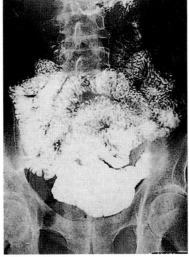

1216

1215 & 1216 X-rays of patient with tropical sprue

The postinfective malabsorption syndrome (also known as tropical sprue) is characterised by chronic steatorrhoea of unknown aetiology, with associated abdominal symptoms, glossitis and anaemia. Fat, bulky faeces are characteristic of this condition. The figures show loss of normal intestinal pattern before treatment (**1215**, left), and then recovery after 3 months of treatment (**1216**, right).

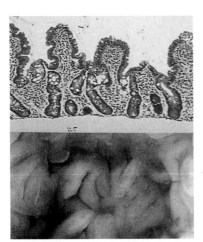

1217 Jejunal biopsy in postinfective malabsorption syndrome

Partial villous atrophy with squat villi are seen in this biopsy from a patient with tropical sprue. The lower figure shows a section of the biopsy seen before fixation. Upper figure shows that the ratio between the villus height and the crypt depth is about 1:0. (*H&E*) × 40)

Endemic bladder stone disease

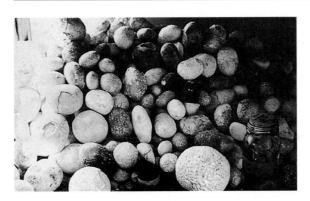

1218 Collection of bladder stones

Bladder stones are very common in children in Thailand, Indonesia and the Middle East. The aetiological factors involved include a low-milk–high-cereal diet, low urinary volume, high ambient temperature and ingestion of certain local vegetables and leaves of forest plants that have a high oxalate content.

Podoconiosis

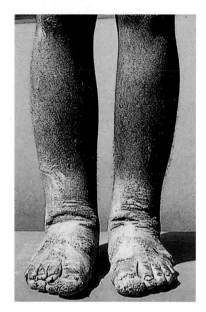

1219 Advanced podoconiosis in an Ethiopian

Podoconiosis ('non-filarial elephantiasis') is a debilitating condition caused by the passage of microparticles of silica and alumino-silicates through the skin of the bare feet of people who walk in terrain characterised by a high content of red laterite of volcanic origin. It is especially prevalent in certain highland areas of Ethiopia and other African countries, but has also been recorded in other continents where such soils occur (such as the high plateau of central Brazil). The cytotoxic microparticles pass into the lymphatics of the foot and lower leg where they become deposited in macrophages. The destruction of the phagocytes serves as a stimulus for excessive collagen formation which culminates in local oedema and fibrosis of the dermis and other tissues. In late cases, such as that shown here, a thickened, leathery, verrucose change develops, while obstruction of the regional lymph nodes gives rise to more generalised lymphoedema in the affected limbs. The disease can be prevented and early changes reversed through the use of appropriate footwear. Treatment of later cases may include compression to reduce the lymphoedema and surgical removal of excessive tissue where indicated.

'Fogo selvagem'

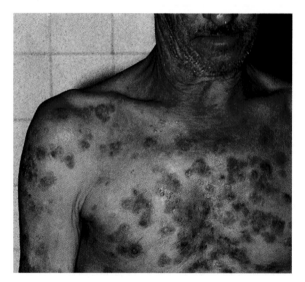

1220 Brazilian man with fogo selvagem

This chronic form of endemic pemphigus foliaceus occurs in a number of localities in central and western Brazil, northern Argentina, Peru, Bolivia and Venezuela. It is commonest in young women in hot, humid rural areas, but about 15% of sufferers are children. The burning sensation in the skin gives rise to the name. It was formerly believed to be caused by massive and repeated bites by the tiny blackfly *Simulium oyapockense* s.l. in the Amazon lowlands but is now recognised to be an autoimmune disease. The flaccid bullae are induced by IgG_4 subclass antibodies. Another, more acute condition known as 'haemorrhagic syndrome of Altamira' is probably caused by the bites of large numbers of *Simulium minusculum* in northern Brazil.

Chapter 9 Nutritional disorders

McClaren D 1992 A colour atlas and text of diet related disorders, 2nd edn. Wolfe Medical, London

McClaren DS, Meguid MM 1988 Nutrition and its disorders. Churchill Livingstone, Edinburgh

Stephenson L 1993 The impact of schistosomiasis on human nutrition. Parasitology 107: S107–S123

Stephenson LS, Latham MC, Adams EJ et al 1993 Weight gain of Kenyan school children infected with hookworm, *Trichuris trichiura* and *Ascaris lumbricoides* is improved following once- or twice-yearly treatment with albendazole. Journal of Nutrition 123: 656–665

Chapter 10 Miscellaneous disorders

Bausch DG, Demby AH, Coulibaly M et al 2001 Lassa fever in Guinea: I. Epidemiology of human disease and clinical observations. Vector Borne and Zoonotic Diseases 1: 269–281

Birtles RJ, Harrison TG, Taylor AG 1993 Cat scratch disease and bacillary angiomatosis: aetiological agents and the link with AIDS. CDR Review 3: review 8, R107–R110

Bösner S 1993 Das Burkitt-Lymphom. Erforschungsgeschichte und Epidemiologie. Basilisken-Presse, Marburg

Braude AI, Davis CE, Fierer J (eds) 1981 Medical microbiology and infectious diseases. WB Saunders, Philadelphia, PA

Demby AH, Inapogui A, Kargbo K et al 2001 Lassa fever in Guinea: II. Distribution and prevalence of Lassa virus infection in small mammals. Vector Borne and Zoonotic Diseases 1: 283–297

Ergönül, Ö 2006 Crimean-Congo haemorrhagic fever. Lancet Infectious Diseases 6: 203-214

McKee KT Jr, LeDuc JW, Peters CJ 1991 Hantaviruses. In: Belshe RB (ed.) Textbook of human virology. Mosby, St Louis, MO, pp 615–632

Peters CJ 1991 Arenaviruses. In: Belshe RB (ed.) Textbook of human virology. Mosby, St Louis, MO, pp 541–570

Peterson AT, Bauer JT, Mills JN 2004 Ecologic and geographic distribution of filovirus disease. Emerging Infectious Diseases 10: 40–47

Price EE 1990 Podoconiosis. Non-filarial elephantiasis. Oxford University Press, Oxford

Richmond JK, Baglole DJ 2003 Lassa fever: epidemiology, clinical features, and social consequences. British Medical Journal 327: 1271–1275

Serjeant GR 1992 Sickle-cell disease, 2nd edn. Oxford University Press, Oxford

Stuart MJ, Nagel RL 2004 Sickle-cell disease. Lancet 364: 1343–1360

Vapalahti O, Mustonen J, Lundkvist Å et al 2003 Hantavirus infections in Europe. Lancet Infectious Diseases 3: 653–660

World Health Organization 1985 Arthropod-borne and rodent-borne viral diseases. Technical Report Series No. 719. WHO, Geneva

World Health Organization 1985 Viral haemorrhagic fevers. Technical Report Series No. 721. WHO, Geneva

Zuckerman AJ, Thomas HC (eds) 1998 Viral hepatitis. Scientific basis and clinical management, 2nd edn. Churchill Livingstone, Edinburgh

INDEX